NEUROANAESTHESIA
PRACTICAL TIPS

EDITORS

DWARKADAS K. BAHETI

MD

Consultant Anaesthesiologist & Pain Physician, Bombay Hospital and Medical Research Centre, Mumbai.

RAJSHREE DEOPUJARI

MD, DA

Consultant Anaesthesiologist, Jaslok Hospital & Research centre, Pedder Road, Mumbai.

FALGUNI R SHAH

MD, DNB, FCPS, DA, MNAMS

Consultant & Coordinator Department of Anaesthesiology Lilavati Hospital & Research Centre, Mumbai.

FIRST EDITION

www.nationalbookdepot.com

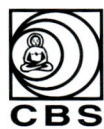

CBS

CBS Publishers & Distributors Pvt Ltd

First Edition   2018

Published by
Raju Shah
THE NATIONAL BOOK DEPOT
Opp. Wadia Children's Hospital, Parel, Mumbai - 400 012.
Tel : (91-22) 2416 5274 / 2413 1362 / 2413 2411 | Fax : 2413 0877
E-mail: nationalbook55@gmail.com
www.nationalbookdepot.com

and

Satish Kumar Jain for
CBS Publishers & Distributors Pvt Ltd
4819/XI Prahlad Street, 24 Ansari Road, Daryaganj, New Delhi - 110 002, India.
Ph: 23289259, 23266861, 23266867 | Fax: 011-23243014
Website: www.cbspd.com | E-mail: delhi@cbspd.com; cbspubs@airtelmail.in
Corporate Office: 204 FIE, Industrial Area, Patparganj, Delhi - 110 092.
Ph: 4934 4934 | Fax: 4934 4935 | E-mail: publishing@cbspd.com; publicity@cbspd.com

ISBN : 978-93-80206-92-9

Printing and Setting by : Neel Graphics, Mumbai

FROM EDITOR'S DESK

Anaesthesiology, as a speciality, has witnessed a revolution in the understanding and applications of technological advances in medicine over the last few decades. It has widened its horizons into super specialities like neuro-anaesthesia, cardiac anaesthesia, paediatric anaesthesia, regional anaesthesia, pain management etc. The physiology, pharmacology, technology, diagnostic modalities etc has also progressed significantly. This has led to the commencement of many training and fellowship programmes in universities & multi-speciality hospitals across the country.

ANACC (Association of Neuro Anaesthesiologists & Critical Care) has made a humble attempt to contribute this book as an educational aid in the training of Post graduates and practicing neuro-anaesthesiologists. "Neuro Anaesthesia: Practical Tips:" explains the basics of Neuro-anaesthesia as well as updates on advanced techniques and technology. We, the practicing anaesthesiologists, felt the need for such a handbook on practical tips in neuro-anaesthesia, as most available books serve as reference books.

We express our heartfelt gratitude to all the contributors, without their efforts, this Herculean task would not have been possible at such a short notice. We have taken utmost care to publish this handbook of highest standard at an affordable price.

We are thankful to our publishers 'The National Book Depot' & their entire team for all the support and assistance.

We, the Editors, sincerely hope that our efforts will benefit all the post graduates and the practicing anaesthesiologists alike. This in turn will improve our patient care and surgical outcomes.

Dwarkadas K. Baheti

Rajshree Deopujari

Falguni Shah

LIST OF CONTRIBUTORS

Aditi S. Tilak
MBBS, MD, DNB, FRCA
Consultant - Global Hospitals, Mumbai.

Amol T. Kothekar
MD, IDCC
Dept. of Anaesthesia, Critical Care and Pain, Tata Memorial Center, Mumbai.

Anil Parakh
MD
Consultant Anaesthesiologist and HOD, Global Hospital, Parel, Mumbai.

Anita N. Shetty
MBBS, DA, MD
Professor, Seth G. S. Medical College and KEM Hospital, Mumbai.

Aparna S. Budhakar
MD, FRCA (LON)
Consultant Anaesthetist, Jaslok Hospital & Research Centre, Mumbai.

Avinash S. Kakde
DNB Anaesthesia
Neuroanaesthesia Fellow, Neuroanaesthesia Dept., Kokilaben Dhirubhai Ambani Hospital, Mumbai.

Bhoomika Thakore
MBBB, DNB Anaesthesia, PDF Neuroanaesthesia
Consultant - P. D. Hinduja Hospital, Mumbai.

Chinmaya P. Bhave
MBBS, DNB Anaesthesiology, PDF Neuroanaesthesiology
Consultant Anaesthesiologist, Dept. of Anaesthesia, Kokilaben Dhirubhai Ambani Hospital, Mumbai.

Divyadarshni Vadivel
MBBS, MD Anaesthesia
Neuroanaesthesia Fellow - Seth G. S. Medical and KEM Hospital, Mumbai.

Dwarkadas K. Baheti
MD
Anaesthesiologist and Pain Physician, Bombay Hospital & Medical Research Centre, Mumbai.

Falguni R. Shah
MD, DNB, FCPS, DA, MNAMS
Consultant Anaesthesiologist and Co-ordinator, Lilavati Hospital & Research Centre,
Ex-Associate Professor, BYL Nair Hospital and TNMC

Joanna Rodrigues
MBBS, MD Anaesthesiology, PDF Neuroanaesthesiology
Consultant - P. D. Hinduja Hospital, Mumbai.

Joseph Monteiro
MD, DA Anaesthesiology
Fellowship Anaesthesia Adden Brooke's Hospital Cambridge University, UK
Consultant - P. D. Hinduja Hospital, Mumbai.

Kalyani A. Sathe
DNB Anaesthesia
Neuroanaesthesia Fellow, Neuroanaesthesia Dept., Kokilaben Dhirubhai Ambani Hospital, Mumbai.

Lalita D. Naik
MD, DA, DGO
Consultant Neuroanaesthesiologist, Dept. of Anaesthesiology, Nanavati Super Specialty Hospital, Mumbai.

Madhavi Desai
DA, DNB
Associate Professor, Dept. of Anaesthesia, Critical Care and pain, Tata Memorial Hospital, Mumbai.

Neeta V. Karmarkar
MBBS, DA, FCPS, DNB Anaesthesiology
Consultant - Nanavati Super Speciality Hospital, Mumbai.

Nikhil S. Chamankar

MBBS, DNB General Surgery, DNB Neurosurgery

Consultant - Jaslok Hospital & Research Centre, Mumbai.

Nirav Kotak

MBBS, MD Anaesthesia

Associate Professor - Seth G. S. Medical and KEM Hospital, Mumbai.

Nitin Bhorkar

MD, DA Anaesthesiology

Consultant, Saifee Hospital, Mumbai.

Pallavi Gaur

MBBS, MD Anaesthesia

Neuroanaesthesia Fellow, Seth G. S. Medical and KEM Hospital, Mumbai.

Pramila Kurkal

MD, DA Anaesthesiology

Consultant - P. D. Hinduja Hospital, Mumbai.

Pratima S. Kothare

MBBS, MD, DNB

Consultant Anaesthesiologist, Dept. of Anaesthesia, Bombay Hospital and Research Centre, Mumbai.

Prerna Gomes

MBBS, MD Anaesthesia

Senior Consultant and Co-ordinator Dept. of Anaesthesia, Jaslok Hospital & Research Centre, Mumbai.

Rajshree C. Deopujari

MD, DA

Senior Consultant - Dept. of Neuroanaesthesia, Jaslok Hospital & Research Centre, Mumbai.

Raghvendra V. Ramdasi

MBBS, MS General Surgery, M.Ch. Neurosurgery

Department of Neurosurgery, Jaslok Hospital & Research Centre, Mumbai.

Rajani M. Ramakrishnan

MBBS, DA, DNB, PDF (Neuroanaesthesia)

Consultant - Jaslok Hospital & Research Centre, Mumbai.

Rajashree Gandhe

MBBS, MD Anaesthesiology

Co-ordinator Neuroanaesthesiology and Programme Director, ISNACC Fellowship, Kokilaben Dhirubhai Ambani Hospital, Mumbai.

Ranjana Das

MD

Consultant Anaesthesia, Dept. of Anaesthesia, Bombay Hospital & Research Center, Mumbai.

Ritu K. Kashikar

DNB, DMRD Radiodiagnosis

Consultant - Jaslok Hospital & Research centre, Mumbai.

Savi J. Kapila

DNB Anaestheisa

Consultant - Jaslok Hospital & Research centre, Mumbai.

Shwetal Goraksha

M.D. Anaesthesia, Post Doctoral Fellowship Neuroanaesthesia (ISNACC)

Consultant - P. D. Hinduja Hospital, Mumbai.

Shrinivas B. Desai

MD Radiology

Consultant - Jaslok Hospital & Research Centre, Mumbai.

Siva S. Chivukula

M. Ch

Dept. of Neurosurgery, Jaslok Hospital & Research Centre, Pedder Road, Mumbai.

Smita D. Sharma

DA, DNB

Consultant Anaesthesiologist, Dept. of Anaesthesia Bombay Hospital & Research Centre, Mumbai.

Smita Thorve

MBBS, DNB General Surgery, DNB Neurosurgery

Dept. of Neurosurgery, Jaslok Hospital & Research Centre, Mumbai.

Sugandha A. Karapurkar

MD, DA

Former Prof. Anaesthesiology, KEM Hospital and Seth G. S. Medical College, Consultant - Breach Candy Hospital, Mumbai.

Swati F. Daftary

DA , MD Anaesthesia

Consultant : Jaslok Hospital & Research Center, Mumbai.

Tasneem Dhansura

MBBS, MD, DNB, PDCC (Cardiac & Neuroanaesthesia)

Consultant - Saifee Hospital, Mumbai.

Vaibhavi Baxi

DA, FCPS, DNB

Consultant - Lilavati Hospital & Research Centre, Mumbai.

Varun Jain

MBBS, MD, DNB, DM (Neuroanaesthesiology)

Assistant Professor

Dept. of Neuroanaesthesia and Critical Care,

All India Institute of Medical Sciences, New Delhi.

Vidhu Bhatnagar

MBBS, MD, DNB, DM (Neuroanasthesia)

Dept. of Anaesthesiology and Critical Care, INHS Asvini, Mumbai.

Vikram S. Karmarkar

MS (GEN) MRCSEd DNB (NS)

Consultant - Neurosurgeon and Asst. Professor, Dept. of Neurosurgery - Bombay Hospital Institute of Medical Sciences, Mumbai.

CONTENTS

CHAPTER 1

APPLIED ANATOMY OF BRAIN AND SPINAL CORD

Raghvendra Ramdasi, Rajshree Deopujari, Siva Chivukula, Smita Thorve, Nikhil Chamankar

Introduction

Neuroanatomy forms the basis of neurological surgery. But knowledge of the anatomy is also a prerequisite for an anaesthetist for the safe practice of anaesthesia.

It is discussed under following headings

A) Embryology

B) Scalp

C) Meninges

D) Ventricles and CSF

E) Surface of the brain

F) Subcortical structures

G) Brainstem

H) Long sensory and motor tracts

I) Blood supply of the brain

J) Cerebellum

A) Embryology

The neural tube

The nervous system develops from the ectoderm of the embryo. The neural plate, a thickening of the ectoderm, is evident 16 days after fertilization, and by 18 days it is indented in the midline (neural groove) with enlargements on either side (neural folds). By 22 days the rostral ends of the neural folds are conspicuously enlarged; they will become the cerebral hemispheres. Fusion of the neural folds begins on Day 22 at a level that will eventually be that of the cervical segments of the spinal cord. Fusion proceeds rostrally and caudally, to form the neural tube. The initially open ends of the tube close on Day 24 (rostral neuropore) and Day 27 (caudal neuropore).

In **anencephaly** the rostral neural tube fails to develop. In **myeloschisis**is, there is failure of closure of the posterior neuropore. In **meningocoele** and **meningomyelocoele** the caudal neuropore closes, but the mesodermal tissues (bone, dermis) dorsal to the spina cord and nerve roots fail to develop. The caudal part of the spinal cord (below segment L2) is originates from pluripotential cells of the caudal cell mass (not the neural tube).

The cephalic end of the neural tube dilates to form three primary brain vesicle (see table)

Primary vesicle	Primary division	Subdivision	Adult structures
Forebrain Vesicle	Prosencephalon (Forebrain)	Telencephalon	Cerebral Hemispheres, Basal Ganglia, Hippocampus
		Diencephalon	Thalamus, Hypothalamus, Pineal Gland, Infundibulum, Pars nervosa of the hypophysis
Midbrain Vesicle	Mesencephalon (Midbrain)	Mesencephalon (Midbrain)	Tectum, Tegmentum, Crus cerebri
Hindbrain Vesicle	Rhombencephalon (Hindbrain)	Metencephalon	Pons, Cerebellum
		Myelencephalon	Medulla Oblongata

B) Scalp

- As per the mnemonic, scalp contains five layers. It has S-Skin, C-or Connective tissue & nerves, A-Galeal Aponeurosis, L-Loose areolar tissue, P-Pericranium.

- Nerve supply
    - Forehead-innervated by supraorbital & supratrochlear nerves(branches of V1 division of trigeminal nerve)
    - Vertex & Lateral scalp-zygomatico-temporal (V2), Temporo-mandibular and auriculo-temporal (V3).
    - Occiput-greater auricular, occipital nerve and C2, C3 cervical nerves.

- Scalp block
    - Ophlamic nerve(anterior scalp) block- supraorbital & supratrochlear nerves are anesthetized at the point of supraorbital foramen. It is palpated on the supraorbital ridge.
    - Lateral scalp & vertex block

      For auriculo-temporal nerve, the injecting needle is inserted between tragus and superficial temporal artery. For zygomatico-temporal nerve needle inserted halfway down the line joining tragus to outer corner of the eye.
    - Greater and lesser occipital nerve block (posterior scalp)

      For greater occipital nerve 2.5 cm lateral to median nuchal line medial to occipital artery and for lesser occipital nerve 2.5 laterally and 1cm caudally needle is inserted.

C) Meninges

The three layers of the meninges are as follows (Fig. 1)

The dura mater is the outermost meningeal membrane.

- Two dural sheets, or reflections, extend into the cranial cavity:
    - The falx cerebri, lying between the two cerebral hemispheres
    - The tentorium cerebelli, lying between the cerebellum and the occipital lobes of the cerebrum and encircling the midbrain.

- Dura is adherent to inner table of skull (no epidural space). It is composed of two fused layers (periosteal and meningeal), which split to form sinuses.

The middle meningeal layer is the arachnoid mater.

- Both the dura and arachnoid surround the brain loosely. It contains arachnoid villi (in superior sagittal sinus) and arachnoid trabeculae which are important in CSF absorption.

- It encloses subarachnoid space containing CSF. It forms many pockets called cisterns

The innermost meningeal layer is the pia mater, which adheres to the surface of the brain, follows vessels and closely follows contours of the brain. This creates a subarachnoid space of variable depth.

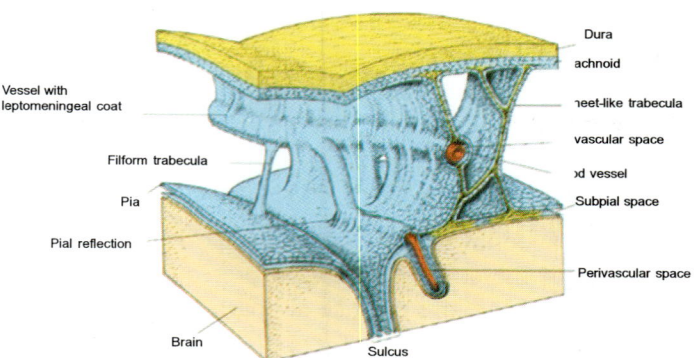

Fig. 1. Shows layers of meninges with arrangement of blood vessels.

Infections

Infections of the meninges (**bacterial meningitis**) may be called **leptomeningitis** because the causative organisms localize to the subarachnoid space and involve the pia and arachnoid. Extension into the dura is called **pachymeningitis**. The patient becomes critically ill with confusion, stupor, neck stiffness [**meningismus**] with or without focal deficits. Patients with **viral meningitis have more indolent course.** Treatment is antibiotics.

Epidural (extradural) hematoma is commonly caused by a skull fracture damaging a major dural vessel (middle meningeal artery most common). The extravasated blood dissects the dura mater off the inner table forming large, lens (lenticular) shaped hematoma. They do not cross suture lines forming its characteristic shape. The patient may be unconscious initially, followed by a lucid interval (the patient is wide awake), and then deteriorate rapidly to death; this is called "talk and die." Treatment is urgent surgical removal.

Subdural hematoma is commonly caused by tearing of bridging veins as a result of trauma. Acute subdural hematomas are commonly seen immediately in younger patient after severe trauma. Chronic subdural hematomas are usually seen in the elderly or in patients on anticoagulation therapy after trivial falls. They may take days or weeks to become symptomatic. This lesion appears "biconcave" and follows the surface of the brain for long distance (not limited by sutures). Treatment is surgery if it is causing mass effect.

Subarachnoid hemorrhage is most commonly caused by trauma. In approximately 75% to 80% o patients with

spontaneous (nontraumatic) subarachnoid hemorrhage is as a result of an intracranial aneurysm. Onset is sudden; the patient complains of a sudden and excruciatingly painful headache ("the worst of my life," "thunderclap," "felt like my head exploded") and may remain conscious, become lethargic and disoriented, or may be comatose. Treatment of an aneurysm is to surgically separate the sac of the aneurysm from the parent vessel (by clip or coil), if possible, and protect against the development o vasospasm.

D) Ventricles and CSF

The brain and spinal cord are suspended weightlessly in the CSF, which acts as a protective cushion for fragile nervous tissue.

Secretion – CSF is secreted by the choroid plexuses of the four ventricles of the brain, largest being those of the lateral ventricles (Fig. 2). It has secretory epithelium enclosing permeable capillary blood vessels.

Lateral Ventricles-Paired C shaped cavity present one in each hemisphere

Divisions:

Body	–	occupies the parietal lobe
Anterior horn	–	extends into frontal lobe
Posterior horn	–	extends into occipital lobe
Inferior horn	–	extends into temporal lobe

Circulation and Absorption

The CSF from lateral ventricles enters the third ventricle through two foramen of Monro. It then travels to fourth ventricle through aqueduct of Sylvius. CSF leaves the ventricular system by a median aperture (foramen of Magendie) into the cisterna magna and two lateral apertures (foramen of Lushka) into the cerebello-pontine angle cistern. In the subarachnoid space CSF flows upward and forward around the brain stem and cerebellum and then around the cerebral hemispheres to the main site of absorption, the arachnoid granulations beside the superior sagittal sinus (Fig. 2).

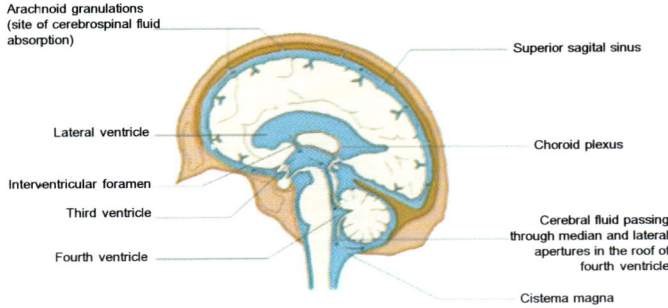

Fig. 2. Shows ventricular system with circulation of the cerebrospinal fluid

Applied anatomy of brain and spinal cord

Non communicating hydrocephalus occurs when there is blockage of flow in the ventricles. It can be because of tumor, clot or congenital aqueductal stenosis.

Communicating hydrocephalus occurs when the flow of CSF through the subarachnoid space or arachnoid granulations is blocked (*e.g.* by pus and scarring in bacterial meningitis, or by blood following haemorrhage into the subarachnoid space. The abnormally large volume of CSF around a shrunken brain (*e.g.* in Alzheimer's disease) is sometimes called **hydrocephalus ex vacuo.**

CSF statistics (lumbar) :

Pressure (recumbent) 10–15 cm of CSF

Cells Less than 3-4 white cells/mm³

Protein 0.15- 0.45 g/l

(15–45 mg/100 ml)

Glucose 2.8–4.2 mmol/l (65%of the blood plasma level in the fasting state)

(50–75 mg/100 ml)

IgG 10–12% of total protein

Chloride 120–130 mmol/l

Cerebrospinal fluid dynamics

The CSF is produced by the choroid plexus ata rate of approximately 0.4 ml per minute. Approximately 500 ml of CSF is produced each day. The total CSF volume is 140 ml; the lateral ventricles contain approximately 25 ml, the spinal cord subarachnoid space 30 ml and the remainder of the fluid is found in the basal cisterns. The fluid is normally clear and colourless; it will appear turbid if it contains more than 400 white blood cells or 200 red blood cells per mm³.

Methods of CSF collection

CSF can be obtained by:

- Lumbar puncture

  The fluid is usually obtained by lumbar puncture. It is performed by palpating the iliac crest; this lies at the L3-4 level. The lumbar puncture can be carried out at this space or at the spaces immediately above or below.

  It is strictly contraindicated in raised ICP

- Cisternal puncture

  Cisternal puncture is performed if the lumbar puncture has failed due to technical difficulties, if there is local skin sepsis or, in some radiology investigations, where it is the preferred route of contrast administration for myelography.

- Cannulation of the lateral ventricle.

  Ventricular puncture is usually only performed as an intraoperative procedure or for temporary reduction of intracranial pressure in an emergency[1,2,4,7].

E) Surface of the brain

The surface of the cerebral hemisphere exhibits a complex pattern of convolutions, or gyri, which are separated by furrows of varying depth known as fissures, or sulci (Fig. 3).

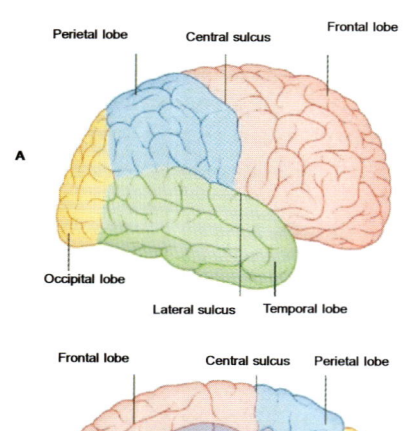

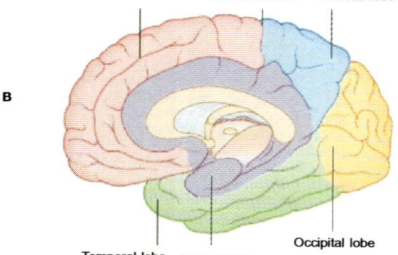

Fig. 3. Shows lateral (A) and medial (B) surface of the brain with demarcation of the lobes

- Frontal Lobe - The frontal lobe is anterior to the central sulcus and above the lateral fissure

- Parietal Lobe - The parietal lobe lies posterior to the central sulcus. On the medial aspect of the hemisphere, its boundary with the occipital lobe is clearly demarcated by the deep parieto-occipital sulcus. The inferior boundary is the posterior ramus of the lateral fissure and its imaginary posterior prolongation.

- Temporal Lobe - The temporal lobe is inferior to the lateral fissure. It is limited behind by an arbitrary line from the preoccipital incisure to the parieto-occipital sulcus.

- Occipital Lobe - The occipital lobe lies behind an arbitrary line joining the preoccipital incisures and the parieto-occipital sulcus

Eloquent Areas of the brain:

The following are the eloquent areas of the respective lobes (Fig. 4).

Frontal Lobe

- The primary motor cortex (MI) corresponds to the precentral gyrus (area 4). The primary motor cortex contains a detailed, topographically organized map (motor homunculus) of the opposite body half, with the head represented most laterally and the legs and feet represented on the medial surface of the hemisphere in the paracentral lobule

- Premotor cortex-Immediately in front of the primary motor cortex lies Brodmann's area 6. The dorsal premotor cortex is probably important in establishing a motor set or intention, contributing to motor preparation in relation to internally guided movement. In contrast, ventral premotor cortex is related more to the execution of externally (especially visually) guided movements in relation to a specific external stimulus.

- Supplementary motor cortex - The supplementary motor area (MII) lies medial to area 6 and extends from the most superolateral part to the medial surface of the hemisphere

- Prefrontal cortex - The prefrontal cortex on the lateral surface of the hemisphere comprises predominantly Brodmann's areas 9, 46 and 45

  It contains auditory and visual associations, and areas for calculating, thinking and decision making.

- Frontal eye field - The frontal eye field lies predominantly within Brodmann's area 8, anterior to the superior premotor cortex. It is responsible for saccadic eye control.

- Broca's area - The motor speech area of Broca lies in the inferior frontal gyrus (Broadmann areas 44 and 45).

Applied anatomy:

- **Fronto temporal dementia,** characterized anatomically by atrophy involving predominantly the frontal and temporal cortices (so-called Pick's bodies)

- **Frontal eye movements in disease** Acute destructive (ischaemic) cerebral hemispheric lesions involving the frontal ('adversive') eye field are well known to produce ipsilateral eye deviation. This is in contrast to an irritative lesion (e.g. a focal seizure), which induces deviation of the head and eyes to the opposite side

Parietal Lobe

- Primary somatosensory cortex-

  The sensory area is located in the postcentral gyrus and is called the **first somatosensory area (SI).** It corresponds to areas 3, 1, 2 of Brodmann.

- **Superior and Inferior Parietal Lobules**

  Posterior to the postcentral gyrus, the superior part of the parietal lobe is composed of areas 5a and 5b (superior parietal lobule) 7a and 7b (inferior parietal lobule). This is essential for the synthesis and interpretation of impulses, appreciation of similarities and differences, interpretation of spatial relationships and two-dimensional qualities, evaluations of variations in form and weight, and localization of sensation.

Applied anatomy

- **Gerstmann's syndrome** consists of finger agnosia, left–right confusion, dysgraphia and dyscalculia. The lesion involves the angular and supramarginal gyri of the dominant side.

- **Nondominant parietal syndrome** - Patients with nondominant parietal lobe lesions have apraxia, hemi-inattention, hemineglect, and denial of disability

- **Temporal lobe**

  The auditory radiations run from the medial geniculate body to the auditory cortex (areas 41 and 42) in the superior surface of superior temporal gyrus. The posterior superior temporal area(sensory speech area) of the dominant hemisphere causes Wernicke's aphasia

Applied anatomy

- **Temporal epilepsy**

  Here patient is experiencing repetitive complex partial seizures (so-called uncinate or psychomotor seizures). Clinically, the seizure focus is presumed to be in the vicinity of the uncus, amygdala or insula in her dominant (left) hemisphere.

- **Occipital lobe**

  The areas concerned with vision are located in the occipital lobe, mainly on the medial surface, both above and below the calcarine sulcus (area 17). Due to its gross appearance it is also called the *striate cortex*. In addition to the striate cortex, supplementary areas include area 18 (*parastriate area*) and area 19 (*peristriate area*). Areas 18 and 19 are responsible mainly for size shape contrast of the images received.

Applied anatomy

- **Anton's syndrome**

  Inability to see because of bilateral injury to the occipital lobes is termed cortical blindness. In rare cases of cortical blindness, patients insist that they can see and confabulate when asked to describe objects in their environment. This disorder is called Anton's syndrome.

- **Awake craniotomy**

  The supratentorial intraaxial lesions (cortical and subcortical) located in the eloquent cortex are best approached by awake craniotomy and cortical mapping[1,2,4,7].

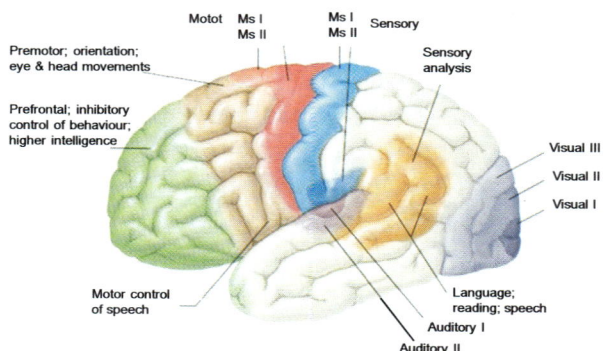

Fig. 4. Shows lateral surface of the brain with eloquent areas

F) Subcortical structures

These include-

- Basal Ganglia
- Diencephalon

The term **basal ganglia** include five structures **caudate nucleus, putamen,** and **globus pallidus** (three large nuclear masses underlying the cortical mantle), the **subthalamic nucleus,** and **substantia nigra.** The globus pallidus is divided into external and internal segments (GPe and GPi). The caudate nucleus and putamen are commonly called the **striatum;** the putamen and globus pallidus are sometimes called the **lenticular nucleus** (Fig. 5).

- The substantia nigra is connected to striatum via dopaminergic nigrostriatal pathway.

- The cerebral cortex projects to the striatum, the striatum to GPi, GPi to the thalamus, and the thalamus back to the cortex, completing a loop. The output from GPi to the thalamus is inhibitory, whereas the output from the thalamus to the cerebral cortex is excitatory.

- The GPe projects to GPi directly and indirectly via subthalamic nucleus.

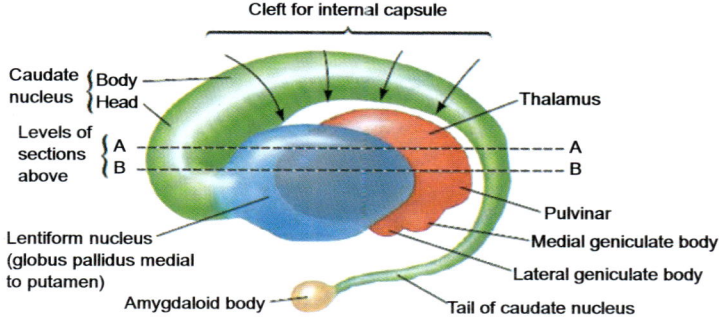

Interrelationship of thalamus, lentiform nucleus, caudate nucleus and amygdaloid body (schema): left lateral view

Fig. 5. Shows basal ganglia and thalamus

Applied anatomy

- ### Disorders of basal ganglia

  Damage to striatum leads to choreoathetosis-Chorea is characterized by rapid, involuntary "dancing" movements. **Athetosis** is characterized by continuous, slow writhing movements. The example is **Huntington disease.**

  Damage to subthalamic nucleus leads to hemiballismus which is flailing, intense, and violent movements occur.

  Damage to nigrostriatal pathway leads to Parkinson's disease which is characterised by rigidity, akinesia, tremor.

- ### Targets for surgery

  GPi – Lesioning or deep brain stimulation (DBS) in this region is used for treating dystonia.

  STN – Lesioning or deep brain stimulation (DBS) in this region is used for treating Parkinson's disease.

Diencephalon

- Epithalamus (includes the pineal gland) - required for diurnal recognition.
- Subthalamus- functionally part of basal ganaglia.
- Hypothalamus
- Thalamus

Hypothalamus

It is situated ventral to thalamus. It regulates temperature, thirst, sexual behaviour, endocrine functions (oxytocin, vasopressin, thyroid and corticotrophin releasing hormone), fight and flight response(sympathetic centre).

Applied anatomy

During operations in the suprasellar region the stretching of hypothalamus or the pituitary stalk lead to diabetes insipedus (DI) characterised by pouring of large dilute urine.

Thalamus

It is situated on either side of third ventricle.(Fig. 5). The thalamus serves primarily as a relay station that modulates and coordinates the function of various systems.

The thalamus is divided by internal medullary lamina into large nuclear groups-medial, lateral, and anterior. The intralaminar nuclei lie scattered along the internal medullary laminae; they essentially comprise a rostral extension of the brainstem reticular formation. These nuclei are primarily concerned with arousal.

a) Anterior - The internal medullary lamina diverges anteriorly, and the anterior nucleus lies between the arms of this Y-shaped structure. The mamillothalamic tract ascends from the mamillary bodies bound primarily for the anterior nucleus of the thalamus, which sends its major output to the cingulate gyrus. The anterior nucleus is part of the limbic lobe and Papez circuit, and it is related to emotion and memory function.

b) The medial nucleus is a single, large structure that lies on the medial side of the internal medullary lamina. Since its position is also slightly dorsal, it is usually referred to as the mediodorsal or dorsomedial (DM) nucleus. The DM has vaguely understood functions, related to cognition, judgment, affect and memory.

c) The lateral nuclear group is subdivided into several component nuclei. The major division is into the dorsal tier and the ventral tier.

- The dorsal tier nuclei consist of the lateral dorsal and lateral posterior nuclei and the pulvinar. These are concerned with extrageniculocalcarine vision.
- The ventral tier subnuclei of the lateral nucleus are true relay nuclei, connecting lower centers with the cortex and vice versa.

- The ventral posterior lateral (VPL) nucleus and ventral posterior medial (VPM) nucleus are the major sensory relay nuclei. The VPL receives the termination of the lemniscal and anterolateral (spinothalamic) sensory pathways for the body; it projects in turn to the somesthetic cortex (Brodmann areas 1, 2 and 3). VPM serves the same function for the head, receiving the trigeminothalamic tracts as well as taste fibers from the solitary nucleus; it projects to the somesthetic cortex.

- The ventral lateral (VL) nucleus coordinates the motor system. The VLo (oralis) receives input from the basal ganglia (globus pallidus), substantia nigra, and VLc (caudalis) from cerebellum (dentate nucleus)The VL then projects to the motor and supplementary motor areas. The ventral anterior (VA) nucleus also receives projections from the globus pallidus, as well as the substantia nigra; it projects primarily to the premotor cortex. It is via VL and VA that the basal ganglia and cerebellum influence motor activity

- Medial geniculate body is connected to auditory and lateral to visual system.

Applied Anatomy

Thalamic Syndrome

Thalamic pain syndrome (Dejerine-Roussy syndrome) is well recognized. The ventral lateral thalamus is most commonly involved. Classic features of the disorder include hyperpathia, hyperalgesia and allodynia.

Thalamotomy

VLo nucleus is ablated stereotactically for writer's dystonia with good control postoperatively.

G) Brainstem

Features of the brainstem

The brainstem consists of the medulla oblongata, pons and midbrain.(Fig. 6).

The brainstem has tectum (dorsally), tegmentum (in between) and base (ventrally).

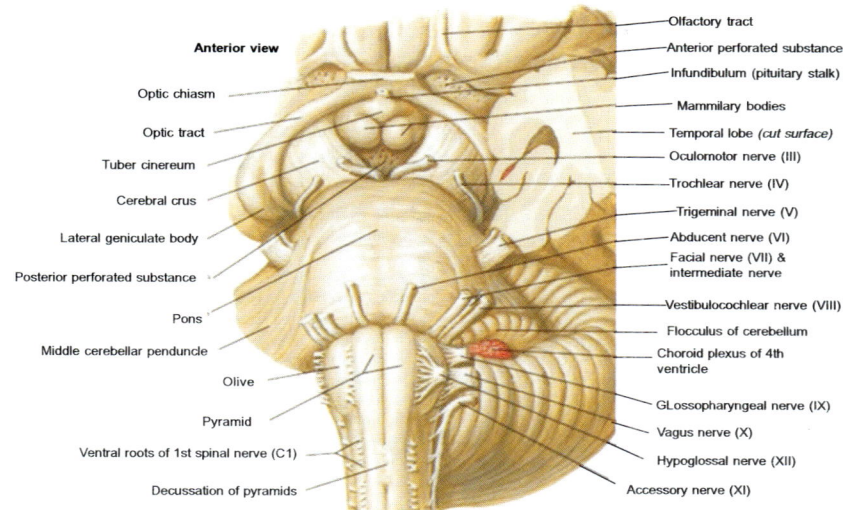

Fig. 6. Shows ventral surface of the brainstem with the cranial nerves

Midbrain:

- Here the tectum consists of superior colliculus (serves visual reflexes) and inferior colliculus (serves hearing)
- Tegmentum at superior colliculus level contains red nucleus (origin of rubrospinal tract) and III nerve nucleus. The IIIrd nerve comes out from ventral aspect in the interpeduncular fossa.
- Tegmentum at inferior colliculus contains crossing of superior cerebellar peduncles and IVth nerve nucleus. The IVth nerve comes out from dorsal aspect (only nerve arising from dorsal aspect) turns in the ambient cistern to reach free edge of the tent.
- The base consists of cerebral peduncle, which consists of the substantia nigra and crus cerebri. The crus cerebri is a continuation of the internal capsule and has descending corticospinal and corticobulbar fibers.

Applied anatomy

Midbrain syndromes

Ventral midbrain syndromes

The lesion is anterior-in the cerebral peduncle-in **Weber's syndrome**, which causes hemiparesis. It is more posterior-in the tegmentum-in **Claude's syndrome**, which causes hemiataxia. In **Benedikt's syndrome** the lesion is more extensive, involving both the tegmentum and the peduncle, which causes hemiparesis with tremor and ataxia of the

involved limbs; Benedikt's is essentially Weber's + Claude's.

Dorsal midbrain (Perinaud's)syndrome

The lesion is posterior near tectal plate. It is commonly caused by pineal tumors. It causes – impaired upgaze; convergence retraction nystagmus; dilated pupils with light near dissociation.

Pons

- The tectum consists of the nonfunctional anterior medullary velum which forms upper roof of fourth ventricle
- The base is rounded and protuberant ("belly" of the pons) and consists of descending corticospinal and corticobulbar fibers admixed crossing of middle cerebellar peduncle (MCP) called basis pontis.
- The tegmentum contains Vth nerve nucleus(comes out from lateral part of upper pons), VIth cranial nerve nucleus (comes out from ventral part near midline for middle part of pons) VIIth & VIIIth cranial nerve nuclei(After looping around the CN VI nucleus, CN VII fibers exit the pons laterally, cross the cerebellopontine angle (CPA) with CN VIII, and disappear into the internal auditory meatus.
- The other important tracts include medial leminiscus (dorsal column sensation) and lateral leminiscus (hearing) and medial longitudinal fasciculus (connecting IIIrd, IVth, VIth cranial nerves)

Applied anatomy

Pontine Syndromes

- **Millard and Gubler** - Millard and Gubler separately described patients with an ipsilateral lower motor neuron facial nerve palsy and contralateral hemiparesis due to a lesion involving the pons

- **Foville syndrome** - Foville described a patient with an ipsilateral lower motor neuron facial palsy and horizontal gaze palsy, with a contralateral hemiparesis.

CPA lesions

The vestibular schwannoma and epidermoid cyst are common CPA lesions presenting with various cranial nerve deficits and warrant surgery.

Medulla

- In the medulla, the tectum consists of the posterior medullary velum forms lower roof of fourth ventricle

- The base consists of the medullary pyramids, which are made up of fibers of the corticospinal tract. At lower level they cross forming pyramidal dicussation.

- The tegmentum of the medulla is conveniently divided into medial and lateral portions.

The **medial medulla** contains the crossing medial leminiscus in a vertical midline position with the MLF capping it posteriorly. The hypoglossal nerve nucleus lies in the midline (comes out from ventral aspect near midline from lower medulla).

The **lateral medulla** contains CN V nucleus, spinothalmic (anterolateral system) fibers,the nuclei of IX to XI crnial nerves. It also contains sympathetic fibers and crossing of inferior cerebellar peduncles (ICP).

Applied Anatomy

Medullary Syndromes

There are two primary medullary syndromes: the lateral (Wallenberg's) and the medial (Dejerine's).

- **Wallenberg syndrome** – Loss of pain and temperature ipsilateral face and contralateral body; decreased ipsilateral corneal reflex; weakness of ipsilateral soft palate; vocal cord and gag reflex, ipsilateral Horner's syndrome; nystagmus; cerebellar ataxia of ipsilateral limbs

- **Dejerine syndrome** - Ipsilateral tongue weakness; contralateral hemiparesis (sparing face); +/- impairment of posterior column function; lateral spinothalamic functions spared

The reticular formation controls the level of consciousness, the cardiovascular system and the respiratory system. It is present throughout.

Brainstem lesions

Localisation

A unilateral brainstem lesion caused by stroke, tumor or multiple sclerosis causes ipsilateral cranial nerve dysfunction, contralateral spastic hemiparesis, contralateral hemisensory loss and ipsilateral incoordination. A bilateral lesion destroys the 'vital centres' that control breathing and the circulation, leading to coma and death.

Brain herniation

The brainstem is vulnerable to pressure at free edge of tent at tentorial notch and

in the foramen magnum (Fig. 7). The supratentorial tumor, bleed, edema can produce

- Uncal herniation - It is caused by displacement of the uncus of the temporal lobe into the tentorial notch. It causes ipsilateral third nerve palsy and contralateral motor weakness.

- Pressure coning - A cone of cerebellar tissue (the tonsil) may descend into the foramen magnum, squeezing the medulla oblongata and causing bilateral cranial nerve dysfunction, quadriplegia, deepening coma and finally apnea—brain stem death.

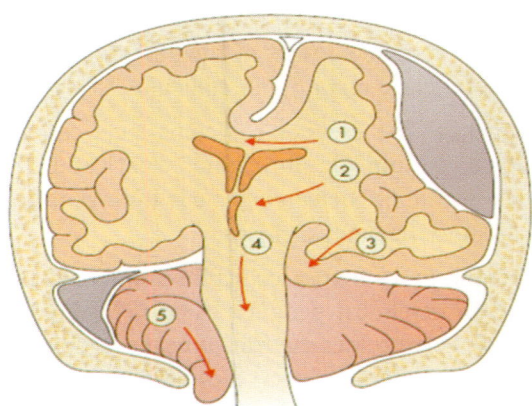

Fig. 7. Shows brain herniations; 1-subfalcine, 2-midline shift, 3-uncal, 4-central, 5 tonsillar

H) Long Sensory and Motor Tracts (Figs. 8–10)

A) Sensory Pathways

The principal direct pathways to the cerebral cortex for touch, vibratory

sense, and proprioception (position sense) are shown in Fig. 8. Fibers mediating these sensations ascend ipsilaterally in the dorsal columns to the medulla, where they synapse in the **gracilus** and **cuneate nuclei**. The second-order neurons from these nuclei cross the midline and ascend in the **medial lemniscus** to end in the contralateral **ventral posterior lateral (VPL) nucleus** and related specific sensory relay nuclei of the thalamus. This ascending system is called the **dorsal column** or **medial lemniscal system.**

Fibers from nociceptors(carrying pain) and thermoreceptors (carrying temperature) synapse on neurons in the dorsal horn.The axons from these neurons cross the midline and ascend in the form of **ventrolateral spinothalamic tract.** Fibers within this tract synapse in the VPL. From VPL nuclei in the thalamus, fibers project to SI and SII. This is the pathway responsible for the **discriminative** aspect of pain, and is also called the **neospinothalamic tract.**

Applied Anatomy

Brown–Séquard Syndrome

A functional hemisection of the spinal cord causes damage to ascending sensory – dorsal column pathway (crosses in medulla), ventrolateral spinothalamic tract (crosses in cord) and descending motor corticospinal tract (crosses in medulla) pathways. It results in ipsilateral weakness; loss of touch, vibration, position and contralateral loss of pain, temperature below that level. This is Brown–Séquard Syndrome.

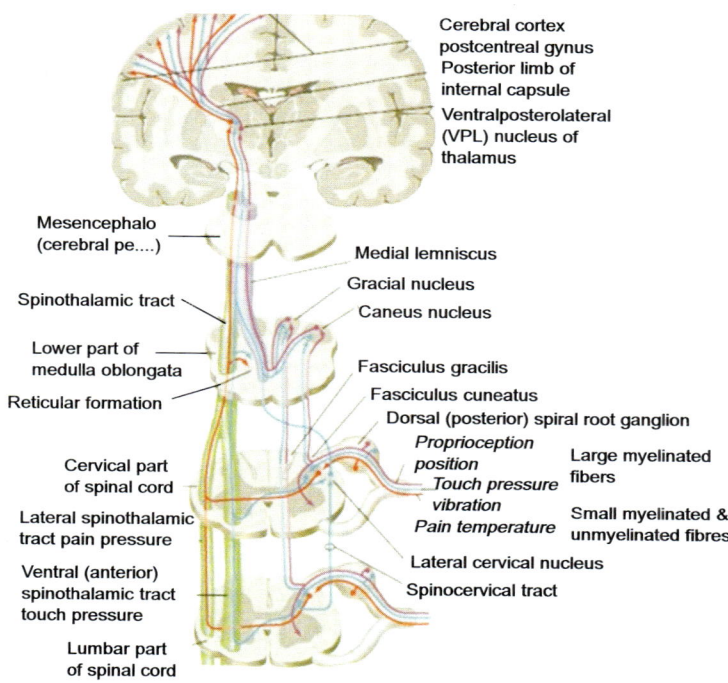

Fig. 8. Shows the sensory system

B) Motor tract

The corticospinal tract (Fig. 9)

This tract originates in the precentral gyrus and passes through the internal capsule. Most (80%) fibers decussate in the pyramids and descend in the lateral white matter of the spinal cord to form the lateral division of the tract which can make monosynaptic connections with spinal motor neurons and control the skilled movements. The ventral division (20%) of the tract remains uncrossed until reaching the spinal cord where axons terminate on spinal interneurons antecedent to motor neurons and coordinate different muscle groups.

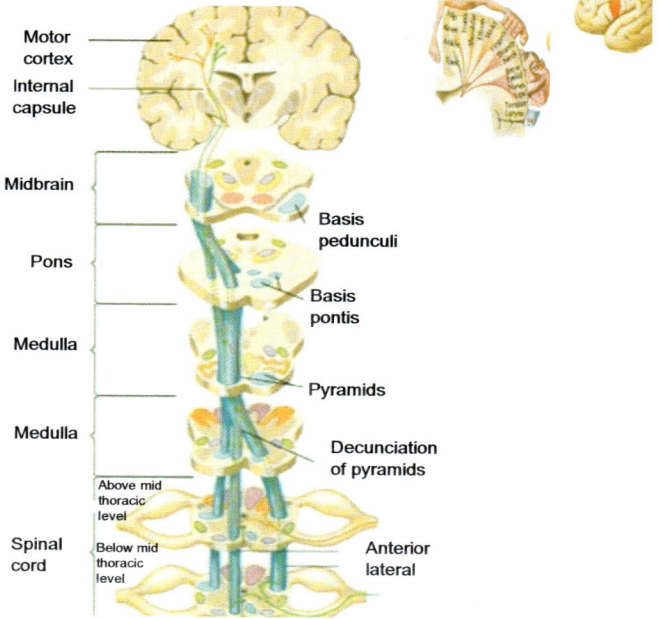

Fig. 9. Shows the pyramidal system

Applied anatomy

The motor system can be divided into lower and upper motor neurons.

Upper motor neurons are those in the cortex and brain stem that activate the lower motor neurons. **Lower motor neurons include anterior horn cells and their** axons which terminate on skeletal muscles.

	Upper motor neuron	Lower motor neuron
Tone	Increased-spasticity	Decreased- flaccidity
Bulk	Normal	Atrophy
Fasciculations	No	Yes
Deep Reflexes	Hyperactive stretch reflex	Hyporeflexia or Areflexia
Plantar reflex	Extensor reflex (Babinski sign)	Absent
xample	Stroke in middle cerebral artery Cervical myelopathy	Poliomyelitis ALS

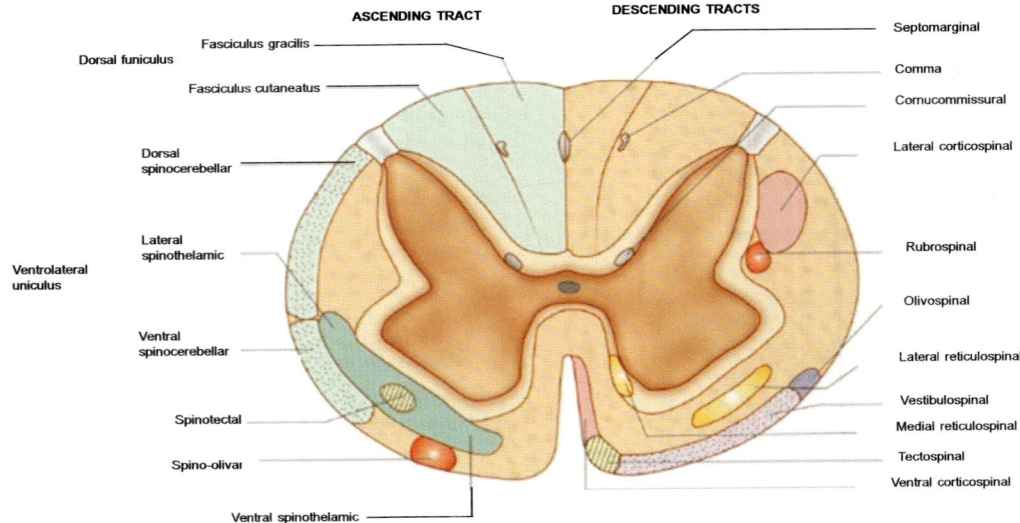

Fig. 10. Shows transverse section of the cervical cord with arrangement of the tracts

C) Brain stem pathways involved in posture and voluntary movement

The pathways are organized such that those innervating the most proximal muscles are located most medially and those innervating the more distal muscles are located more laterally

- **Medial brain stem pathway**

  The medial brain stem pathways, which work in concert with the ventral corticospinal tract, are the pontine and medullary reticulospinal, vestibulospinal, and tectospinal tracts. They terminate predominantly on interneurons and long propriospinal neurons in the ventral horn to control axial and proximal muscles

- **Lateral brainstem pathway**

  The main control of distal muscles arise from the lateral corticospinal tract, but neurons within the red nucleus of the midbrain cross the midline and project to control distal limb muscles of upper limb. This rubrospinal tract excites flexor motor neurons and inhibits extensor motor neurons.

Applied anatomy

- **Decerebration**

  A complete transection of the brain stem between the superior and inferior colliculi cause the brain stem pathways to function independent of their higher brain structures. This is called a **midcollicular decerebration.** The inputs from the cortex (corticospinal and corticobulbar tracts) and red nucleus (rubrospinal tract),to distal muscles of the extremities are interrupted. This leads to the dominance of the excitatory reticulospinal pathways (primarily to postural extensor muscles) resulting in hyperactivity in extensor muscles in all four extremities which is called **decerebrate rigidity.**

Causes

This resembles what ensues after **supratentorial lesions** in humans cause uncal herniation. This is as a result of large tumors or a hemorrhage in the cerebral hemisphere

- **Decortication**

  Removal of the cerebral cortex produces **decorticate rigidity** characterized by flexion of the upper extremities at the elbow and extensor hyperactivity in the lower extremities. The flexion can be explained by rubrospinal excitation of flexor muscles in the upper

extremities; the hyperextension of lower extremities is due to the same changes that occur after midcollicular decerebration.

Causes

Decorticate rigidity is seen on the hemiplegic side in humans after hemorrhages or thromboses in the internal capsule.

I) Blood supply of the brain

A) Arterial Supply

The brain is supplied by two sets of arteries–**internal carotid and vertebrobasilar arteries** (Fig. 11)

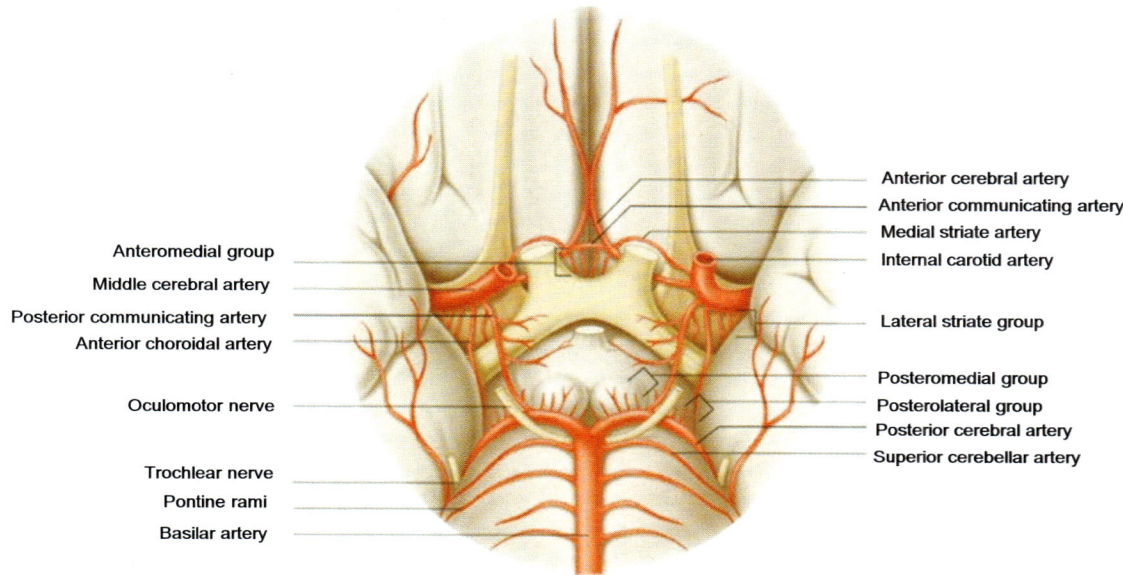

Fig. 11. Shows circle of Willis

a) Internal carotid artery

Each internal carotid artery arises in the neck at the level of C4 vertebra

Branches of the Cerebral Part (Intracranial Part):

- **Ophthalmic artery:** It supplies the orbit and its contents.

- **Anterior choroidal artery:** It runs backwards close to the optic tract and supplies the visual pathway, internal capsule and midbrain and forms the choroid plexus of the inferior horn of lateral ventricle.

- **Posterior communicating artery:** This also runs backwards and anastomoses with the posterior cerebral artery, a branch of the basilar artery.

It divides in to anterior cerebral artery and middle cerebral artery.

- **Anterior cerebral artery** it supplies medial half of orbital surface of the frontal lobe containing medial

olfactory gurus and bulb (Orbital branch), anteroinferior part of the frontal lobe (frontopolar branch),1-2 cm of superior surface and entire medial surface of the frontal and the parietal lobes including the paracentral lobule, cingulate gyrus, corpus callosum and the precuneus of the parietal lobe (callosomarginal and pericallosal branches).

Applied anatomy – effects of occlusion of anterior cerebral artery

Paralysis (or weakness) of muscles of the leg and foot of the opposite side (by involvement of the upper part of the motor area) Loss (or dulling) of sensations from the leg and foot of the opposite side (by involvement of the upper part of the sensory area) Sense of stereognosis is impaired (by involvement of parietal lobe) Personality changes (by involvement of frontal lobe) (Fig. 12).

- **Middle cerebral artery** - It supplies lateral half of orbital surface of frontal lobe (orbital branch). The frontal and parietal branches supply remaining superolateral surface of frontal (precentral, middle, and inferior frontal gyri) and parietal lobe (postcentral gyrus, inferior parietal lobule, and superior parietal lobule). The temporal branches supply the lateral surface of the temporal lobe excluding the inferior temporal gyrus but including the temporal pole

Applied anatomy-effects of occlusion of middle cerebral artery

It causes hemiplegia and loss of sensations on the opposite half of the body. The face and arms are most affected. Foot and leg are spared. Aphasia (by involvement of Broca's and Wernicke's areas in dominant side) Homonymous hemianopia on the opposite side (by involvement of optic radiation) (Fig. 12).

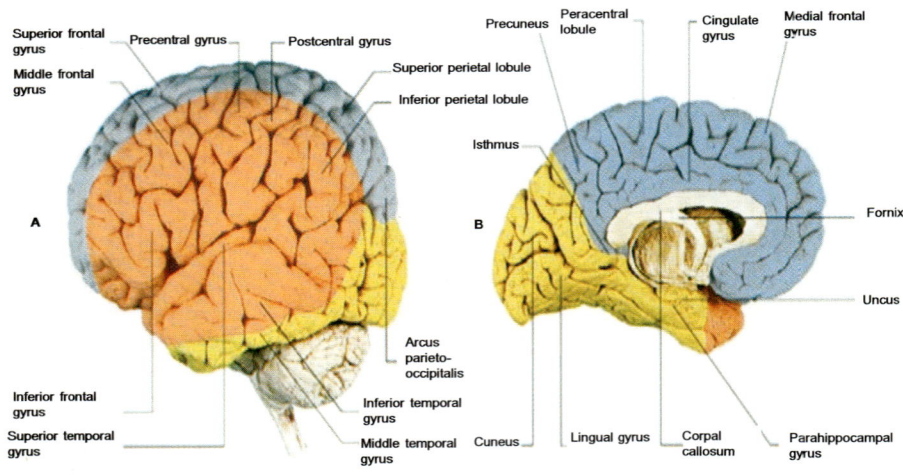

Fig. 12. Shows vascular territories of anterior cerebral artery (blue), middle cerebral artery (orange), posterior cerebral artery (yellow)

b)   Vertebro–basilar system

i)   Vertebral artery

Each vertebral artery is a branch of the first part of the subclavian artery in the neck. Two vertebral arteries ascend up and unite at the pontomedullary junction to form the basilar artery. The basilar artery runs in the basilar sulcus of the pons and at the pontomesencephalic junction divides into two posterior cerebral arteries.

- **Anterior spinal artery:** It supplies the medial part of the medulla oblongata and then descends to supply the spinal cord after fusing opposite one.

- **Posterior spinal artery:** It descends to supply the spinal cord.

- **Posterior inferior cerebellar artery:** It supplies the dorsolateral part of the medulla oblongata, posteroinferior part of the cerebellum and the choroid plexus of the fourth ventricle.

- **Medullary branches:** These branches supply directly medial part of the medulla oblongata.

ii)   Basilar artery

Anterior inferior cerebellar artery: It supplies the anteroinferior part of the cerebellum.

Labyrinthine artery: It supplies the inner ear.

Pontine branches: These paramedian branches dip into the pons and supply the basilar part of the pons.

Superior cerebellar artery: It supplies the superior surface of the cerebellum and midbrain.

Posterior cerebral arteries: They supply the occipital lobes of the cerebrum, deep white matter, basal nuclei, diencephalon and the choroid plexus of the third ventricle and the lateral ventricle.

Applied anatomy

1.   Effect of blockage of vertebrobasilar artery

The loss of blood supply to brainstem ranges from blockage of small perforator leading to brainstem syndrome to entire vertebrobasilar artery leading to fatal outcome.

2. Effects of occlusion of posterior cerebral artery

The loss of cortical supply results in contralateral homonymous hemianopia with macular sparing. This sparing is explained by its dual blood supply from middle and posterior cerebral artery (Fig. 12).

Circle of Willis

The circle of Willis is an arterial anastomotic circle present in the interpeduncular cistern (Fig. 11).

Formation

The anterior communicating artery(ACOM), which connects the right and left anterior cerebral arteries(ACA), forms anterior part of the circle anterior cerebral artery forms the anterolateral part on each side. The lateral part is formed by the termination of internal carotid artery on each side. The circle is completed posteriorly by the bifurcation of basilar artery into the right and left posterior cerebral arteries. Posterolaterally, the posterior communicating artery is the connecting between the internal carotid and posterior cerebral arteries.

Applied anatomy

Berry Aneurysm

Berry aneurysm is a localized dilatation on one of the arteries due to congenital muscular weakness. The most common sites of berry aneurysm are the junction of anterior ACA and ACOM. Rupture of berry aneurysm may cause life-threatening subarachnoid hemorrhage.

B) Venous drainage of the brain

- Venous drainage of the brain involves deep veins, superficial veins and dural venous sinuses.
- Deep cerebral veins drain into the great cerebral vein, which is continuous with the straight sinus (Fig. 13).
- Superficial veins empty principally into the superior sagittal sinus (SSS) and the cavernous sinus.
- One of the most prominent superficial vein sylvian vein is connected to superior sagittal sinus through superior anastomotic vein (vein of Trolad) and to transverse sinus through inferior anastomotic vein (vein of Lebbe) (Fig. 14).
- The superior sagittal sinus and straight sinuses meet at the confluence of the sinuses called as "Torculli Heterophilli"
- Venous blood flows, via the transverse sinus and sigmoid sinus, into the internal jugular vein.
- The **emissary veins** connect the extracranial venous system with the intracranial venous sinuses. They drain from the scalp, through the skull, into the larger meningeal veins and dural venous sinuses

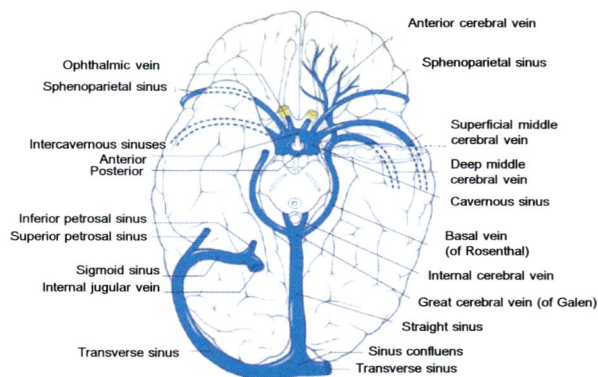

Fig. 13. Shows the deep venous system at the base of the brain

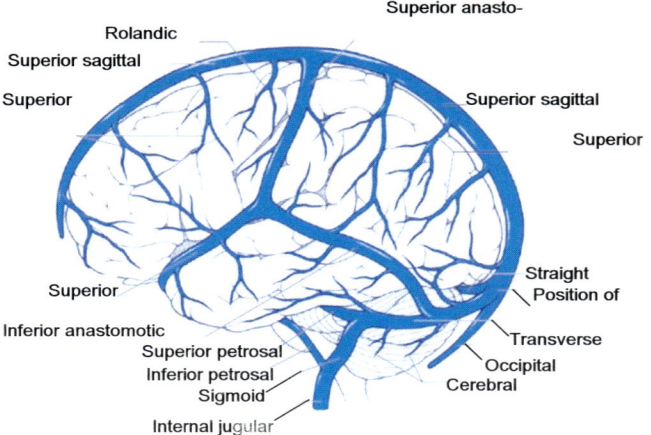

Fig. 14. Shows the superficial venous system

Applied Anatomy

- **Air embolism**

  Venous pressure in the cranial system is negative as compared to the atmosphere. Small opening even in the emissary veins during craniotomy in sitting position sucks air in and leads to air embolism. Preloading with fluids, applying bone wax, copious irrigation in the surgical field and continuous aspiration through central line can prevent and treat the same.

- **Venous infarct**

  Except for anterior one third of the superior sagittal sinus rest of the venous system has no collateral circulation. So thrombosis of any vein or sinus because of dehydration, prothrombotic state leads to hemorrhagic brain infarction. It presents as severe headache and convulsion. Hydration with antithrombotic is the treatment of choice.

J) Cerebellum

External features of the cerebellum

- The cerebellum controls the maintenance of equilibrium, posture and muscle tone and it coordinates movement. It operates at an unconscious level.

- The cerebellum is connected to the medulla, pons and midbrain by the inferior, middle and superior cerebellar peduncles, respectively.

- The cerebellum consists of a midline vermis and two laterally located hemispheres.

- Anatomically, the cerebellum is divided into anterior, posterior and flocculonodular lobes.

Internal structure of the cerebellum

- Internally, the cerebellum consists of a surface layer of cortex, highly convoluted to form folia, beneath which lies white matter.

- Within the white matter lie cerebellar nuclei (fastigial, globose, emboliform and dentate).

- The nuclei are the origin of cerebellar efferent fibres.

Functional anatomy of the cerebellum

- The archicerebellum corresponds to the flocculonodular lobe and fastigial nucleus. Its principal connections are with the vestibular and reticular nuclei of the brainstem and it is concerned with the maintenance of equilibrium.

- The paleocerebellum corresponds to the vermis and paravermal area, together with the globose and emboliform nuclei. It receives fibres from the spinocerebellar tracts and projects to the red nucleus of the midbrain.

- The neocerebellum corresponds to most of the cerebellar hemisphere and the dentate nucleus. It receives afferents from the pons and projects to the ventral lateral nucleus of the thalamus.

Applied Anatomy

Cerebellar lesions cause incoordination of the upper limbs (intention tremor), lower limbs (cerebellar ataxia), speech (dysarthria) and eyes (nystagmus).

Vermian lesions cause truncal ataxia and hemispheric lesions cause appendicular ataxia.

CONCLUSION

The knowledge of the anatomy is a prerequisite for an anaesthesiologist to safely navigate an unstable neurological patient through the travails of surgery and anaesthesia.

REFERENCES

1. Mancall E, Brock D editors. GRAY ' S Clinical Neuroanatomy. 1st ed. Philadelphia:Elsevier; 2011.

2. Singh I, Bhuiyan P, Rajgopal L, Shyamkishore K editors. Textbook of Human Neuroanatomy. 10th ed. New Delhi: Jaypee Publication; 2014.

3. Crossman AR, Neary D editors. Neuroanatomy:An Illustrated Colour Text. 5th ed. Philadelphia:Elsevier; 2015.

4. Estomih M, Gregory G, Peter D editors. Fitzgeralds's Clinical Neuroanatomy and Neuroscience. 7th ed. Philadelphia: Elsevier; 2015.

5. Winn RH. editor.Neurological Surgery. 7th ed. Philadelphia:Elsevier; 2017.

6. Greenstein B, Greenstein A. Color Atlas of Neuroscience.1st ed. New York: Thieme; 2000.

7. Netter FH, Craig JA, Perkins J, Hansen JT, Koeppen BM editors. Atlas of Neuroanatomy and Neurophysiology. Special edition. New York: ICON; 2002

8. Lee T, Mukundan SJ editors. Netters's Correlative Imaging Neuroanatomy.1st edition. Philadelphia: Elsevier Saunders; 2015.

9. Spetzler R, Kalani YM, Nakaji P, Yagmurlu K editors. 1st edition Color Atlas Of Brainstem Surgery. Stutgart, Germany:Thieme; 2017.

MULTIPLE CHOICE QUESTIONS

1. **Fusion of the neural folds begins on**
   a. Day 22
   b. Day 23
   c. Day 24
   d. Day 21

2. **Supraorbital & Supratrochlear nerves are branches of**
   a. V1
   b. V2
   c. V3
   d. Facial nerve

3. **Thunderclap Headache is seen in**
   a. SDH
   b. EDH
   c. SAH
   d. Contusions

4. **Recumbent CSF pressure is**
   a. 10-15 cms of water
   b. 10-15 mm of Hg
   c. 5-10 cms of water
   d. 5-10 mm of Hg

5. **Brocas area corresponds to Brodmanns area**
   a. 40 and 41
   b. 41 and 42
   c. 42 and 43
   d. 44 and 45

6. **Which of the following is not a part of Gertsmanns Syndrome**
   a. Agnosia
   b. Left-right confusion
   c. Dysgraphia
   d. Dysmetria

7. **STN is used as a target to treat which disease**
   a. Parkinsons Disease
   b. Dystonia
   c. Alzheimers Disease
   d. None of the Above

8. **Internal Carotid Artery begins at the level of**
   a. C2
   b. C3
   c. C4
   d. C5

9. **Foville Syndrome includes all of the following except**
   a. Ipsilateral lower motor neuron facial palsy
   b. Horizontal gaze palsy
   c. Vertical and horizontal gaze palsy
   d. Contralateral hemiparesis.

10. **Which of the following Brodmanns Areas is not included in the Primary Somatosensory area.**
    a. 1
    b. 2
    c. 3.
    d. 4

APPLIED PHYSIOLOGY OF THE BRAIN AND SPINAL CORD

Pramila Kurkal, Bhoomika Thakore

Introduction

The normal adult skull can be considered as a bony box of fixed volume and it contains brain, blood and cerebrospinal fluid (CSF). An understanding of how these components interact is essential in managing normal patients and those with intracranial pathology.

Brain[1,2]

- Accounts for 2% of total body weight
- Has a high metabolic rate and receives approximately 15% of cardiac output
- Has virtually no stores of glucose and utilizes 20% of the oxygen, and 25% of the glucose used by the whole body at rest
- Approximately 60% of the brain's energy consumption supports electrophysiological function, rest is consumed by the brain for cellular homeostatic activities
- Loss of consciousness ensueswithin seconds of ischemia, with permanent brain damage occurring within 3–8 min of insufficient blood supply

Cerebral blood flow [CBF][1,3]

- Is 750 ml/min- 15% of cardiac output
- The global CBF in adults is approximately 50 ml/100 g/min:
  - Grey matter [neuronal cell bodies & synapses]- 75ml/100g/min.
  - White matter [fiber tracts] - 20 ml/100g/min.
- The global CBF of children is approximately 95 ml/100g/min- higher than that of adults
- Infants have a slightly lower CBF than adults (40 ml/100 g/min).
- Spinal cord blood flow has been less extensively studied:
  - The gray matter has a rate of 60 ml/100 g/min
  - The white matter a rate of 20 ml/100 g/min
- Two types of local CBF modulation: [Fig 1]
  1. Phasic response-
     - Fast and transient

- Regulated by substances released from neurons- NO, K^+, vasoactive intestinal peptide
2. Tonic response-
   - Slow and long lasting
   - Regulated by metabolites of arachidonic acid from astrocytes- prostaglandin E2, hydroxy and epoxy satreinooic acids

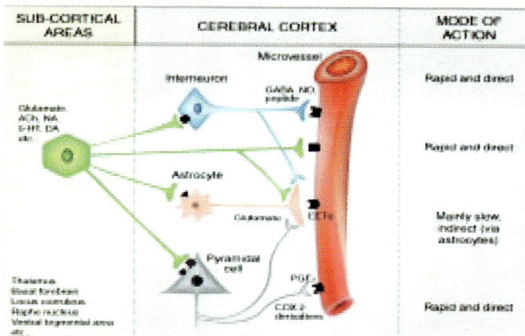

Fig. 1. Cerebral blood flow modulation

- When CBF falls to less than 10-23ml/100g/min- physiological electrical function of the cell begins to fail → "ischemic penumbra"
- Below 8 ml/100g/min irreversible cell death - ionic membrane transport failure occurs

Cerebral metabolic rate of O_2 [$CMRO_2$][1,2,3]

- Cerebral metabolic rate of awake young adults is 3.5 ml O_2/100 g/min or 5.5 mg glucose/100 g/min
  - 60%- electrical activity (signaling)
  - 40%- cellular homeostasis
- Children have a higher metabolic rate, i.e., 5.2 ml O_2/100 g/min

CBF – $CMRO_2$ coupling[1]

- Changes in CBF and metabolism tend to follow each other- local or global increases in metabolic demand are met rapidly by an increase in CBF and substrate delivery and viceversa - often referred to as flow-metabolism coupling [Fig. 2].

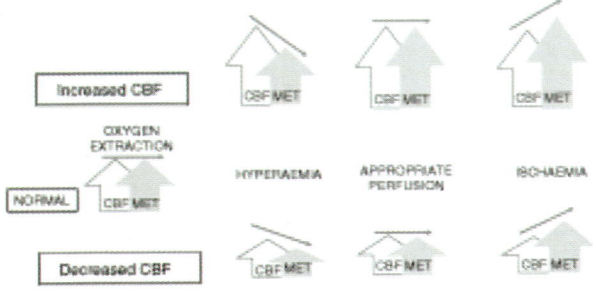

Fig. 2. CBF and CMR Coupling

- These changes are thought to be controlled by several vasoactive metabolic mediators including hydrogen ions, potassium, CO_2, adenosine, glycolytic intermediates, phospholipid metabolites and morerecently, nitric oxide (NO) [Fig. 3].

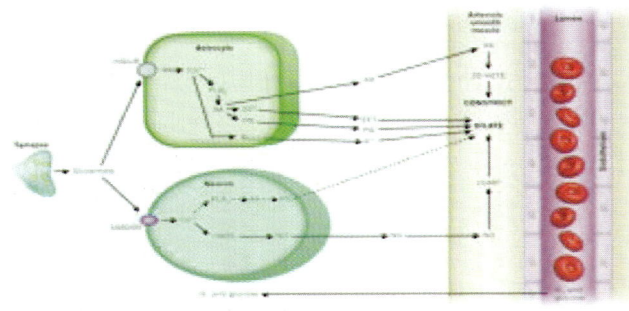

Fig. 3. Mechanisms of coupling.

Cerebral Perfusion Pressure[1,2,3]

- CPP is effective pressure that drives blood flow to the brain
- CPP = MAP - ICP or CVP (whichever is greater)
- Normal CPP = 80-100 mmHg
- Normal ICP = 5-12mmHg
- Moderate to severe increases in ICP (>30mmHg) can significantly compromise CPP and CBF even in the presence of normal MAP
- CPP and EEG [Fig 4]

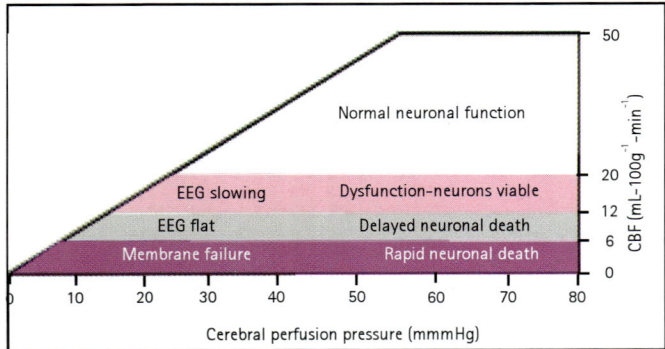

Fig. 4. Between CPP, CBF, EEG and Viability of neurons

- <50 slowing of EEG
- 25-40 Flat EEG
- <25 results in irreversible brain death

Autoregulation[1,2,3]

- Defined as- Intrinsic activity of the organ to maintain a constant blood flow despite changes in perfusion pressure/MAP
- Cerebral vasculature rapidly adapts to changes in CPP by adjusting its resistance:
  - ↑ CPP causes cerebral vasodilation→ ↑CBF
  - ↑ CPP causes cerebral vasoconstriction→ ↑CBF
- In normal individuals CBF is autoregulated to maintain blood flow between MAP 50-150 mmHg [Fig. 5]

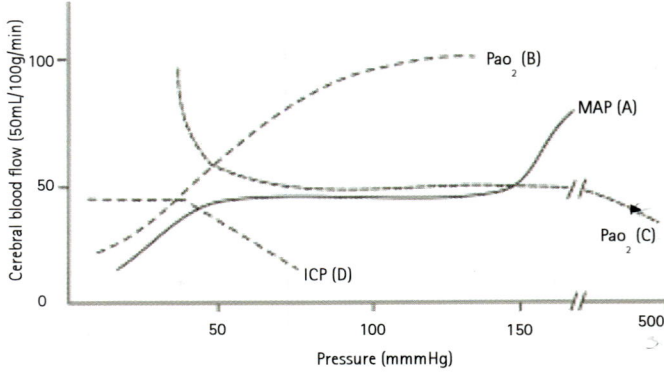

Fig. 5. Autoregulatory limits.

- Beyond these limits blood flow becomes pressure dependent [Fig 6]

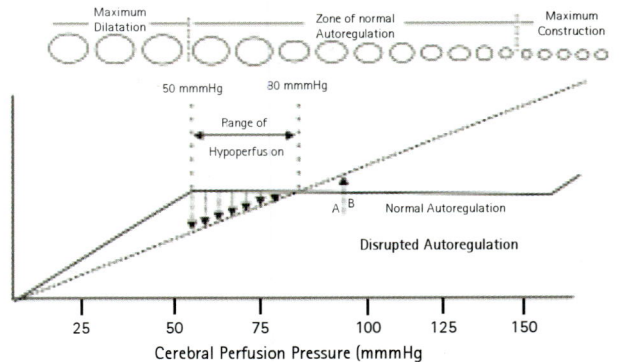

Fig. 6. CBF and CPP.

- Pressure above 150-160mmHg can disrupt BBB causing cerebral edema
- Dysregulation can occur in pathologic states: In traumatized or ischemic brain, or following vasodilator agents (volatile agents and sodium nitroprusside)
  - As arterial pressure rises – CBF rises → increase in cerebral volume
  - As pressure falls - CBF falls → reduces ICP, but induces an uncontrolled reduction in CBF

Mechanisms of Autoregulation

1. Pressure/ myogenic

- Arterioles dilate or constrict in response to changes in BP and ICP in order to maintain a constant CBF
- "Myogenic theory"- vascular smooth muscle within cerebral arterioles intrinsically contract to stretch thereby regulating pressure

2. Metabolic

- Arterioles dilate in response to potent chemicals that are by-products of metabolism such as:
  - Lactic acid
  - Carbon dioxide
  - Pyruvic acid
- CO_2 is a potent vasodilator
  - Increased CO_2 / decreased BP $\rightarrow$ vasodilatation
  - Decreased CO_2/increased BP $\rightarrow$ vasoconstriction

3. Neurogenic

- Autonomic- sympathetic adrenergic receptors seen in cortical layers IV and V

  -$\beta_1\beta_2$ and α_2 ("dilators") and, α_1 ("constrictor") receptors
- Overall sympathetic system plays minor role, unlike in non-cerebral vascular beds
- 5-HT- potent "constrictor," antagonized by NO
- Neuropeptide Y- "vasoconstriction"
- Vasoactive intestinal polypeptide (VIP) and peptide histidine isoleucine (PHI) - "vasodilators"
- Substance P, neurokinin A, calcitonin gene-related peptide histamine H_2-"vasodilatory" esp. substance P
- Autonomic system and neurochemical control of CBF in general is a minor control
- Overall, myogenic and metabolic autoregulation most important

Extrinsic mechanisms

1. Respiratory Gas Tension- CO_2

- CBF directly proportionate to $PaCo_2$ between tension of 20-80mmHg [Fig 5] - each 1 mm Hg $\uparrow$ or $\downarrow$ leads 2-4% $\uparrow$ or $\downarrow$ in CBF
- Co_2 crosses BBB but H^+ does not, so acute metabolic acidosis has little effect on CBF
- Children have less cerebral reactivity to CO_2 changes
- Although the CBF changes in response to $PaCO_2$ alteration occur rapidly, they are not sustained

- In spite of the maintenance of an elevated arterial pH, CBF returns to normal over 6 to 8 hours because cerebrospinal fluid (CSF) pH gradually normalizes as a result of the extrusion of bicarbonate
- Acute normalization of $PaCO_2$ results in a significant CSF acidosis (after hypocapnia) or alkalosis (after hypercapnia)
- The former results in increased CBF with a concomitant intracranial pressure (ICP) increase that will depend on the prevailing intracranial compliance and the latter conveys the theoretic risk of ischemia
- Steal Phenomenon[4]
  - If local autoregulation is impaired and $PaCO_2$ increases, vessels in surrounding normal brain will dilate
  - Vessels in the abnormal area are already maximally dilated due to loss of autoregulation
  - Vascular resistance will be decreased in surrounding normal brain; blood will be shunted away from abnormal areas, resulting in further hypoxia
- Inverse Steal/ Robin Hood Phenomenon[4]
  - Opposite may occur as $PaCO_2$ is decreased by hyperventilation
  - Vessels in surrounding normal brain will vasoconstrict; vessels in the damaged or abnormal area of brain are already maximally dilated and are unable to constrict
  - Because of the vasoconstriction in normal brain, vascular resistance increases, shunting blood into the abnormal area

2. Respiratory Gas Tension- O_2

- Low arterial oxygen tension has profound effects on cerebral blood flow
- When it falls below 50 mmHg (6.7 kPa), there is a rapid increase in CBF and arterial blood volume [Fig 5]

3. Temperature

- Hypothermia decreases both CMR and CBF
- For every 10°C increase in temperature, CMR doubles
- CMR decreases by 50% if temp of the brain falls by 10°C
- Temperature reduction beyond that, at which EEG suppression first occurs, does produce a further decrease in CMR [Fig 7]

Applied physiology of the brain and spinal cord

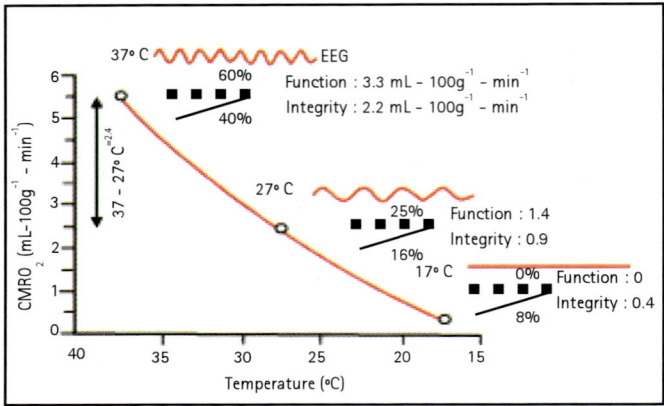

Fig. 7. Effect of temperature on CMR and EEG.

4. Viscosity

- Blood viscosity can influence CBF
- Hematocrit is the single most important determinant of blood viscosity
- In healthy subjects, hematocrit variation within the normal range (33-45%) probably results in only trivial alteration of CBF
- Beyond this range, changes are more substantial:
  - ↓ in hematocrit → ↓ viscosity → ↑ CBF
  - ↓ O_2 carrying capacity
  - ↑ hematocrit → ↑ viscosity → ↓ CBF

Intracranial pressure[2,5]

- Monroe-Kellie Doctrine:
  - The cranial vault is a rigid structure with fixed volume
    a) Brain 80%
    b) Blood 12%
    c) CSF 8%
  - Any increase in one component must be offset by an equivalent decrease in another, to prevent rise in ICP
- ICP normally is 10mmHg and less
- IC compliance is determined by measuring the change in ICP in response to change in intracranial volume
- Initially increases in volume are well compensated until it reaches a point where further increase can cause rise in ICP
- Compensatory mechanisms:
  - Displacement of CSF from cranial to spinal compartment
  - Increase in CSF reabsorption
  - Decrease in CSF production
  - Decrease in cerebral blood volume

- Intracranial Hypertension:
  - Defined as a sustained increase in ICP above 15mmHg
  - Uncompensated increases in tissue or fluid within the rigid cranial vault produce sustained ICP elevations
  - If ICP exceeds 30 mmHg, CBF progressively decreases [Fig 5] and vicious circle is established: ischemia causes brain edema, which increases ICP hence more ischemia
  - Cycle continues – patient dies of progressive neurological damage or catastrophic herniation [Fig. 8]

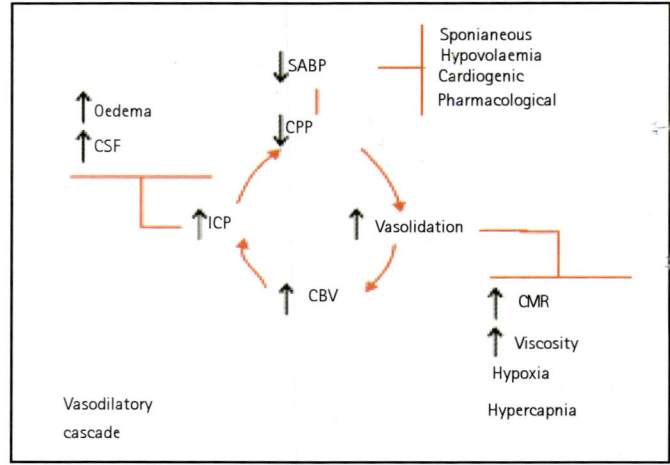

Fig. 8. Vasodilatory cascade.

Cerebrospinal Fluid [CSF][4,5]

- **Functions:**
  - Provide mechanical protection
  - Maintain a stable extracellular environment for the brain
  - Remove some waste products
  - Nutrition
  - Convey messages [hormones/releasing factors/ neurotransmitters]

- **Production**
  - 70 % CSF produced in choroid plexuses of lateral, third and fourth ventricles
  - Produced at rate of 500 cc/day or approximately 20cc/hour (0.3-0.5 cc/kg/hr)
  - Eliminated by being absorbed into the arachnoid villi → dural sinus → jugular system
  - The secretion of fluid by the choroid plexus depends on the active Na^+ transport across the cells into the CSF

- The electrical gradient pulls along Cl^- and both ions drag water by osmosis
- The CSF has lower K^+, glucose and much lower protein than blood plasma, and higher concentrations of Na^+ and Cl^-
- The production of CSF in the choroid plexuses is an active secretory process and not directly dependent on the arterial blood pressure
- Other sources of CSF production- from capillary ultra filtrate [Virchow-Robin spaces]
- Additionally some produced from metabolic H_2O production

- **Absorption**
  - CSF is reabsorbed into the blood of the venous sinuses via the arachnoidal villi- absorption is directly related to the CSF pressure in the cranial cavity
  - Hydrostatic pressure in subarachnoid space > pressure in dural sinuses
  - Typical hydrostatic values of CSF are 150 mm H_2O (11 mm Hg) in subarachnoid space vs. about 70 mm H_2O (5 mm Hg) in dural sinuses.
  - Arachnoid villi are one-way valves that open when the hydrostatic pressure of CSF in the subarachnoid space is about 1.5 mm Hg greater than venous hydrostatic pressure in the dural sinuses (i.e., passive process)
  - Other modes of absorption- lymphatics and trans ependymal flow

Blood/ Brain- Blood/ CSF barriers[4]

- The blood brain barrier (BBB) is the specialized system of capillary endothelial cells that protects the brain from harmful substances in the blood stream, while supplying the brain with the required nutrients for proper function [Fig 9].

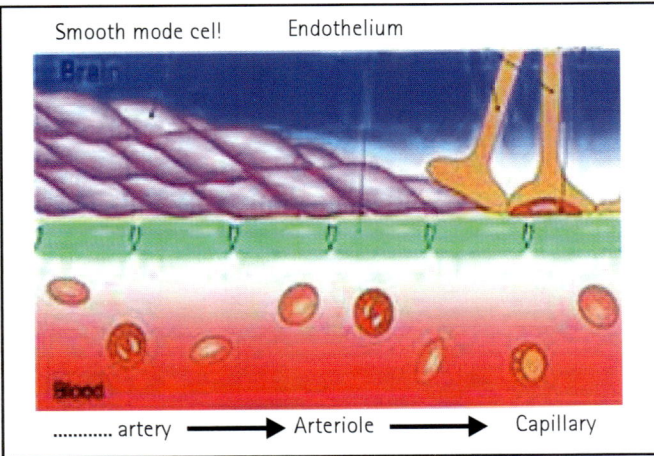

Fig. 9. Blood Brain Barrier

- Formed by the non-fenestrated capillaries and to much lesser degree, the astrocytic foot processes → keeps out most macromolecules
- The blood CSF barrier consists of "Tight" junctions at the ependymal level and fenestrated junctions at the choroidal capillaries
- The choroid plexus is composed of fenestrated capillaries and an epithelial (ependymal) covering, which reverts from "tight" to moderately "open" at the base -- not as strenuous of barrier as blood/brain [Fig 10].

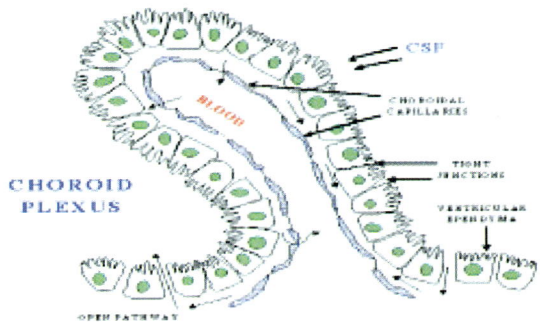

Fig. 10. Blood CSF Barrier

- Circumventricular organs:
  - Are midline structures bordering the 3rd and 4th ventricles
  - They are barrier deficient areas- recognized as important sites for communicating with the CSF and between the brain and peripheral organs via blood-borne products
  - CVO's include:
    1. The pineal gland
    2. Median eminence
    3. Neurohypophysis
    4. Subfornical organ and Sub commissural organ
    5. Area post rema
    6. Organum vasculosum of the lamina terminalis
    7. Choroid plexus

Spinal cord[5]

- Limited studies describing determinants of spinal cord blood flow
- Spinal cord blood flow [SCBF] values vary from 10 to 20 mL/100 g/min for white matter and from 41 to 63 mL/100 g/min for gray matter
- Autoregulation maintained between 60-120mmHg MAP

- CO_2 reactivity similar to the brain- hypercapnia $\rightarrow$ vasodilatation and vice versa
- SCBF stable between 10-50 mmHg of CO_2, beyond 50 mmHg $\rightarrow$ marked rise in SCBF
- Hypothermia decreases the SCBF but no proven benefit in spinal cord injury

CONCLUSION

- Management of the patient for neurosurgery requires a good understanding of the inter-relationships of neurophysiology, pathophysiology and pharmacology
- The main aim is to maintain CPP and CBF to meet the metabolic demands after a neurological insult and prevent secondary brain injury

REFERENCES

1. P. Patel, J.Drummond. Cerebral physiology and the effects of anesthetics and techniques. In: Ronald D. Miller, editor. Miller's Anesthesia, 8th Edition. Elsevier, Inc; 2015: p 387-422

2. Alifia Tameem, Hari Krowidi : Continuing education in anaesthesia, Critical care and pain 2013; 13 (4): 113-118

3. L.D. Mishra. Cerebral blood flow and anaesthesia: A review, Indian J. Anaesth. 2002; 46 (2) : 87-95

4. Shailendra Joshi, William Young. Cerebral and Spinal cord blood flow. In: James E. Cotrell, William L. Young, editors. Cottrell and Youngs Neuroanesthesia 5th Edition. Elsevier, Inc; 2010: p 17- 59

5. M. Sethuraman. Neurophysiology. In: Hemanshu Prabhakar editor. Essentials of neuroanesthesia 1st Edition, Academic press London: Elsevier Inc; 2017: p 62- 90

MULTIPLE CHOICE QUESTIONS

1. **The brain accounts for ... of total body weight and receives ... of cardiac output:**
   a. 4%, 20%
   b. 3%, 25%
   c. 2%, 15%
   d. 2%, 10%

2. **The global cerebral blood flow in adults is:**
   a. 60ml/100g/min
   b. 50/ml/100g/min
   c. 75ml/100g/min
   d. 20ml/100g/min

3. **The $CMRO_2$ of adults is:**
   a. 3.5mg glucose/100g/min
   b. 5.2mg glucose/100g/min
   c. 2.5mg glucose/100g/min
   d. 5.5mg glucose/100g/min

4. **All of the following are true regarding CPP except:**
   a. CPP = MAP - ICP or CVP (whichever is greater)
   b. Normal CPP = 80-100 mmHg
   c. CPP is effective pressure that drives blood flow to the brain
   d. CPP ? 50mmHg results in irreversible brain death

5. **Which statement regarding autoregulation is true:**
   a. ↑ CPP causes cerebral vasoconstriction→ ↓ CBF
   b. CBF is autoregulated to maintain blood flow between MAP 60 -120 mmHg
   c. ↓ CPP causes cerebral vasoconstriction → ↓ CBF
   d. Neurogenic mechanism of autoregulation plays the most important role

6. **Regarding respiratory Gas Tension- CO_2 and CBF – all are true except:**
   a. CBF directly proportionate to $PaCo_2$ between tension of 20-80mmHg
   b. Each 1 mm Hg ↑ or ↓ leads to 2-4% ↑ or ↓ in CBF
   c. Each 1 mm Hg ↑ or ↓ leads to 1- 2% ↑ or ↓ in CBF
   d. Co2 crosses BBB but H^+ does not, so acute metabolic acidosis has little effect on CBF

7. **Temperature, viscosity and autoregulation – which statements are true**
   a. Hypothermia decreases both CMR and CBF
   b. CMR increases by 50% if temp of the brain falls by 10°C
   c. For every 10° C decrease in temperature, CMR doubles
   d. ↓ in hematocrit → ↓ viscosity → ↑ CBF

8. **Compensatory mechanisms for ICP maintenance include:**
   a. Decrease in CSF reabsorption
   b. Increase in CSF production
   c. Displacement of CSF from cranial to spinal compartment
   d. Decrease in cerebral blood volume

9. **All of the below are true except:**
   a. CSF maintains a stable extracellular environment for the brain
   b. Produced at rate of 350 cc/day or approximately 10cc/hour
   c. Produced at rate of 0.3-0.5 cc/kg/hr
   d. Eliminated by being absorbed into the arachnoid villi → dural sinus → jugular system

10. **Which of the following is true:**
    a. The pituitary gland is a circumventricular organ
    b. Spinal cord autoregulation maintained between 50-150mmHg MAP
    c. CO_2 reactivity of spinal cord similar to the brain- hypercapnia → vasodilatation and vice versa
    d. Hypothermia increases the SCBF and has shown benefit in spinal cord injury

CHAPTER 3

EFFECTS OF ANAESTHETIC AGENTS AND OTHER DRUGS ON CEREBRAL PHYSIOLOGY

Bhoomika Thakore, Rajani M. Ramakrishnan

Introduction

A basic knowledge of the effects of anaesthetic drugs and techniques on cerebral circulation metabolism and intracranial pressure, both in normal as well as pathological conditions, is important for both- safe neuroanesthetic practices and understanding effects of any neuro protection offered by these agents.

The major properties of drugs used in neuroanaesthesia should be:

(i) To provide adequate tissue perfusion to the brain and spinal cord

(ii) Provide adequate surgical conditions, i.e., relaxed brain

(iii) Rapid post operative recovery of consciousness to enable early neurological assessment

(iv) Good analgesic effect

(v) Non epilepticogenic

(vi) Minimal interference with neuromodality monitoring and advantageous effect on cerebral haemodynamics

(vii) No systemic adverse effect

This chapter will focus on the pharmacological considerations in relation to neurosurgical procedures.

Intravenous anaesthetics:[1,2,5]

Globally all intravenous [IV] Induction Agents (except ketamine) cause:

- Reduction in cerebral blood flow [CBF] and cerebral metabolic rate [CMR]
- Slowing of surface EEG [Fig. 1]

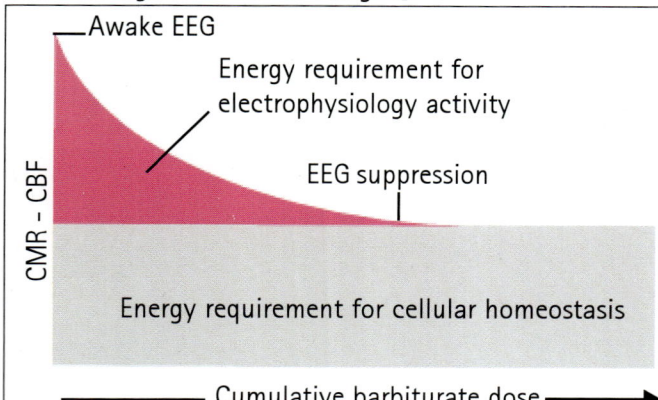

Fig. 1. EEG response to increasing doses of barbiturates

- Deep Level: Burst suppression pattern
- Extremely deep level: Isoelectric pattern

Barbiturates

- Dose dependent reduction in CBF & CMR
- Metabolism related with brain's electrical activity is mainly suppressed
- $CMRO_2$ decrease → vascular resistance increase → CBF decrease → intracranial pressure decrease
- Cerebrovascular autotregulation and vasoreactivity to CO_2 are preserved
- Thiopentone protects brain from incomplete ischemia:
  - Suppression of CMR
  - Free radical scavenging
  - Redistribution of CBF
  - Decreases ATP consumption
- Significant reduction in spinal cord blood flow [SCBF], autoregulation intact in the range of 60-120 mmHg

Propofol

- Primarily reduces CMR → vasoconstriction → decrease CBF & ICP - more in regions implicated in regulation of arousal, performance of associative functions and autonomic control
- Decreases CBF > CMR
- Fentanyl + propofol → ablates increase in ICP at intubation
- CO_2 responsiveness and autoregulation preserved
- Minimal interference with electrophysiological monitoring, including MEP
- Decreases local spinal cord metabolism in both gray and white matter
- Offers brain protection:
  - CMR suppression
  - Attenuates changes in ATP, Ca^{++}, Na^+ and K^+
  - Antioxidant action by inhibiting lipid peroxidation

Etomidate

- Parallel reductions in CBF and CMR
- Regionally variable; more in forebrain
- Reactivity to CO_2 and autoregulation preserved
- Concerns:
  - Adrenocortical suppression
  - Seizure activity
  - Involuntary muscle activity

Ketamine

- Antagonist at NMDA receptor
- Limited use in neuroanesthesia:
  - Increase in CBF (but not when used with other sedatives)
  - Increase in ICP (but not when used with other sedatives)
  - Increase in CMR (particularly in Limbic structures)
  - Cerebral protection via NMDA antagonism in animal studies
- Anaesthetic drugs (diazepam, midazolam, propofol, isoflurane) have been shown to blunt or eliminate increase in the ICP effect of ketamine.

Table 1: Summarises the effects of IV Anaesthetic Drugs

	Propofol	Thiopentone	Etomidate
	Most widely used	IMP agent in neurocritical care ↓↓ ICP	Cardiovascular stable drug
CBF	↓	↓	↓
CMR	↓	↓	↓
ICP	↓	↓	↓
Auto-regulation	+	+	+
Response to CO_2	+	+	+

Inhalational Anaesthetic Agents[1,2,5]

- All inhalational agents are cerebral vasodilators and augment the CBF
- Decrease the MAP → decrease CPP [dose dependent manner]
- Decrease cerebral activity → reduce CMR
- Effect at different MAC [Fig. 2]

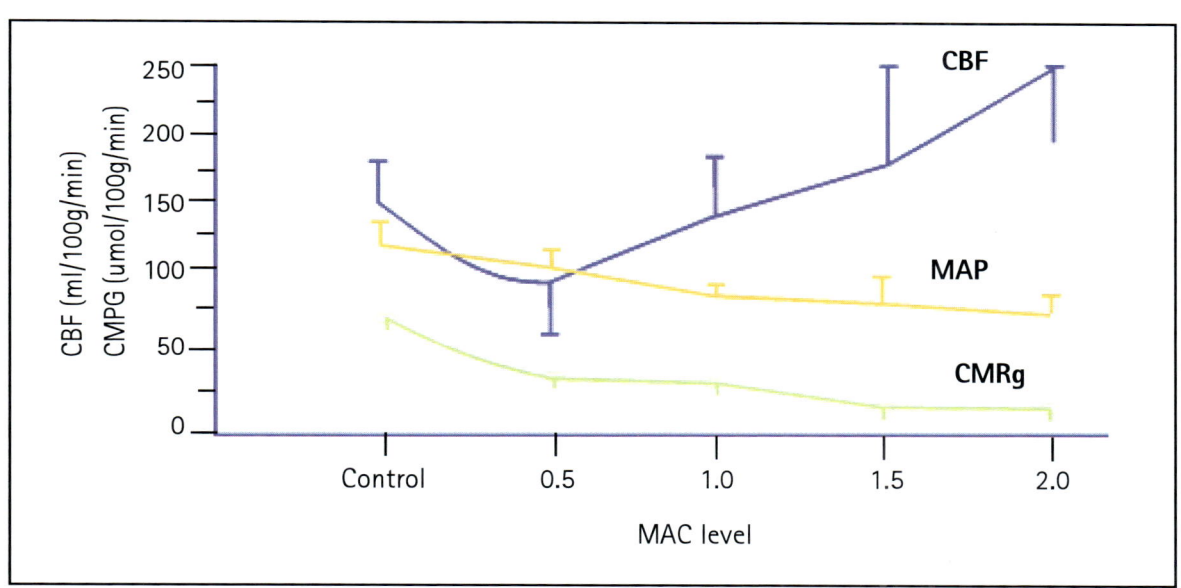

Fig. 2. CBF, MAP and CMR response at different MAC

- At 0.5 MAC - CMR suppression predominates → net effect CBF decreases
- At 1 MAC - CMR suppression = Vasodilatation → CBF unchanged
- Beyond 1 MAC - CMR reduced but vasodilatory effect predominates → CBF increases
- Autoregulation
  - >0.5 MAC: Impaired autoregulation
  - Blood flow passively follows MAP- ischemia or luxury perfusion with edema or hemorrhage more likely

- Cerebrovascular response to $PaCO_2$: Maintained
- Order of vasodilatory potency:

  Halothane >> Enflurane > Desflurane = Isoflurane > Sevoflurane
- The vasodilator effects usually appear rapidly than the effects on $CMRO_2$. The CBF falls to near prevolatile agent levels 2.5 to 5 hrs later
- If antecedent lowering of CMR by drugs/disease, then vasodilator effect may predominate

Effects of anaesthetic agents & other drugs on cerebral physiology

Halothane

- CBF - dramatic increase in CBF with a simultaneous modest reduction in CMR
- CMR - suppression is less compared to other agents
- Produces isoelectricity in EEG at MACs >4

Enflurane

- CBF - dramatic increase in CBF with a simultaneous modest reduction in CMR
- Potentially epileptogenic and hypocapnoea potentiates this effect
- Seizure activity increases brain metabolism by as much as 400%
- Avoid: if seizure predisposition and h/o occlusive cerebrovascular disease with hypocapnoea in high doses

Isoflurane

- CBF - increases CBF; but to a lesser extent
- CMR - decreases $CMRO_2$ and maximal reduction is attained simultaneously with EEG suppression at clinically relevant concentrations [1.5-2.0 MAC]
- The institution of hyperventilation , simultaneous with its introduction can prevent increase in ICP (which may occur with normocarbia)
- At both 1 MAC and 2 MAC, SCBF ↑ and autoregulation attenuated.

Sevoflurane

- Reduce CBF
- Reduce $CMRO_2$ by 38% at 1 MAC
- Max at EEG suppression- At 1.5-2.0 MAC
- Has small potential to evoke epileptiform activity ; use with caution in patients with epilepsy

Desflurane

- Reduce CBF
- Decrease $CMRO_2$ by 22% at 1 MAC
- In general, the effect of Isoflurane, Desflurane and Sevoflurane on CBF are modest

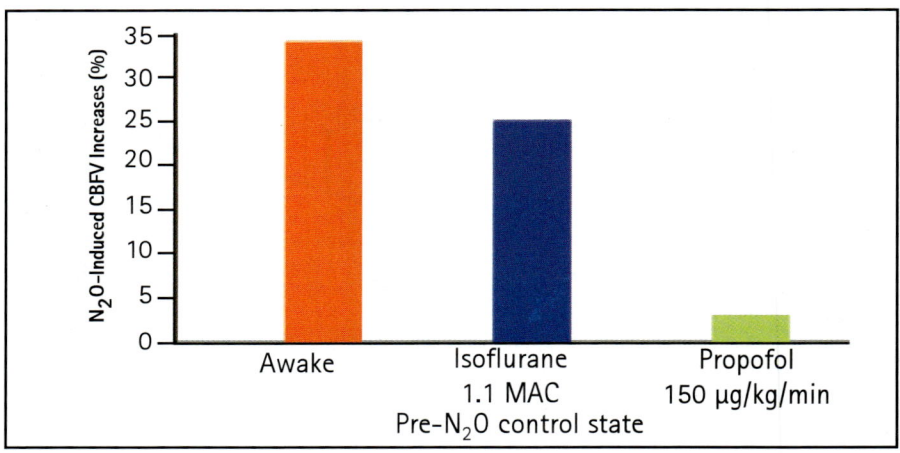

Fig. 3 Nitrous Oxide

Nitrous Oxide

- Can cause significant increase in CBF, CMR & ICP [sympathoadrenal stimulating effect]
- Most extensive increase when used alone
- With IV agents or hypocapnia: CBF effect considerably reduced [Thiopentone, Propofol, benzodiazepines, narcotics]
- With Volatile Agents: CBF increase is exaggerated
- It should be avoided in cases, where a closed intracranial gas space may exist, since it can enter and expand it [pneumocephalus, VAE]
- CBF response to CO_2 preserved
- Autoregulation maintained
- ↑ spinal cord's utilisation of glucose
- No uniform agreement reached on its effect on CMR

Table 2 : Summary of effects of inhalational agents

	Isoflurane	Desflurane	Sevoflurane
CBF	MAC < 0.6 (minimal) > 0.6 : ↑	MAC < 0.6 (minimal) > 0.6 : ↑	MAC < 1: no change > 1 : ↑
$CMRO_2$	↓	↓	↓
ICP	↑	↑↑	↑ (MAC > 1.5)
Autoregulation	Impaired MAC > 1	Impaired MAC > 1	Impaired MAC > 1.5
CO_2 Responsiveness	+	+	+
Others		• Sympathetic stimulation (BP & CPP)	• IAA of choice • Safe in seizure prone pts if hyperventilation avoided & MAC < 1.5

Narcotics[2,3,5,6]

- Helps attenuation of pressure response because of ET intubation, suction, skull pin application
- Improved intra-op haemodynamics with rapid emergence
- Narcotics have minimal adverse effects on CBF, $CMRO_2$ and ICP as long as ventilation is maintained & it is within clinical doses
- In higher doses it progressively decreases both CBF & $CMRO_2$
- All opioids maintain or preserve autoregulation & CO_2 reactivity
- Morphine [due to histamine release] can cause an increase in ICP secondary to autoregulatory induced vasodilatation after a reduction in MAP → should be given in a manner avoiding sudden reduction in MAP
- Fentanyl has been the narcotic of choice for most neuroanesthetics
- Recent times Remifentanil has become a popular choice for many procedures:
  - Short context-sensitive half time
  - Provides good analgesia
  - Prompt awakening of the patient immediately post surgery to evaluate neurological status.

Naloxone

- Narcotic antagonist
- Has little effect on CBF & ICP when given in titrated doses

- In large doses causes arrhythmias, hypertension & intracranial haemorrhage

Benzodiazepines

- Modest reduction in CBF
- The reduction attained is intermediate between that caused by
  - Narcotics (modest)
  - Barbiturates (substantial)
- They can produce respiratory depression → increase in $paCO_2$, hyperventilation at induction counteracts the effect
- Maintains autoregulation
- Preserves vasoreactivity to CO_2
- Increases seizure threshold – used as antiepileptic

Flumazenil

- Highly specific, competitive benzodiazepine antagonist
- Reverses the CBF, CMR, ICP lowering effects of BZD
- Overshoot phenomenon may occur
- Avoided or used cautiously to reverse BZD sedation in patients with impaired intra-cranial compliance

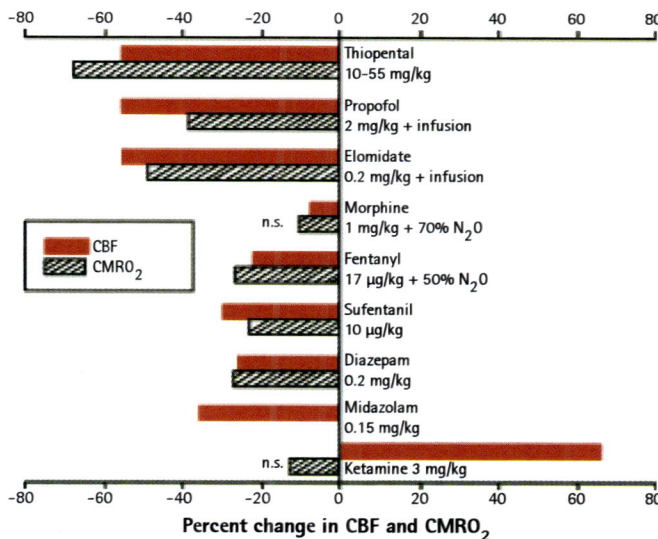

Fig. 4. *Effect of Different Drugs on Cerebral Physiology*

Neuromuscular Blocking Agents

- Neuromuscular blocking agents do not cross the blood brain barrier [BBB]- lack direct action on brain
- The cerebral effects are secondary to:
  - Histamine release
  - Systemic hemodynamic changes
  - Action of metabolites

Depolarizing Neuromuscular blocking agent:

Succinylcholine[2,3,5,7]

- It increases ICP (≤ 5 mmHg) and CBF secondary to:
  - Muscle fasciculations
  - An increase in muscle spindle afferent activity & EEG activity
  - The venous stasis in the jugular caused by fasciculations of the neck muscles
- These effects are transient, modest and can be prevented by pretreatment with small doses of NDMR.
- It can cause exaggerated release of K^+ in certain conditions like closed head trauma, cerebrovascular accidents, hemiparesis
- The benefit of a rapid, reliable onset and recovery from muscle relaxation makes it choice of relaxant in emergency situations like full stomach & anticipated difficult airway
- Maintains cerebral autoregulation & CO_2 reactivity

Non Depolarizing Muscle Relaxants[2,3,5]

- All NDMR have little or no effects on CBF, $CMRO_2$ & ICP
- No clinical effects on CO_2 reactivity & cerebral autoregulation

Pancuronium

- Large doses cause hypertension & tachycardia $\rightarrow$ increase CBF & ICP

Atracurium

- Can cause histamine release with large bolus doses $\rightarrow$ hypotension & decrease in CBF
- It is metabolized by ester hydrolysis & Hoffmann elimination $\rightarrow$ useful in patients with renal or liver dysfunction
- It does not accumulate & is suitable for prolonged infusions
- A metabolite of atracurium called laudanosine can cross BBB & induce seizure but not clinically relevant

Cisatracurium

- Newer analogue of atracurium
- Produces less toxic metabolite & histamine release with no dependence on hepatic & renal metabolism $\rightarrow$ very useful for neurosurgery procedures with patients in whom liver metabolism is affected by use of long term anticonvulsants

Vecuronium

- Maintains hemodynamic stability
- Can cause bradycardia when combined with large doses of narcotics for induction
- Produces active metabolites & not suitable for prolonged infusions

Rocuronium

- Has a rapid onset of relaxation with large doses
- Relatively stable hemodynamics
- Excellent drug of choice in neurosurgery patients where succinylcholine is contraindicated & rapid sequence induction is required

Dexmedetomidine[2,4,5,8]

- It is a relatively new intra venous drug gaining popularity in neuroanesthesia and neurocritical practice
- It is highly selective alpha 2 adreno receptor agonist
- Produces dose dependent sedation, anxiolysis and analgesia (involving spinal and supra spinal sites) without significant respiratory depression
- Decreases the anaesthetic requirement
- Good haemodynamic stability due to sympatholytic properties during the intra operative period
- There are limited data available on the effect of dexmedetomidine on cerebral physiology:
  - It decreases CBF and $CMRO_2$
  - Impairs autoregulation
  - At low doses transiently decreases the ICP, at high doses ICP unchanged
  - It has neuro protective effects as shown in variety of invivo and invitro studies, mechanism are not clear
  - It has minimum effects on sensory or motor evoked potentials $\rightarrow$ can be used safely in surgeries requiring neuro physiological monitoring
  - It has minimum effects in EEG $\rightarrow$ has a rapid onset and offset of sedation without respiratory depression $\rightarrow$ proves effective and safe for awake craniotomies

Table 3 : Antihypertensives[2,3,4]

Drugs	NOA	Dose	Side Effects
Sodium Nitroprusside (SNP)	Arteriolar and venous smooth muscle dilatation	0.5–10 µg/kg/min	Rebound hypertension, tachycardia, CN toxicity
Nitroglycerine (NTG)	Venous dilatation	5–10 µg/min	Reflex tachycardia
Hydralazine	Direct arteriolar smooth muscle dilator	0.1–0.2 mg/kg	Reflex tachycardia
Esmolol	β receptor blockade	0.15–1 mg/kg and then 50–300 µg/kg/min	Bronchospasm,exacerbation of heart failure
Labetalol	β > α blockade	5–20 mg and then 2 mg/min	

Table 4:

Drugs	CBF	CPP	ICP	Autoregulation	CO_2 Reactivity
Sodium Nitroprusside	?	?	+	?	?
Nitroglycerine	?	?	+	–	?
Esmolol	0/–	?	?	?	0
Labetalol	0	?	?	?	0
Nimodipine	+	+	–	+	–

Vasodilators

(Sodium Nitro Prusside [SNP], Nitroglycerine [NTG]. Hydralazine)

- They cause direct smooth muscle relaxation of cerebral vasculature → increase CBV, ICP and cause cerebral oedema in dose related fashion
- Usually avoided in patients with decreased intracranial compliance, can be used once the dura is opened
- Good options for achieving acute titration of blood pressure, particularly in severe hypertension or when other drugs fail to control the blood pressure adequately

Alpha and beta blockers

- Have little or no effect on CBF ad ICP
- They are most common anti hypertensives used in neuro surgical patients
- Treat hypertension as well as complications of the increased sympathetic response like tachyarrythmias, MI and immune suppression
- Esmolol is ultra short acting beta blocker suitable for rapid intervention in the treatment of tachyarrythmias in the peri-operative period and is generally given as continuous IV infusion
- Metoprolol has a longer half life and is used in patients with acute MI

- Labetalol is an alpha and beta blocker commonly used in neurosurgical patients for control of peri-op hypertension as it does not increase ICP

Calcium channel blockers

- These agents are of little use in hypertensive emergencies because of their long duration of action and potential to cause cerebral vasodilatation
- Nicardipine is a calcium channel blocker which causes reductions in MAP with minimal effect on cardiac output
- It attenuates cerebral autoregulation & also reduces CO_2 reactivity

Lignocaine[2,4,5,9]

- Lignocaine is a Na^+ channel blocker and commonly used as an adjuvant in neuroanesthesia
- Shows dose related reductions in CBF & $CMRO_2$ with non-seizure inducing doses
- Its clinical effects depends on blood concentration → at low doses it cause sedation but at higher doses causes seizures
- At clinical doses of 1.5mg/kg intravenous, it blunts stress response & increase in ICP during endotracheal intubation, suctioning, pinning or skin incision in patients undergoing craniotomy

- Maintains cerebral autoregulation & CO_2 reactivity
- Shows neuroprotective properties in animals,although not been seen in severe ischaemic conditions

Steroids[2,3]

- Steroids are routinely used in neurosurgery for lowering ICP caused by localized cerebral oedema around brain tumour

- Mechanism for beneficial effect not known but may be due to decreased CSF formation by 50% & decreased resistance to absorption & stabilization of capillary membrane
- In Traumatic Brain Injury [TBI], steroids has been associated with an increased risk of death
- In acute spinal cord injury use of steroids not shown to improve long term motor function

Table 5 : Anticonvulsants[2,5]

Drug	Dose/dosing frequency	Remarks	Therapeutic level Mcg/ml	Adverse effects
Phenytoin	300-400 mg/d (3-6 mg/kg, adult; 4-8 mg/kg, child); od-bid	Loading dose : 20 mg/kg @ < 50 mg/min infusion Cardiac monitoring check BP	10-20	Gum hyperplasia Lymphadenopathy Hirsutism Osteomalacia Hyperglycemia Dizziness Ataxia Incoordination
Carbamazepine	600-1800 mg/d (15-35 mg/kg, child); bid-qid	Start low and increase slowly Oral form only	6-12	Aplastic anemia Leukopenia Hyponatremia
Valproate	750-2000 mg/d (20-60 mg/kg); bid-qid	Start 15 mg/kg/day Increment weekly 5-10 mg/kg/day	50-100	Hepatotoxicity Thrombocytopenia Hyperammonemia Pancreatitis
Levetiracetam	1000-3000 mg/d; bid		20-60	Sedation Fatigue Incooradination Psychosis

- They are widely used in the periop course of surgical patients either for prophylaxis or therapeutic reasons especially who have epilepsy, head trauma or craniotomy
- Seizures can exacerbate the effects of ischemia which can worsen the neurological outcome
- CBF, $CMRO_2$ & intracellular Ca^{++}, excitatory neurotransmitters like glutamate increase during seizures
- Long term use induces liver enzymes and increases the requirements of anaesthetic drugs especially NMBD

OSMOTIC AGENTS
Mannitol[2,3,4]

- It is a primary drug for therapeutic brain dehydration & effective method of decreasing raised ICP
- It is given in dose of 0.25-1g/kg over 10-15 minutes

- Mainly acts by creating an osmotic gradient between plasma & brain when BBB is intact → reduction in brain water, brain volume & ICP
- It has a biphasic effect on ICP with infusion:
  - ICP may transiently increase,presumably because of vasodilatation of cerebral vessels in response to the sudden increase in osmolality
  - Subsequent decrease in ICP is achieved by movement of free water from the brain interstitial spaces into the vasculature
- ICP decreases also due to improved rheology of RBC → improves cerebral circulation
- Can cause transient increase in serum omolality, electrolyte abnormalities & rebound increase in ICP
- If serum osmolality > 320mmol/kg, it is seldom effective

Effects of anaesthetic agents & other drugs on cerebral physiology

Hypertonic saline[2,4,9]

- Its action on cerebral physiology is similar to manitol
- Administration of 5ml/kg of 3% HS provides same osmolar load as 1g/kg of mannitol
- Equiosmolar doses of HS & mannitol shows similar effects on brain dehydration & decrease in ICP in pts with TBI
- HS is not associated with diuresis or hypotension → beneficial in hemodynamically unstable or hypovolemic patients and patients with heart disease

Diuretics[2,3]

- Loop diuretics decreases ICP & brain oedema when used alone in large doses (1mg/kg) or in combination with mannitol in smaller doses
- Mechanism of reduction of ICP by Frusemide is unknown
- May reduce CSF formation & water penetration across the blood–brain barrier without increasing CBV or blood osmolality

CONCLUSION

- A good understanding of the effects of various drugs on the cerebral physiology will help provide ideal conditions for the growing minimally invasive and functional neurosurgical procedures
- Knowledge and expertise of the anaesthetist may directly influence patient's outcome

REFERENCES

1. P. Patel, J.Drummond. Cerebral physiology and the effects of anesthetics and techniques. In: Ronald D. Miller, editor. Miller's Anesthesia, 8th Edition. Elsevier, Inc; 2015: p 387-422.

2. TakefumiSakabe,Mishiya Matsumoto.Effects of anesthetic agents and other drugs on cerebral blood flow,metabolism,and intracranial pressure. In:James E.Cotrell ,William L.Young,editors.Cotrell and Youngs Neuroanesthesia 5th Edition.Elsevier,Inc;2010:p78-94.

3. Arun k Gupta. Opioids and other adjuvants.In:Arun k Gupta,Adrian W Gelb editors.Essentials of neuroanesthesia and neurointensive care.1st Edition.Elsevier, Inc;2008:p51-63.

4. P.Ganjoo,I.Kapoor.Neuropharmacology.In:Hemanshu Prabhakar editor.Essentials of neuroanesthesia 1st Edition,Academic press London:Elsevier Inc; 2017: p104-115.

5. Rosemary Hickry,Effects of Anesthesia on cerebral and spinal cord physiology.In: James E Cotrell editor. Handbook of Neuroanesthesia.5th Edition.2012: p20-31.

6. Herrick IA,Gelb AW,Manninen PH et al: Effects of fentanyl,sufentanil and alfentanil on brain retractor pressure,AnesthAnalg 1991; 72:359-363.

7. Lanier WL,Iaizzo PA,Milde JH:Cerebral blood flow and afferent muscle activity following IV succinyl choline in dogs,Anesthesiology Rev 1987;14: 60-66.

8. Drummond JC, Dao AV, Roth DM et al:effect of dexmedetomidine on cerebral blood flow velocity,cerebral metabolic rate and carbon dioxide response in normal humans, Anesthesiology 2008; 108:225-232.

9. Butterworth JF, StrchartzGR.Molecular mechanisms of local anesthetics: a review.Anesthesiology 1990;72:722-34.

10. FranconyG,Fauvage B,Falcon D et al:Equimolar doses of mannitol and hypertonic saline in the treatment of increased intracranial pressure, Crit care Med 2008; 36: 795-800.

MULTIPLE CHOICE QUESTIONS

1. **Which opioid should be avoided in neuroanesthesia**
   a. Morphine
   b. Fentanyl
   c. Pethidine
   d. Remifentanil

2. **The following agents decreases CBF/CMRO2 & ICP except**
   a. Dexmedetomidine
   b. Propofol
   c. Etomidate
   d. Nitrous oxide

3. **The following statements regarding osmotic agents to lower intracranial pressure are true except:**
   a. They create an osmotic gradient between plasma & brain
   b. Mannitol& HTS can cause hypernatremia
   c. In a situation of low blood pressure, mannitol is preferred
   d. Treatment goals for osmotic agents includes osmolality 310-320mosm/l

4. **All the following regarding the use of dexmedetomidine as an adjuvant for neurosurgical procedures are true except**
   a. Reduces the stress response to layrngoscopy
   b. Reduces post op pain
   c. Useful for awake craniotomies
   d. Has a context sensitive half life similar to remifentanil

5. **All the following are true about effects of inhalational anesthetics on CBF except**
   a. Isoflurane & sevoflurane are the ideal volatile anesthetics for neurosurgery
   b. Desflurane is recommended for space occupying lesions
   c. Induction doses of sevoflurane (1.5-2MAC) causes epileptiform seizures in some patients
   d. Volatile agents abolish CO_2 reactivity of CBF

6. **Which of the following statements concerning the cerebral effects of barbiturates is true?**
   a. Barbiturate coma produces greater cerebral protection than hypothermia to 17 degree celcius
   b. Barbiturates decreases the cerebral metabolic rate for oxygen by decreasing CBF
   c. SSEP & EEG are equally sensitive to suppression by barbiturates
   d. When administered in doses sufficient to produce an isoelectic EEG, barbiturates decreases the CMR for O_2 by 50%

7. **The following increases cerebral blood flow**
   a. Ketamine
   b. Propofol
   c. Mannitol
   d. Cisatracurium

8. **Which is the ideal relaxant of choice in neurosurgical patients**
   a. Succinyl choline
   b. Vecuronium
   c. Atracurium
   d. Rocuronium

9. **All are true regarding barbiturates except:**
   a. Effective anti- convulsant activity
   b. Reduction of free radical formation
   c. Causes hypertension and cerebral vasodilatation
   d. Reduced ATP depletion

10. **Ideal anti-hypertensive in neuro is**
    a. Calcium channel blockers
    b. Alpha and beta blockers
    c. Nitroglycerine
    d. Sodium nitroprusside

CHAPTER 4

ANAESTHETIC MANAGEMENT OF SUPRATENTORIAL SURGERIES

Rajashree Gandhe, Chinmaya Bhave, Kalyani Sathe, Avinash Kakde

Introduction

Supratentorial compartment is the largest in the intracranial space and is separated from the infratentorial compartment by tentorium cerebelli, a dural projection.

Supratentorial surgeries encompass wide variety of procedures which include tumor resection, aneurysm surgery, arteriovenous malformation excision, functional neurosurgery, hematoma evacuation and abscess drainage.

Embryology

At around the fourth week of gestation, the superior part of the neural tube differentiates into the prosencephalon (forebrain), mesencephalon (midbrain) and rhombencephalon (hindbrain). The prosencephalon differentiates into rostral-telencephalon from which cerebral hemispheres arise and the caudal-diencephalon which gives rise to thalamus and hypothalamus[1].

Anatomy

Roof of supratentorial compartment is formed by calvarium and the floor by tentorium cerebelli. Supratentorial compartment consists of the cerebral hemispheres and diencephalon. Cerebral hemispheres are separated in the midline by falx cerebri and are interconnected by corpus callosum. Cerebral hemispheres encase lateral ventricles and diencephalon encase third ventricle. Each cerebral hemisphere has frontal, parietal, temporal and occipital lobes. Diencephalon consists of thalamus and hypothalamus.

Supratentorial compartment is supplied by supraclinoid portion of internal carotid artery and its anterior and middle cerebral, ophthalmic, posterior communicating and anterior choroidal branches; the components of circle of Willis (Fig.1); basilar apex and posterior cerebral arteries[2]. Venous drainage of cerebral hemispheres is into superior and inferior sagittal sinuses.

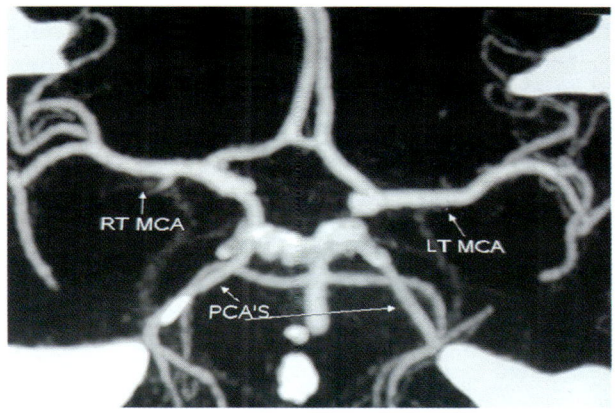

Fig. 1 : Circle of Willis

Diseases of supratentorial compartment

Pathologic processes within the supratentorial compartment include various tumors, hematomas, abscesses, arteriovenous malformations and aneurysms.

Intracranial tumors

They may be primary or secondary (metastatic). Most common primary tumors are meningiomas (Figs.2 & 3), glioma, glioblastoma, and astrocytoma. Most common sources of metastatic tumors are from breast, colorectal, kidney, lung and melanoma.

Hematomas

Hematomas may be epidural, subdural or intracerebral. They usually occur as result of trauma, uncontrolled hypertension, rupture of arteriovenous malformation and aneurysms. Patients on antiplatelet therapy are at higher risk for development of intracerebral hematoma.

Abscesses

Abscesses may occur as a direct spread from adjacent sites such as middle ear (temporal lobe), paranasal sinuses (frontal lobe) or by hematogenous spread from distant locations such as heart, lungs and teeth. Rarely infective organisms may also present as space occupying lesion like neurocysticercosis.

ANESTHETIC CONSIDERATIONS

Preoperative anesthetic assessment

Patients with supratentorial lesions may present with variety of symptoms based on their location, extent and their effect on intracranial pressure. Patient can present with various levels of consciousness ranging from drowsiness to coma. Other symptoms include headache, nausea and vomiting (due to raised ICP), seizures (space occupying lesions), limb weakness (lesions involving eloquent cortex), speech or visual disturbances (lesions involving fronto-temporal and occipital lobes respectively). Patients' Glasgow Coma Scale (GCS) score and any preexisting neurological deficit should be documented. Patient with co morbidities like hypertension and diabetes mellitus need to be optimized prior to elective surgeries. Chronic hypertension leads to shift of auto regulation curve to the right so blood pressure should be controlled to maintain adequate perfusion pressure. Uncontrolled blood sugar can worsen neurological outcome. Patient with ischemic heart disease should be evaluated with necessary investigations such as electrocardiogram and echocardiography. Specialist consultation can be considered in indicated cases.

CT and MRI imaging should be reviewed for size, location and vascularity of tumor and any evidence of midline shift.

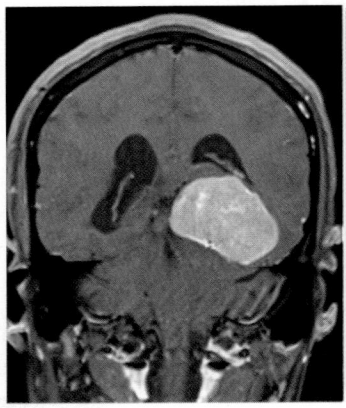 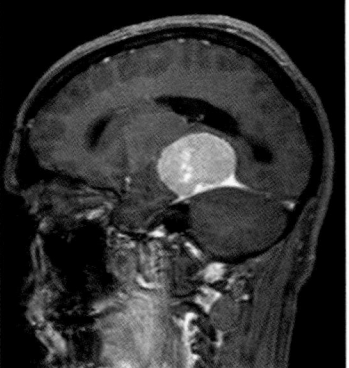

Coronal Section   *Sagittal Section*

Fig. 2 & 3 : MRI showing tumor

All patients must be kept nil per oral minimum eight hours prior to elective surgery. Patients should be evaluated for their preoperative medications. Patient may be receiving IV mannitol for raised intracranial pressure, which can lead to electrolyte disturbances and hypovolemia. Patient receiving inj. Dexamethasone for reducing peritumor edema may have elevated blood sugars. As mentioned earlier elevated blood sugars can be associated with worse neurological outcome. In patients who are on antiplatelet or anticoagulant medications, surgery should be deferred as per guidelines. In case of emergency, patient should be

transfused with appropriate blood products preoperatively to avoid uncontrolled bleeding during surgery. Patients with supratentorial lesions are often on antiepileptic and steroid medications which should be continued perioperatively. Antacids (Inj. Pantoprazole 40 mg) should be considered on the day of surgery.

Pre-anaesthetic assessment is not complete without explaining the plan of anaesthesia to the patient and obtaining consent of the patient. In the elective neurosurgical cases, discussion with the neurosurgeon about positioning of the patient, approach to the lesion and its vascularity or any expected difficulties plays a very important role in the success of surgery.

Monitoring

ASA standard monitoring like electrocardiography, pulse oximetry, non invasive blood pressure and capnography should be done. Invasive arterial blood pressure monitoring is indicated in intracranial surgeries or as dictated by the patient's comorbid conditions. Invasive blood pressure monitoring helps in detecting abrupt hemodynamic changes that might compromise cerebral perfusion pressure (CPP) and also facilitate arterial blood gas analysis. Additional monitors include core temperature monitor to ensure normothermia, blood glucose to ensure glycaemic control and Foley's catheter for measurement of urine output, especially in patients receiving mannitol and in long duration surgeries.

Specific monitoring includes evoked potentials like SSEP and MEP, neuromuscular blockade, ICP, CBF, Jugular venous oximetry ($SjvO_2$) and depth of anaesthesia.

Precordial Doppler and Transesophageal echocardiography can help in detecting venous air embolism, especially in surgeries requiring sitting position and patient with right to left intra cardiac shunts.

Anaesthetic management

Anesthetic management of patients with supratentorial lesions should aim towards

1. Providing excellent operating conditions and to minimize secondary brain injury while preserving the uninjured brain.

2. Rapid recovery of the patient to help neurological assessment in the immediate postoperative period.

3. Adequate pain relief, prevention of postoperative nausea and vomiting and thus ensuring hemodynamic control in the postoperative period.

This involves basic understanding of the neuropathophysiology and neuropharmacology.

Neuropathophysiology

As per Monroe Kelly doctrine, skull has a fixed volume formed by brain tissue (80%), cerebrospinal fluid (10%) and cerebral blood volume (10%). Any increase in one of these must be compensated by corresponding decrease in the other to maintain intracranial pressure (ICP). Compensatory mechanisms to prevent rise in ICP are a) Decrease in intracranial blood volume, b) Shift of CSF to spinal canal and c) Increase absorption of CSF[3]. When these compensatory mechanisms are exhausted there is sudden rise in ICP and this may lead to cerebral ischemia and brain herniation (Fig. 4).

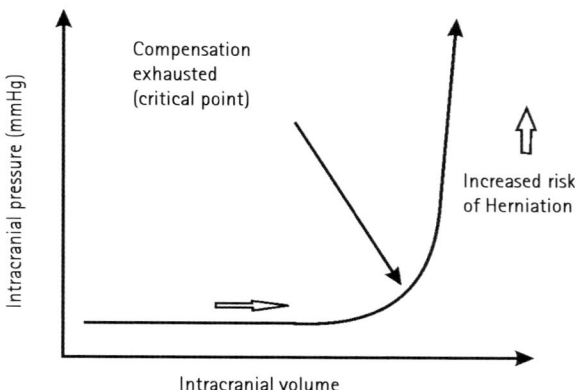

Fig. 4 : Intracranial volume versus pressure curve

ICP is a critical determinant of cerebral perfusion pressure (CPP). The normal ICP measured in the horizontal position is 5-15 mmHg. ICP is considered abnormal when levels exceed 15-20 mmHg[4].

CPP is the difference between mean arterial pressure (MAP) and intracranial pressure. [CPP=MAP-ICP]. Normally CPP is auto regulated over a mean arterial pressure range of 65-150 mmHg[5].

Cerebral blood flow (CBF) is normally tightly maintained by the process of autoregulation. Normal CBF ranges from 45-55 ml/100 gm/min, with grey matter having higher flow than white matter (75-85 ml/100 gm/min and 20 ml/100 gm/min respectively)[5].

As per the concept of flow-metabolism coupling CBF parallels cerebral metabolism. Cerebral metabolic requirement of oxygen (CMRO$_2$) is a measure of cerebral metabolism.

Vasodilatation cascade suggests that whenever CPP decreases there is cerebral vasodilatation with subsequent increase in CBV and ICP.

Vasoconstriction cascade proposes that increase in CPP can lead to reduction in CBV and hence ICP.

There is a linear relationship between PaCO2 and cerebral blood flow between 20 mmHg and 80 mmHg. Every 1mmHg rise in PaCO2 increase CBF by 2 to 4%[6].

Neuropharmacology

According to flow metabolism coupling, blood flow to brain areas depends on the brain activity. Various anesthetic drugs affect the brain neurophysiology by affecting CMR, CBF and ICP.

Inhalational agents

Inhalational volatile anesthetic agents cause cerebral vasodilatation which leads to increase CBF which in turn leads to increase in ICP (direct mechanism). These agents also lead to decrease in CMR which will decrease CBF in brain (indirect mechanism). Ultimately changes in CBF depend on minimum alveolar concentration (MAC) value of inhalational agent. Usually MAC below 1 does not increase CBF.

Nitrous oxide acts as neuro stimulant and increases CBF, CMR and ICP and should be avoided. Halothane is the most potent in these effects and should be avoided. Other volatile agents have following sequence in affecting ICP and CBF. Desflurane> Isoflurane > Sevoflurane[7].

Enflurane should be avoided due to its epileptogenic potential.

Intravenous agents

Dexmedetomidine, an alpha 2 agonist can be used as a premedication agent. It has analgesic, sympatholytic and sedative effect at the same time preserving intracerebral hemodynamics.

Propofol and Thiopental sodium are good intravenous induction agents in neuroanaesthesia as both decrease CBF and CMR. Both these agents decrease ICP, maintain autoregulation and CO2 reactivity.

Propofol causes peripheral vasodilatation and hypotension which may lead to decrease CPP. Etomidate may be used as it preserves cerebral perfusion due to its stable hemodynamic profile.

Ketamine increases CMR, ICP and CBF. For these reasons, Ketamine is avoided as an induction agent. But there are newer studies stating a neuroprotective role of Ketamine due to its antagonistic action at NMDA receptors.

Neuromuscular blocking agent

These agents do not cross blood brain barrier and have no effect on cerebral hemodynamics. Succinylcholine can cause mild increase in ICP because of fasciculations.

Opioids

Opioids do not have any direct effect on CBF or cerebral autoregulation. Opioids should be used in preinduction carefully as they can cause respiratory depression which can lead to hypoxia and hypercarbia further increasing ICP.

Remifentanil has a specific consideration due to its very short context sensitive half life.

Osmotic agents

Mannitol is most commonly used osmotic agent to reduce ICP. It increases blood osmolality relative to that of brain and draws water from brain extracellular fluid (ECF) to vascular compartment. Action of mannitol depends on intact blood brain barrier (BBB). In case of disruption of blood brain barrier, mannitol enters brain and can worsen cerebral edema. Dose of mannitol is 0.5 -1 g/kg intravenous and its action starts in 10-15 minutes with peak effect at 1 hour.

Hypertonic saline is used in refractory cases of raised ICP or as an alternative to mannitol. Dose of 3% hypertonic saline is 3 ml/ kg intravenously.

Glucocorticoids

Dexamethasone is the most commonly used steroid for vasogenic edema caused by brain tumors. Blood sugars should be monitored as even a single dose can increase blood sugars drastically which can increase risk of infection, extent of cerebral injury and worsens neurological outcome.

Diuretics

Loop diuretics like furosemide can decrease ICP by their diuretic action and reduction in CSF production. Electrolytes should be monitored as diuretics can cause electrolyte disturbances and hypovolemia.

Anaesthetic management

Patients are taken for elective surgery after confirming adequate fasting; obtaining written, informed consent and confirming routine preoperative medications. Routine monitors are attached and patients are adequately preoxygenated. Sedative premedications should be given in the operation theatre under direct supervision as they can cause respiratory depression, upper airway obstruction, resulting in hypercarbia and hypoxia which is detrimental to patient with raised ICP. The authors premedicate with Inj. Dexmedetomidine intravenous loading dose for 10 minutes and then maintenance dose. In addition, intravenous Midazolam 0.03-0.05 mg/kg, Glycopyrrolate 0.002 mg/kg and Fentanyl 1-2 mcg/kg is given.

Two large bore intravenous accesses are established. Central venous access may be established if there is risk of excessive blood loss or air embolism or the need to use vasopressors. Intravenous Isotonic fluids are administered at 2 ml/kg during fasting period and continued intraoperatively as per requirement.

Induction of anaesthesia

Anaesthesia induction is done with intravenous Propofol 2-2.5 mg/ kg and muscle relaxation for tracheal intubation is achieved with 0.5-1mg/kg intravenous Atracurium. Cisatracurium may be preferred over Atracurium as it does not cause histamine release. In patients with ischemic heart disease, induction with intravenous Etomidate at 0.2 mg/kg is preferred because of its stable hemodynamic profile. Hemodynamic response to laryngoscopy is attenuated by additional boluses of Propofol, Fentanyl, Esmolol or Lignocaine. Patients are intubated with adequate size endotracheal tube (preferably flexometallic) and its position is confirmed.

Positioning

Application of a three pin head holder is a painful stimulus causing hemodynamic and CNS stimulation, which needs to be minimized. This can be achieved by bolus doses of Fentanyl and Propofol and pin site local infiltration. Scalp block can be given post induction to attenuate pinning response and to maintain stable hemodynamics. It also decreases need of intraoperative opioids and provides postoperative analgesia[8].

Positioning for surgery requires co-ordination between neurosurgical and anaesthesia team. The optimal position is the position which allows easy surgical access, minimizes cardiovascular and respiratory compromise and prevents neurological injury. Supratentorial surgeries are done in supine, lateral or prone position and their variants (Park bench and Concorde). Eyes and pressure points are adequately taped and padded. Endotracheal tube position is reconfirmed. The excessive flexion and lateral rotation of neck should be avoided as this can cause jugular venous compression affecting venous drainage and causing an increase in ICP.

Maintenance

Anaesthesia is maintained with either inhalational agents, intravenous anaesthetic agents or a combination of both depending on patients' preoperative neurological status. The authors prefer a combination of 0.5-1.0 MAC of Sevoflurane in air oxygen mixture with intravenous infusions of Propofol (1mg/kg/hour), Dexmedetomidine (0.3-0.5 mcg/kg/hour), Fentanyl (1-2 mcg/kg/hour) and Atracurium (0.5 mg/kg/hour). Ventilation should be adjusted to maintain normocapnia. Normothermia is ensured using forced air warming blankets, warm intravenous fluids and a temperature monitoring probe. Urine output should be continuously monitored. Mechanical calf compression or compression stocking should be used to minimize the risk of venous thromboembolism.

Intraoperative neuroprotection is achieved by a) adequate depth of anaesthesia, b) mild hyperosmolarity (mannitol/ hypertonic saline), c) brief mild hyperventilation (PaCO$_2$ 32-35 mmHg), d) normotension, e) normovolemic and f) mild hyperoxia. Additionally head end elevation upto 30°, minimum PEEP to maintain low intrathoracic pressure and lumbar drainage of CSF may also be useful.

Blood loss should be replaced with adequate cross matched blood and blood products. Anti-epileptics, analgesics and antiemetics should be administered perioperatively. Adequate hemostasis should be confirmed prior to closure.

Emergence

Decision regarding early versus delayed extubation depends on multiple factors. Patients with poor preoperative neurological status, those with prolonged duration of surgery (more than six hours), massive intraoperative blood loss or fluid shifts should be ventilated postoperatively. All other patients must be extubated at the end of procedure to allow early neurological assessment and provide a baseline for continuing neurologic follow up. Emergence is associated with hemodynamic and ICP responses. These need to be curtailed with the use of antihypertensives like Labetalol (0.5-1mg/kg), Esmolol (1mg/kg) to minimize incidence of postoperative hematomas and ensure smooth extubation. The targeted neurological examination should be performed prior to shifting patient to intensive care unit.

POSTOPERATIVE COMPLICATIONS

Delayed emergence

It is defined as failure to regain expected level of consciousness within 20-30 minutes of pharmacologically adequate cessation of anesthesia[9]. Medical causes like seizures, metabolic and electrolyte disturbance should be ruled out. CT or MRI may be required to detect bleeding, ischemia or cerebral edema.

Pain

Post craniotomy pain may be treated using multimodal analgesia in the form of scalp block, superficial cervical plexus block, intravenous opioids, Paracetamol or non steroidal anti inflammatory drugs (NSAID's).

Nausea and vomiting

It can lead to hypertensive responses and raised ICP and should be minimized with antiemetic medications.

Seizures

Airway should be protected during an episode of seizure. Hemodynamics should be maintained. Intravenous Midazolam 0.2 mg/kg (maximum dose 10 mg) and

antiepileptic boluses (Fosphentyoin, Levetiracetam, and Sodium valproate) should be administered. Antiepileptic levels should also be checked simultaneously.

SPECIFIC CONSIDERATIONS

Tumors

Anesthetic and surgical implications may change based on the tumor type. Meningiomas are generally benign, highly vascular tumors with high chances of local recurrence. Complete excision is usually the goal lead to prolonged surgery duration and intraoperative blood loss. Gliomas on the other hand are not so demanding. Tumor location is also important, not only from the point of view of positioning and surgical access but tumors in eloquent areas may require special monitoring like evoked potentials, electrocorticography or awake techniques and anaesthesia needs to be tailored accordingly.

Abscess

Generally, solitary abscess is amenable to treatment by surgery while multiple abscesses are treated by medical management. Administration of appropriate antibiotics as per their sensitivity and steroids to reduce peri-abscess edema (risk of reduction of antibiotic penetrance) are important during treatment of cerebral abscess. Prophylactic antiepileptics are also often required as incidence of seizures is high in these patients. Echocardiography should be done in congenital heart disease patients for detection of shunts or septal defects.

Intracranial hematomas

These are extradural, subdural or intracerebral and may require emergency decompression due to raised ICP. Traumatic hematomas may be associated with additional cervical spine injury or other life threatening injuries which also need to be addressed. History should include medication history especially antiplatelet and anticoagulant treatment and investigations and blood products need to be requested accordingly.

Awake craniotomy

It is done for functional neurosurgery (Deep Brain Stimulation for Parkinsonism) and for tumors or epileptic foci located in eloquent cortex[10,11] (Fig. 5 a & b). Three types of anaesthetic techniques can be used for awake craniotomies 1) scalp block and pin site local anesthetic infiltration, 2) conscious sedation and 3) asleep-awake-asleep technique[10,11]. Cooperative and motivated patients who have no language barriers or anticipated airway problems are candidates for awake craniotomies. Preoperative counselling by the anaesthesiologist helps to relieve anxiety and preparing patients for the surgery. Thorough airway assessment and equipment for securing airway at any stage of the procedure are essential[12]. Rescue airway equipment like laryngeal mask airway, nasopharyngeal airway must be ready in cases of airway emergencies. Authors prefer conscious sedation technique with infusion of intravenous Dexmedetomidine which is supplemented with scalp block for analgesia and comfort of patient.

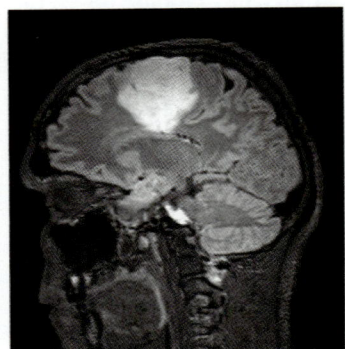 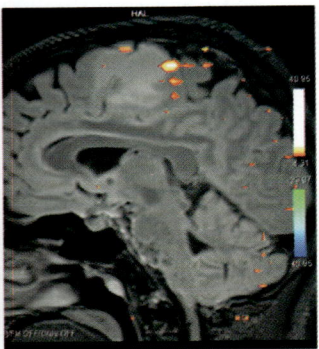

(a) Eloquent cortex lesion   *(b) Functional MRI showing relation of tumor and motor cortex.*

Fig. 5 : a & b.

CONCLUSION

Successful anaesthetic management of supratentorial surgeries requires a thorough understanding of the relationship between anatomy, pathophysiology and pharmacology.

Mainstay of neuroanaesthesia management includes, optimization of the patient, documentation of preoperative neurological status, provision of ideal operating conditions, minimizing secondary brain injury, preserving the uninjured brain and allowing early postoperative recovery to help neurological assessment.

Postoperative comfort and hemodynamic stability should be achieved by ensuring adequate control of pain, nausea and vomiting.

REFERENCES

1. Collins P (ed). Embryology And Development. In: Williams PL(late), Bannister LH, Berry MM, Collins P, Dyson M, Dussek JE et al (eds.), *Gray's anatomy,* 38th ed, New York, Churchill Livingstone; 1995. p 217-22.

2. Rhoton AL, The supratentorial arteries, Neurosurgery, 2002, volume 51 [suppl 1]: 53.

3. Zweifel C., Hutchinson P, Czosnyka M. Intracranial pressure In: Matta BF, Menon DK, Smith M. (eds.), *Core topics in Neuroanaesthesia and Neurointensive care.* Cambridge University Press, Cambridge; 2011. p 45-7.

4. Sulek CA. Intracranial pressure In: Cucchiara RF, Black S, Michenfelder JD (eds.), Clinical Neuroanesthesia, 2nd ed., New York, Churchill Livingstone Inc; 1998. p 75.

5. Patel PM, Drummond JC, Lemkuil BP. Cerebral physiology and the effects of anesthetic drugs In: Miller RD (ed), Miller's Anesthesia, 8th ed., Canada, Elsevier Saunders; 2015. p 389-90.

6. Rahimi E, Manninen PH. Routine craniotomy for supratentorial masses In: Mongan PD, Soriano SG, Sloan TB (eds.), A practical approach to Neuroanesthesia, China, Lippincott Williams and Wilkins; 2013. p 38.

7. Dinsmore J, Anaesthesia for supratentorial surgery In: Matta BF, Menon DK, Smith M (eds.), *Core topics in Neuroanaesthesia and Neurointensive care.* Cambridge University Press, Cambridge; 2011.p 165.

8. Osborn I, Sebeo J. "Scalp Block" During Craniotomy: A Classic Technique Revisited. J Neurosurg Anesthesiol. 2010;22(3):p187-94.

9. Bruder NJ, Ravussin P, Schoettker P. Supratentorial masses: Anesthetic consideration In: Cottrell JE, Patel P (eds.), Cottrell's and Patel's Neuroanesthesia, 6th ed., USA, Elsevier; 2017. p 201.

10. Bilotta F, Rosa G. 'Anesthesia' for awake neurosurgery. Curr Opin Anaesthesiol. 2009;22:560-65.

11. Skucas AP, Artru AA. Anesthetic Complications of Awake Craniotomies for Epilepsy Surgeries. Anesth Analg. 2006;102:882-7.

12. Bindu B, Bithal PK. Anaesthesia and deep brain stimulation. J Neuroanaesthesiol Crit Care 2016;3:200.

MULTIPLE CHOICE QUESTIONS

1. **Cerebral hemispheres are separated in the midline by**
   a. Corpus Callosum
   b. Tentorium Cerebelli
   c. Falx Cerebri
   d. Calvarium

2. **Cerebral autoregulation curve is shifted to the right by**
   a. Hypoxia
   b. Chronic hypertension
   c. Intravenous anaesthetic agents
   d. Bronchial asthma

3. **Secondary brain injury can be caused by all except**
   a. Hypercapnia
   b. Hypotension
   c. Hypothermia
   d. Raised intracranial pressure (ICP)

4. **Each mmHg increase in PaCO2 will increase cerebral blood flow (CBF) by**
   a. 1%
   b. 2%
   c. 8%
   d. 12%

5. **Which of the following is the most sensitive means to detect venous air embolism**
   a. Electroencephalography
   b. Transesophageal Echocardiography
   c. Mass spectrometry
   d. Jugular oximetry

6. **Signs and symptoms of raised intracranial pressure (ICP) are**
   a. Headache
   b. Papilloedema
   c. Nausea and vomiting
   d. All of the above

7. **ASA standard monitors include all except**
   a. Pulse oximetry
   b. Capnography
   c. Noninvasive blood pressure
   d. Precordial Doppler

8. **Average cerebral blood flow (CBF) ranges from**
   a. 45-55ml/100g/min
   b. 75-85ml/100g/min
   c. 150-200ml/100g/min
   d. 65-95ml/100g/min

9. **Ketamine**
   a. Decreases cerebral blood flow
   b. Increases cerebral blood flow
   c. Reduces cerebral metabolic rate
   d. Decreases intracranial pressure

10. **36 year old female is anaesthetized for resection of temporal lobe tumour. Preoperatively patient is lethargic and disoriented. After induction of general anaesthesia, which of the following would be the most appropriate drug to control haemodynamic response to direct laryngoscopy and intubation?**
    a. Esmolol
    b. Nitroglycerine
    c. Hydralazine
    d. Sodium Nitroprusside

CHAPTER 5

ANAESTHESIA FOR POSTERIOR FOSSA SURGERY

Anil Parakh, Aditi Tilak

Introduction

Posterior fossa surgery faces difficult challenges to both anaesthesiologists and surgeons due to the peculiarities observed from an anatomical and physiological point of view. It also requires the patient to be put in a specific position prior to surgery. The intraoperative goals are to facilitate surgical access, minimize nervous tissue trauma and maintain respiratory and cardiovascular stability. To achieve these goals, a thorough knowledge of anatomy and pathology, preoperative history and neurological assessment, image findings, proper positioning, adequate intraoperative monitoring and management, and timely treatment of adverse effects is essential for favourable outcome.

ANATOMY

The posterior fossa is the deepest cranial fossa and is surrounded by the dorsum sellae and basilar portion of the occipital bone (clivus) anteriorly, the petrosal and mastoid components of the temporal bone laterally and the dural layer (tentorium cerebelli) superiorly and the occipital bone posteriorly and inferiorly. The foramen magnum in the occipital bone is the largest opening of the posterior fossa. The posterior fossa contents include the hindbrain (cerebellum, pons, medulla), the lower cranial nerves, venous sinuses (sigmoid, occipital, transverse). The Aqueduct of Sylvius connecting the 3rd and 4th ventricles is a very narrow CSF pathway susceptible to obstruction. Pathologies in the posterior fossa therefore often cause hydrocephalus.

PATHOLOGY

Pathologies in the posterior cranial fossa requiring surgical intervention can be classified as:[1]

- Tumours – Medulloblastoma (commonest), cerebellar astrocytoma, brainstem glioma, ependymoma, choroid plexus papilloma, dermoid tumours, haemangioblastomas, metastasis, Cerebellopontine angle tumours like acoustic neuroma, schwannoma, gliomas, glomus jugulare tumours, meningioma.
- Vascular malformations – Aneurysms, arteriovenous malformations, haematomas, cerebellar infarctions.
- Cysts – Epidermoid/arachnoid.

- Cranial nerve lesions – Trigeminal neuralgia, hemifacial spasm, glossopharyngeal nerve neuralgia.
- Craniocervical anomalies – Atlanto-occipital/ atlantoaxial instability, arnold chiari malformation.

PREOPERATIVE MANAGEMENT

CLINICAL PRESENTATION: Posterior fossa space occupying lesions often present with hydrocephalus and signs and symptoms of raised intracranial pressure. Headache, vomiting, drowsiness and visual disturbances are common. Cranial nerve dysfunction, such as VI or IV nerve palsy, causes disorders of ocular motility. Bulbar symptoms may be seen with involvement of lower cranial nerves. Ataxia occurs with involvement of cerebellum.

The preoperative clinical status plays a role in planning postoperative management. Patients with bulbar dysfunction are at greater risk of aspiration pneumonitis. They may need a period of elective ventilation and thorough assessment of cough and gag reflex prior to a trial of extubation.

ASSESSMENT

- Thorough history of co-morbidities especially of cardiovascular and respiratory system must be noted. The cardio-respiratory status decides how well the patient will tolerate unusual surgical positions. In case of severe coronary artery disease, carotid disease, pre existing hemodynamic instability, alternatives to sitting position may be sought.
- Raised intracranial pressure of dangerous proportions require preoperative surgical management in the form of external ventricular drainage or a shunt procedure.
- Investigations must be ordered as per patient's co-morbidities and institutional protocol. Routine blood investigations, X-Ray chest, ECG are standard requirements. Cardiac evaluation as deemed necessary for risk stratification and trans-oesophageal echocardiography to rule out patent foramen ovale in case of planned surgery in sitting position are ordered in our institution.
- Simple preoperative interventions such as attention to hydration can be useful to blunt the adverse consequences of positioning.

INTRAOPERATIVE MANAGEMENT

General principles of neuroanaesthesia should be followed during anaesthesia induction and maintenance. Care should be taken to avoid severe changes in heart rate and blood pressure, hypoxia, hypercapnia, light plane of anaesthesia leading to coughing and raised intracranial pressure.

Induction of anaesthesia may be done using opioids like fentanyl to blunt the intubation response and titrated doses of propofol. Combinations of propofol/remifentanil versus sevoflurane/remifentanil for maintenance of anaesthesia are found to be comparable[2].

The use of Nitrous oxide for maintenance of anaesthesia is considered controversial for several reasons. Because of its tendency to expand gas filled spaces it is often implicated in pneumocephalus.[3] The other concern is that it might increase the size of venous air emboli due to its greater solubility in blood than nitrogen.

There have been studies evaluating the development of pneumocephalus after posterior fossa surgery which show that techniques with and without nitrous oxide carry similar incidences of pneumocephalus.[4] There is no significant difference in the amount of air accumulated with any anaesthetic technique. However nitrous oxide must be avoided if surgical re-exploration becomes necessary during the first fourteen postoperative days because intracranial air is absorbed only slowly[5].

Regarding venous air embolism, nitrous oxide itself does not increase the risk of venous air embolism.[6] but it must be discontinued immediately if air embolism is suspected to minimise the volume and consequences.

POSITIONING

Posterior fossa surgery can be carried out in number of unusual positions. Sitting, prone positions, rarely the lateral position or modification of these are used.

Sitting position:

Advantages of sitting positions: The sitting position provides optimal access to midline structures and improves surgical exposure, anatomical orientations and venous drainage from the surgical field. The gravitational drainage of the blood, cerebrospinal and irrigating fluids provides cleaner operating field. The sitting position also requires less cerebellar retractions hence reduces the postoperative cerebellar swelling and helps preservation of cranial nerves. The other advantages of sitting position includes better access to tracheal tube, central line, hands and chest wall, better ventilation, less facial and airway swelling, less intracranial pressure and better observation of motor response of cranial nerves stimulation while intra-operative monitoring.

Disadvantages of sitting position: The sitting position is associated with more haemodynamic instability particularly when patient is already hypovolaemic due to use of diuretics or mannitol for high intracranial pressure, increased risk of venous air embolism, paradoxical air embolism, pneumocephalus, quadriplegia due to extreme neck flexion and macroglossia.

Contraindications of sitting position:

Absolute
- Patent ventriculo-atrial shunt
- Cerebral ischaemia when upright and awake

Relative
- Severe hypotension/hypertension
- Severe cervical canal stenosis
- Severe autonomic neuropathy
- Extremes of age

How sitting position is given

The back is tilted up gradually and hips flexed to a maximum of 90°. Pillows are placed below the knees and thighs to elevate the legs and maintain a degree of flexion to avoid overstretching the tendons and nerves. The upper arms should be well supported to avoid stretching of brachial plexuses due to the weight of the arms. The head is supported in a head holder. The neck is flexed with at least two finger breadth distances between the chin and sternum. Ideally the head holder should be attached to the back portion of the table rather than the portion under the thighs or legs. This will permit lowering of the head and CPR without taking the patient out of the head holder (Fig.1 A). The head holder attached to thigh portion of the table should be avoided (Fig. 1B).

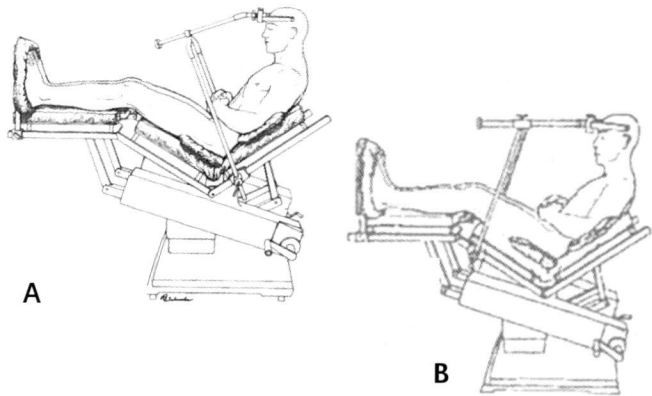

A

B

Fig.1: Sitting Position. In A, the head holder support is correctly positioned such that the head can be lowered without the necessity of first detaching the head holder. In B, with the support attached to the thigh portion of the table, should be avoided.
(From Martin JT. Positioning in Anesthesia and Surgery. Phildephia,WBSauunders.1988)

Position must be given in a slow gradual manner to allow compensation for changes in cardiac output and venous return.

Although controversial due to its association with complications, various studies have found the incidence of these to be comparable to other positions such as prone[7,8], hence sitting position continues to be used with varying incidences worldwide

Alternative positions

Prone position: Prone position is the traditional and most suited position for the midline approach during infratentorial craniotomies. The head is supported in the midline by Mayfield tongs. Support the thorax with firm bolsters which are placed under the patients sides from clavicle to iliac crest. This allows the belly to hang free and increases ventilation while preventing aorto-caval compression. Breasts are placed medial and cephalad. It is ensured that genitals are not compressed. Mirror is used to see the facial structures after the patient is given prone position.

This position carries a lower risk of venous air embolism but does not eliminate it entirely. The head is still above the level of the heart. Surgical access is inferior to that obtained in the sitting position. There is increased risk of postoperative visual loss due to variety of mechanisms including ischaemic optic neuropathy and retinal artery thrombosis. Similar haemodynamic changes are anticipated as in sitting position. These are attributed to venous pooling in the lower extremities and decreased venous return. There is higher surgical blood loss and more chances of blood transfusion[9].

Lateral position: Lateral position can be given in unilateral lesion excision surgery. Special attention should be given to take care of lower arm and all the pressure points.

Three-quarter prone position: This is the combination of lateral and prone position and used in far lateral approach, by placing the patient sufficiently superiorly on the operating table such that the dependent arm is hanging over the edge of the table and secure with sling. The trunk is rotated 15° from lateral position into the semiprone position and supported by pillow. The ipsilateral shoulder is pulled inferiorly. This position has less incidence of venous air embolism.

Park bench position: This is a modification of lateral position. The head is turned around 30° facing down with maximum flexion of the neck. The back is also elevated. The upper arm is positioned along the lateral trunk and the upper shoulder taped towards the table. The lower extremities should be slightly flexed and a pillow placed between the legs[10].

Anaesthesia for posterior fossa surgery

MONITORING

Standard non-invasive monitoring ECG, pulseoximetry, NIBP and capnography after intubation are instituted.

Invasive arterial pressure monitoring is indicated for beat to beat measurement of blood pressure. This is especially useful during positioning. The transducer is zeroed at the skull level so cerebral perfusion pressure can be estimated. Routine use of central venous catheter is recommended. The tip of the catheter is positioned at the junction of the superior vena cava and right atrium. It is then useful to confirm the presence of intravascular air in case of venous air embolism and also for evacuation of the air as a therapeutic measure.

Since venous air embolism is a concern, special monitoring is indicated for timely detection of the same. Techniques include precordial doppler, transoesophageal echocardiography, pulmonary artery catheter, fractional excretion of N2 and oesophageal stethoscope.

Neurophysiological monitoring is used to monitor integrity of vital neurological structures, detect cerebral hypoperfusion and depth of anaesthesia. Somatosensory evoked potentials are used to monitor spinal cord dysfunction. Brain stem auditory evoked potential monitoring helps preserve hearing by detecting damage to the VIII cranial nerve and auditory pathways. Electromyography and motor evoked potentials are other modes of cerebral function monitoring.

COMPLICATIONS AND THEIR MANAGEMENT

1. **Haemodynamic changes** - Sitting position is associated with marked decrease in venous return due to pooling of blood in the lower limbs. This causes decreased cardiac output and hypotension.

   The degree of hypotension that is labelled significant is different in studies by different authors. However a decrease in mean arterial pressure by > 10% or a decrease in systolic pressure by >20% was observed to have an incidence of 5%-32%.[11,12] Vasodilatation caused by intravenous and inhalational agents and decreased venous return caused by positive pressure ventilation further aggravates the cardiovascular instability. In the sitting position, there has been observed a decrease in mean arterial pressure, right atrial pressure, cardiac index and an increase in systemic vascular resistance index.[13]

   The extent of haemodynamic changes is influenced by the speed of positioning, volume loading of patients pre-positioning and the use of accessory devices to improve venous return. Slow and gradual change in position is recommended. All measures must be undertaken to avoid dehydration in subjects. Fluid loading with colloids/crystalloids at induction, before positioning is desirable. Calf pumps and compression stockings will encourage venous return from lower limbs.

Invasive blood pressure monitoring allows beat to beat monitoring of blood pressure. Vasoactive drugs like ephedrine/phenylephrine along with fluid boluses are useful to prevent dangerous fall in blood pressure.

2. **Venous air embolism–** Venous air embolism is a risk in any surgical procedure where open vascular channels are above the level of the heart. This is especially important to remember in neurosurgery due to the presence of non collapsible venous channels like the diploic veins and dural sinuses. These channels remain open due to attachment to the skull or dura. Development of sub-atmospheric pressure in open veins causes entrainment of air in the vascular system. The incidence of venous air embolism is widely variable in studies and case series. It is reportedly between 15%-76%.[14,8] This variation can be attributed to the difference in sensitivities and specificities of the various diagnostic modalities.

Pathophysiology: Air enters the vascular system from the cerebral veins and finally enters the right atrium or ventricle. The morbidity and mortality are directly related to the volume and speed of air entrainment. The volume of air that is lethal is dependent on the body size. The adult lethal volume is described as 200-300 ml.[15] Rate of entrainment is also important as the pulmonary circulation can compensate to a certain extent for the presence of intravascular gas.

A large or rapid entrainment is capable of, causing an air lock, decreasing the right ventricular output. It increases the right heart pressures, decreases the cardiac output, causing myocardial ischaemia, dysrhythmias and cardiovascular collapse.

At the microcirculatory level, bubbles of air can cause activation of endothelial cells leading to complement activation, release of cytokines, reactive oxygen molecules. The mechanical obstruction and local hypoxia produces reflex vasoconstriction[9].

Intra-operatively venous air embolism manifests as cardiorespiratory compromise. A sudden decrease in EtCO2 and an increase in EtN2 are seen due to increased dead space. There may be an increase in airway pressures and rarely an audible wheeze in case of severe bronchospasm. Desaturation is a late sign. Hypotension and elevated central venous pressure are common cardiovascular manifestations. ECG changes with right heart strain pattern are expected. The classic mill wheel murmur indicates a near terminal event. Cardiac arrest is the most serious effect of venous air embolism. Neurological sequelae become obvious postoperatively. Stroke/delayed awakening can be due to cerebral hypoxia secondary to cardiac compromise or due to paradoxical air embolism.

Monitoring

*   **Transoesophageal echocardiography –** This is the most sensitive modality for detection of intracardiac air. It permits detection of venous and paradoxical air embolism. It can detect as little as 0.02ml/kg of air administered by bolus injection[16,] however it is invasive compared to other available tools, requires specialised training to be useful and detects even microbubbles that may not be clinically significant[9].

*   **Precordial Doppler –** This being a noninvasive monitoring, has good sensitivity in detecting clinically significant volumes of air in circulation. The probe is placed in the right parasternal area. The position is confirmed by injecting agitated saline through the right atrial catheter and listening to the characteristic change in signal.

*   **End tidal N2 –** EtN2 is more efficient than EtCO2 in detecting intravascular air. Changes in EtN2 occur 30-90 seconds earlier than EtCO2[17]. However not all anaesthetic monitors are capable of measuring N2 levels. Concurrent use of N2O limits its use.

*   **End tidal CO2 –** Sudden significant fall in EtCO2 is a useful early sign of venous air embolism when there is no advanced monitoring available. It is a routinely used monitor.

*   **Pulmonary artery catheter –** Pulmonary artery catheter can be used to detect elevated right heart pressures. It is slightly more sensitive than EtCO2 for venous air embolism detection. However it is an invasive procedure that carries its own risks and morbidity. Its use in patients with no significant cardiovascular indications is hard to justify. It is not as useful as a right atrial catheter for aspiration of intracardiac air.

*   **Right atrial catheter –** An appropriately placed right atrial catheter aids both diagnosis and treatment of venous air embolism. The tip of the catheter must be placed at the junction of the right atrium and superior vena cava. The correct position of the tip of the catheter should be confirmed either by fluoroscopy or ECG.

A combination of a few diagnostic tools is recommended to increase the yield of venous air embolism detection[16]. No monitor can substitute for the anaesthesiologists vigilance. A high index of suspicion is required for timely diagnosis and treatment.

Management

Venous embolism is best prevented or at least detected promptly to prevent serious morbidity.

Prevention is by careful positioning so that the lower limbs are elevated, adequate hydration to maintain vascular filling pressures and judicious use of positive end expiratory pressure.

Positive end expiratory pressure although advocated previously is currently controversial. It increases the haemodynamic disturbance while having questionable benefits in preventing air embolism.[18]

Vigilant monitoring and prompt action on suspicion of venous air embolism are of paramount importance.

Treatment is supportive

- Inform the surgeon immediately. They are expected to flood the field with saline to prevent further air entrainment.
- Give 100% oxygen. Stop the use of N2O immediately.
- Tilt further the foot end of the operating table higher than heart (Trendelenburg)
- Aspirate the right atrial catheter. This confirms the diagnosis, removes a possible airlock and reduces the cardiorespiratory consequences of intravascular air.
- Provide appropriate cardiovascular support. Treat hypotension, arrhythmias as per standard guidelines.
- Bilateral compression of jugular veins to increase the intracranial venous pressure which increase the venous bleeding from the surgical site veins hence help surgeon to identify the culprit veins and prevent further entrapment of air.
- Institute prompt CPR in case of cardiovascular collapse.
- Make the patient supine if all above measures to prevent the venous embolism fails.

Paradoxical air embolism: Entry of air in the systemic circulation is possible after venous air embolism. As already established venous air embolism increases right sided pressures. If the right atrial pressures exceed left atrial pressures in the presence of intracardiac defect such as patent foramen ovale, air bubbles may reach systemic circulation. Here they have the potential to cause myocardial/cerebral ischaemia.

The incidence of patent foramen ovale is 10%-23% on screening by transoesophageal echocardiography.[19] Although the exact incidence of paradoxical air embolism is not known it is seen to occur in the more severe of venous embolism grades.[20] So prompt treatment of venous air embolism seems like a good strategy to prevent paradoxical embolisms. The incidence of paradoxical air embolism is not as frequent as may be expected given the frequency of venous air embolism and patent foramen ovale. But given its significant complications such as potential for myocardial and cerebral ischaemia, it warrants thorough investigation.

3. **Pneumocephalus** – Entry of air into a closed cranial space is almost an inevitable consequence of intracranial surgery. It occurs due to decrease in the volume of the contents of the cranial cavity intraoperatively. Various measures undertaken to reduce the intracranial pressure such as administration of mannitol, hyperventilation, head elevation leading to CSF drainage under gravity, better venous drainage, all contribute to decreased intracranial volume.

   After dural closure when supine position is given CSF and blood reaccumulate. There is some degree of cerebral oedema postoperatively. In this situation the accumulated air behaves like a space occupying lesion. Sufficient volumes of air can produce tension pneumocephalus which is a life threatening complication.

   Clinical features include confusion, headache, convulsions, delayed awakening following anaesthesia, neurological deficit. Diagnosis requires high degree of suspicion. Early CT scan aids diagnosis.

   Treatment includes high flow oxygen and neuromonitoring in a suitable environment. Tension pneumocephalus warrants surgical intervention such as burr hole to aspirate the air.

4. **Brainstem injury** – During surgical manipulation nearby brainstem structures may get damaged due to retraction, trauma or ischaemia. More dangerous is injury to circulatory/respiratory structures. It manifests as rhythm disturbances, bradycardia, tachycardia, hypotension or hypertension. Any sudden haemodynamic changes warrant informing the surgeon to prevent further injury. Administration of drugs to alter the rate and rhythm as primary management of these disturbances must be avoided as it is an important sign of potential brainstem injury.

5. **Quadriplegia** – It is a rare complication of posterior fossa surgery. Mechanism is thought to be pressure on the spinal cord and extreme flexion of the cervical spine. Pre-existing cervical spine disorders like cervical stenosis, spondylosis further increase the risk. Severe hypotension may have a role to play by compromise of regional cord perfusion.

6. **Macroglossia** – Neck flexion decreases the anteroposterior diameter of the neck and pharynx. With simultaneous use of oral endotracheal tube,

transoesophageal probe, temperature probe and bite block there is crowding. It compromises perfusion of the soft palate, pharynx and base of the tongue. Swelling may develop due to obstruction to venous and lymphatic drainage. Post extubation, reperfusion further increases oedema. Failure to maintain a patent upper airway can lead to respiratory failure.

Strategies to reduce the risk of macroglossia include use of a small size transoesophageal echo probe, using a bite block rather than oral airway and keeping at least 2 finger breadth distance between the chin and sternum at the time of positioning to maintain the pharyngeal diameter.

Postoperative Management: Preoperative neurological status and perioperative course will decide the plans of extubation. If patient is preoperatively neurologically intact and surgery is uneventful, extubation can be done but patient should be closely monitored for neurological deterioration. Patients with mild venous air embolism can also be extubated. During extubation hypertension and coughing should be avoided to prevent haematoma formation hence proper care

should be taken for pain and PONV management. Patients with severe preoperative cranial nerves involvement, tension pneumocephalous, intracranial haemorrhage, severe venous air embolism, brain stem handling and delayed emergence should be electively ventilated.

CONCLUSION

Posterior fossa surgeries present a unique set of challenges to the anaesthetist. Majority of these are associated with surgery in sitting position. Careful positioning will help minimise the risk of complications such as cervical spinal cord injury, brainstem injury and macroglossia. Gradual changes in position will attenuate haemodynamic disturbances. The risk of venous and paradoxical air embolism must be borne in mind and use of special monitoring equipment to detect these at early stage is advisable. Considerations of the patient's preoperative and co-morbid status and the intraoperative course is essential at the time of extubation. While catastrophic complications are rare, anaesthetist's vigilance and timely intervention can change the outcome.

REFERANCES

1. Duffy C. Anaesthesia for posterior fossa surgery. In: Matta BF, Menon DK, Turner MJ, eds. Textbook of Neuroanaesthesia and Critical Care. London, Greenwich Medical Media Ltd, 2000; 269–80.

2. J. R. Sneyd, C. J. H. Andrews, T. Tsubokawa; Comparison of propofol/remifentanil and sevoflurane/remifentanil for maintenance of anaesthesia for elective intracranial surgery. *Br J Anaesth* 2005; 94 (6): 778-783.

3. Schirmer CM, Heilman CB, Bhardwaj A. Pneumocephalus: Case illustrations and review. Neurocrit Care. 2010;13:152–8.

4. Hernandez-Palazon J, de la Rosa-Carrillo VN, Tortosa JA, Martínez-Lage JF, Lopez F, Poza M. Anesthetic technique and development of pneumocephalus after posterior fossa surgery in the sitting position. Neurocirugia. 2003 Dec 31;14(3):216-21.

5. Porter JM, Pidgeon C, Cunningham AJ. The sitting position in neurosurgery: a critical appraisal. British journal of anaesthesia. 1999 Jan 1;82(1):117-28.

6. Losasso TJ, Muzzi DA, Dietz NM, Cucchiara RF. Fifty percent nitrous oxide does not increase the risk of venous air embolism in neurosurgical patients operated upon in the sitting position. Anesthesiology. 1992 Jul;77(1):21-30.

7. Orliaguet GA, Hanafi M, Meyer PG, Blanot S, Jarreau MM, Bresson D, et al. Is the sitting or the prone position best for surgery for posterior fossa tumours in children?. Pediatric Anesthesia. 2001 Sep 1;11(5):541-7.

8. Rath GP, Bithal PK, Chaturvedi A, Dash HH. Complications related to positioning in posterior fossa craniectomy. Journal of clinical neuroscience. 2007 Jun 30;14(6):520-5.

9. Cottrell JE, Patel P. Cottrell and Patel's Neuroanesthesia E-Book. Elsevier Health Sciences; 2016 Aug 24.

10. Rozet I, Vavilala MS. Risks and benefits of patient positioning during neurosurgical care. Anesthesiology clinics. 2007 Sep 30;25(3):631-53.

11. Black S, Ockert DB, Oliver Jr WC, Cucchiara RF. Outcome following posterior fossa craniectomy in patients in the sitting or horizontal positions. Anesthesiology. 1988 Jul;69(1):49-56.

12. Matjasko J, Petrozza P, Cohen M, Steinberg P. Anesthesia and surgery in the seated position: analysis of 554 cases. Neurosurgery. 1985 Nov 1;17(5):695-702.

13. Buhre W, Weyland A, Buhre K, Kazmaier S, Mursch K, Schmidt M, et al. Effects of the sitting position on the distribution of blood volume in patients undergoing neurosurgical procedures. British journal of anaesthesia. 2000 Mar 1;84(3):354-7.

14. Papadopoulos G, Kuhly P, Brock M, Rudolph KH, Link J, Eyrich K. Venous and paradoxical air embolism in the sitting position. A prospective study with transoesophageal echocardiography. Acta neurochirurgica. 1994 Jun 1;126(2):140-3.

15. Toung TJ, Rossberg MI, Hutchins GM. Volume of air in a lethal venous air embolism. Anesthesiology: The Journal of the American Society of Anesthesiologists. 2001 Feb 1;94(2):360-1.

16. Mirski MA, Lele AV, Fitzsimmons L, Toung TJ. Diagnosis and treatment of vascular air embolism. Anesthesiology: The Journal of the American Society of Anesthesiologists. 2007 Jan 1;106(1):164-77.

17. Matjasko J, Petrozza P, Mackenzie CF. Sensitivity of end-tidal nitrogen in venous air embolism detection in dogs. Anesthesiology. 1985 Oct;63(4):418-23.

18. Giebler R, Kollenberg B, Pohlen G, Peters J. Effect of positive end-expiratory pressure on the incidence of venous air embolism and on the cardiovascular response to the sitting position during neurosurgery. British journal of anaesthesia. 1998 Jan 1;80(1):30-5.

19. Guggiari M, Garen-Colonne C, Fusciardi J, Viars P. Early detection of patent foramen ovale by two-dimensional contrast echocardiography for prevention of paradoxical air embolism during sitting position. Anesthesia & Analgesia. 1988 Feb 1;67(2):192-4.

20. Mammoto T, Hayashi Y, Ohnishi Y, Kuro M. Incidence of venous and paradoxical air embolism in neurosurgical patients in the sitting position: detection by transesophageal echocardiography. Acta anaesthesiologica scandinavica. 1998 Jul 1;42(6):643-7.

MULTIPLE CHOICE QUESTIONS

1) **Which of the following is not a content of the posterior cranial fossa?**
   a. Pons
   b. Sigmoid sinus
   c. Tentorium cerebelli
   d. Aqueduct of Sylvius

2) **Commonest indication for securing airway in preoperative period for patients with posterior fossa pathology is**
   a. Raised intracranial pressure
   b. Ataxia
   c. Visual disturbances
   d. Bulbar symptoms

3) **Adult lethal volume of air in case of venous air embolism is**
   a. 50 ml
   b. 75 ml
   c. 100 ml
   d. 300 ml

4) **The morbidity and mortality following venous air embolism depends upon all the following except**
   a. Depth of anaesthesia
   b. Rate of entrainment
   c. Volume of air
   d. Body size

5) **Which of the following is the most sensitive modality for detecting venous air embolism?**
   a. Precordial Doppler
   b. PA catheter
   c. Transthoracic echocardiography
   d. Transoesophageal echocardiography

6) **First line of treatment for post craniotomy pneumocephalus is**
   a. Administration of mannitol
   b. Burr hole
   c. Hyperventilation and anticonvulsants
   d. High flow O_2 and neuromonitoring

7) **Which of the following is an absolute contraindication for sitting position craniotomy?**
   a. Severe cervical canal stenosis
   b. Cerebral ischaemia in an awake and upright patient
   c. Autonomic neuropathy
   d. Patent foramen ovale

8) **Sign of venous air embolism is**
   a. Sudden decrease in $EtCO2$
   b. Sudden decrease in $EtN2$
   c. LV strain pattern
   d. All of the above

9) **Which of the following is not a treatment modality in case of venous air embolism?**
   a. Flood the field with saline
   b. Expedite the surgery
   c. Use vasopressors
   d. Bilateral jugular venous compression

10) **Caution should be exercised while extubating posterior fossa craniotomy patients immediately post surgery in case of**
   a. Mild venous air embolism
   b. Preoperative low GCS
   c. Intraoperative blood transfusion
   d. All of the above

CHAPTER 6

ANAESTHESIA FOR PITUITARY SURGERIES

Madhavi Desai, Amol Kothekar

Introduction

Pituitary is a master endocrine gland. A multidisciplinary teamwork of an endocrinologist, anaesthesiologist, neurosurgeon, and intensivist during the peri-operative period is required for successful outcome of pituitary surgeries.

Functional Anatomy[1]

Pituitary weighs approximately 500-900 mg and measures 15 x 10 x 5 mm in size. The anterior pituitary lobe (adenohypophysis) is glandular, and forms 2/3rd of the gland. Developmentally, it originates from Rathke's pouch from oral-ectoderm. Posterior lobe (neurohypophysis) develops from neural crest cells of the neural ectoderm. Functionally, anterior and posterior lobes are two separate units secreting different hormones, and having different feedbacks. Adenohypophysis synthesizes Growth hormone (GH), Prolactin, Thyroid stimulating hormone (TSH), Follicle stimulating Hormone (FSH), Leuitinizing hormone(LH), Adrenocorticotropic stimulating Hormone (ACTH) and β-endorphin. The posterior pituitary itself does not synthesize any hormones. It has the axonal terminals of neurons of hypothalamus which store and release oxytocin and vasopressin/antidiuretic hormone (ADH) directly into the systemic vasculature. These hormones are synthesized in the paraventricular and supraoptic nuclei of the hypothalamus. The anterior and posterior pituitary lobes receive blood supply from bilateral superior hypophyseal and inferior hypophyseal arteries respectively; both being the terminal branches of anterior carotid arteries. The venous drainage of the pituitary is via hypophyseal portal veins into the cavernous sinus.

Surgical anatomy[1,2]

The pituitary gland is situated within saddle shaped sella turcica of the sphenoid bone and is enveloped by dura. Superiorly it is covered by the diaphragm sellae, which is a fold of dura mater that separates subarachnoid space from the pituitary. The infundibulum passes through the diaphragm sellae and connects the hypothalamus to pituitary. The pituitary fossa is limited posteriorly by the clivus of the sphenoid, and anteriorly and inferiorly by the sphenoidal air sinuses. Third ventricle, hypothalamus and optic chiasm lie superiorly to pituitary; whereas cranial nerves III, IV, V,and VI, cavernous sinus and the internal carotid arteries are lateral to it. The optic chiasm is 2-5mm from pituitary. Internal carotid arteries are at a distance of 3-7 mm from the pituitary (Fig. 1).

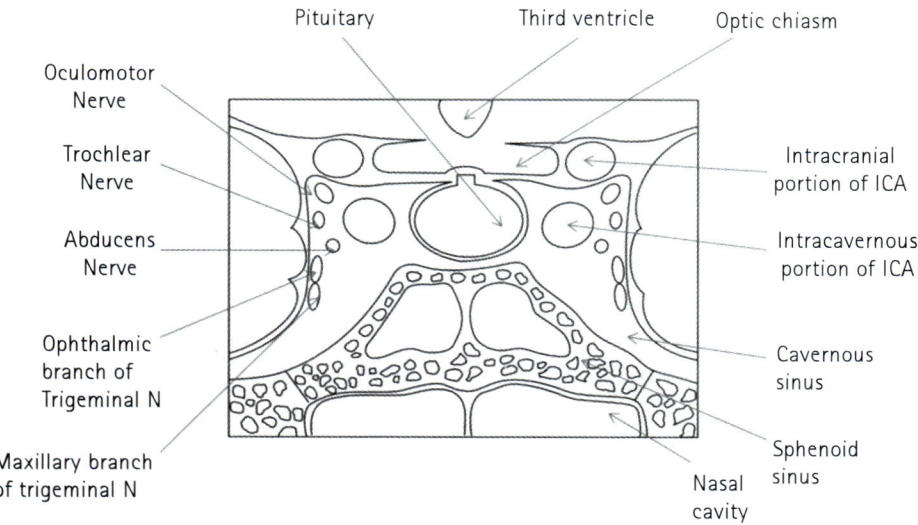

Fig. 1 : Surgical anatomy of pituitary gland

Sellar, parasellar lesions

- Pituitary Tumours : About 10% of all primary brain tumors are pituitary tumours[1,3]. While most of the tumours originate from adenohypophysis; tumours of neurohypophysis are rare.

  Pituitary adenomas could be either secreting or nonsecreting tumours. Depending upon their size, they are classified as macroadenomas (> 1 cm) or microadenomas (< 1 cm).

  Secreting tumours are Prolactinomas, Growth Hormone secreting tumours, ACTH secreting tumours, and rarely TSH secreting tumour. Clinical features are related to the secretion of hormones. Macroadenomas may exhibit features of mass effect as well. (explained later in the text).

  Nonfunctional (null cell) tumours account for 20% pituitary tumours: These tumours do not secrete hormones. Symptoms are either due to mass effect or due to panhypopituitarism following the compression of the gland.

- Pituitary Apoplexy: It is an abrupt and occasionally catastrophic occurrence of acute hemorrhagic infarction of the pituitary gland resulting in panhypopituitarism. This is an endocrine and neurosurgical emergency which is treated with intravenous fluids and hydrocortisone replacement, and urgent decompression.

- Rathke'scleft /cyst: Rathke's pouch is the place where the anterior and posterior lobes meet. It closes early in fetal development, but a remnant often persists as a cleft. Occasionally, this remnant gives rise to a large cyst called the Rathke's cleft cyst.

- Craniopharyngioma: 1-5% of primary brain tumours are craniopharyngiomas, observed in children between ages of 10-14 years or in adults in 50s. They are relatively benign (WHO grade I) neoplasms that typically arise from Rathke's cleft anywhere along the infundibulum from the floor of the third ventricle to the pituitary gland.

Presenting symptoms: Pituitary lesions may have varied presentation[1]

- Mass effect: headache, hemianopia with compression of optic chiasm, and raised intracranial pressure if third ventricle is compressed leading to hydrocephalus.

- Hormonal hypersecretions: Cushing's disease, Acromegaly.

- Hormonal hyposecretions: due to pituitary apoplexy and pituitary infarction.

- Few may have nonspecific presentation.

- Asymptomatic: 10-12% of Pituitary adenomas are picked up as an incidental finding during MRI brain performed for some other reason. They are known as Incidentalomas.

Hormone hypersecretion syndromes : Among these most relevant for perioperative anaesthesia concerns are briefly described here:

- Hypersecretion of GH[1,4,5]: Manifests clinically as changes in physical characteristics (bone and soft tissues) and its systemic effects (cardiovascular, respiratory and endocrine).

  - Physical manifestations: Bony proliferation lead to prognathism, malocclusion of teeth. Soft tissues changes are thickening of skin, hands, palms and feet causing carpal tunnel syndrome, thickening of the pharyngeal and laryngeal tissues causing obstructive sleep apnoea (OSA), hypertrophy of the peri-epiglottic region, calcinosis of the larynx leading to narrowing of the glottic opening, injury to the recurrent laryngeal nerve resulting in hoarseness of voice. OSA is observed in 70% of the acromegalic patients.

  - Endocrine manifestations: Diabetes mellitus and adrenocorticotrophic hypersecretion. It could be a component of Multiple endocrine neoplasia type 1 (MEN1) involving neoplasm of the parathyroid gland, islet cells of the pancreas, and pituitary gland. Patients with MEN I may present with hypercalcaemia.

  - Cardiovascular manifestations:

  i) Hypertension is seen in almost 40% of patients

  ii) Left Ventricular Hypertrophy (LVH) is observed is observed in normotensive as well as hypertensive acromegalics

  iii) Cardiomyopathy with poorly compliant left ventricle and diastolic dysfunction may develop due to interstitial myocardial fibrosis. This ventricle needs higher ventricular filling pressures. The ventricular dysfunction may not return to normal after treatment of pituitary.

  iv) Right ventricular dysfunction secondary to pulmonary hypertension due to long standing OSA

  v) Supraventricular and ventricular arrhythmias due to interstitial myocardial fibrosis[6]

  - Respiratory manifestations: Upper airway obstruction, OSA, Lung proliferation leading to bronchiectasis

- ACTH secreting adenomas[4,5]

  - Cardiovascular manifestations:

  i) Hypertension is seen in almost 50% of patients - due to increased endogenous corticosteroids causing increased cardiac output, hepatic angiotensinogen and angiotensin II receptor. Increased renin-angiotensin activity increases circulating plasma volume.

   ii) LVH with strain pattern-LVH may revert within 1 year after treatment of adenoma.

- Respiratory manifestations: 33% patients have OSA, 18% patients have severe OSA.
- Obesity related: truncal obesity, gastroesophageal reflux
- Diabetes mellitus in 60%
- Other: Osteoporosis in 40% patients, Myopathy, skin fragility

- TSH secreting pituitary tumours causing hyperthyroidism are rare

Preoperative Evaluation

- *General:* Hemoglobin, renal function test, electrolytes, glucose, serum calcium
- *Neurological:* Symptoms and signs of raised ICP, Optimetry for bitemporal hemianopia
- *Cardiovascular:* BP, ECG may show LVH, arrhythmias secondary to interstitial myocardial fibrosis[6]. Dobutamine stress test is in relevant in cases especially having ST- T changes in a presence of diabetes mellitus. few authors recommend 2D-ECHO for all patients of pituitary adenomas to investigate for diastolic dysfunction and for prognostication of cardiomyopathy [3, 4]
- *Respiratory:* Clinical evaluation of upper airway for obstruction, sleep apnoea. X-ray chest
- *Endocrine:* thyroid panel, plasma cortisol, ACTH, IGF[1], testosterone, FSH, and prolactin. Patient may have amenorrhea due to hypersecretion of FSH. It is good practice to rule out pregnancy before elective surgery. Females presenting with amenorrhea should undergo pregnancy test.
- *Airway:* Difficult airway may be encountered even in patients with Mallampati I and II because of macroglossia and thickening of pharyngeal and laryngeal tissues. Indirect laryngoscopy is indicated in a patient with hoarseness of voice to rule out involvement of recurrent laryngeal nerve.

Preoperative preparation

Preoperative steroids[4] : Should be administered with endocrinologist's concordance.

- Routine hydrocortisone therapy for all patients is not necessary.

- Patients with panhypopituitarism may not have effective oral absorption. Therefore, they are supplemented with intravenous hydrocortisone.
- Patients with Cushing's are given preoperative dexamethasone instead of hydrocortisone because it does not interfere with postoperative serum cortisol levels. Alternatively, steroid are avoided in preoperative period, and hydrocortisone is started postoperatively, either when patient is symptomatic for adrenal insufficiency or based on postoperative serum cortisol levels.

- **Antibiotic prophylaxis:** Trans-nasal Pituitary surgery is considered a clean-contaminated wound. Currently there are no evidence-based guidelines regarding prophylactic antibiotics. Commonly cephalosporins are given for 24 hours or less.[7]

- Blood sugar management with intravenous insulin.

- **Inform patient regarding postop nasal packing** and need of mouth breathing in immediate postop period.

Surgical approach[1,3]

- *Transcranial sub-frontal approach:* This is preferred for giant or invasive suprasellar lesions, and for small children for the lesions where transphenoid exposure would be inadequate. It involves standard risks associated with craniotomy e.g bleeding, ischaemia of frontal lobes with bifrontal retraction.

- *Microscopic trans-septal trans-sphenoidal approach:* using a sublabial trans-septal approach. This was the gold standard till 1990s.

- *Endoscopic transnasal transphenoidal approach:* presently 95% of the pituitary surgeries are performed using this approach[8] in view of more cosmetic, lower hospital stay and lower incidence of diabetes insipidus (DI). However, recent meta analysis has shown no difference in the incidence of CSF leak, visual complications, meningitis, hypopituitarism, DI or cranial nerve injury with the endoscopic approach as compared with microscopic sublabial approach[9].

Position is supine with head fixed on pins to give 'cock robin' position. The head is turned to the patient's right with the bridge of the nose parallel to the floor. Endoscopic endonasal incision is created on the anterior wall of the sphenoid sinus. Sphenoid bone is fractured to provide entry into the sphenoid sinus. The sellar floor is then penetrated, and a durotomy is performed to visualize the sellar region.

Intraoperative anaesthesia management

- *Objectives of anaesthesia:*

  - Avoid sudden inadvertent movements of the patient whose head is clamped on Mayfieldclamps. Also, such movements are not desirable and in view of surgery in vicinity of major intracranial vascular structures (ICA, cavernous sinus)

  - Fast track recovery from anaesthetics for

    i) Safe extubation in presence of pre-existing difficult airway

    ii) Early postoperative neurological assessment.

- Good surgical field ensuring haemodynamic stability of the patient

- Wide bore intravenous access and long extension tubings for drug administration as this is a "long distance anaesthesia". Anaesthesia workstation is at the foot end of the patient.

- Preparation of nose for transphenoidal approach: Xylometazoline nasal drops 10-15 min before induction of anesthesia and infiltration of nasal mucosa of with saline/2% lignocaine with adrenaline (1 in 200,000) just before starting surgery. Hypertensive response is frequently observed during nasal preparation[5]. This response may be exaggerated in patients with Cushing's disease[4,5].

- *Induction:*

  Preoxygenation and apnoic oxygenation during conduct of intubation.

  Fentanyl or remifentanil are opioids of choice to avoid opioid induced respiratory depression in postoperative period.

  Propofol is preferred over thiopentone for fast track recovery. Succinylcholine may be indicated in view of difficult intubations.

- *Airway concerns at Induction:*

  - *Mask ventilation:* Can be difficult in Acromegalic patients because of macroglossia and, thick pharyngeal soft tissues. Patient may require oral airway. Important to note that LMA insertion and placement also could be difficult in them. Compared with acromeaglic, patients with Cushings may not have difficult mask ventilation.

  - Mallampati and Modified Mallampati have poor prediction of difficult intubation in acromegalics. Video laryngoscopes may have good role.

  - Awake fiberoptic intubation is indicated in patients with anticipated difficult mask ventilation and difficult intubation.

- *Maintenance:* Oxygen + Air/Nitrous oxide with or without inhalational agents. Desflurane and sevoflurane are preferred in view of desired rapid emergence. Propofol infusion in sedation dose 25-50 mic/kg/min or dexmedetomidine infusion 0.2-0.5 mic/kg/hr controls the hypertensive response during nasal endoscopy and sphenoid fracture. These are good choice for early recovery from anaesthesia for extubation.

- The use of propofol and/or dexmedetomidine has reduced the use of nitroglycerine or sodium nitroprusside in pituitary surgeries. Blood pressure reduction should not be more than 20% from the baseline mean arterial pressures (MAP) to prevent the secondary ischaemic insult to brain and hypoperfusion of the vital organs.

  Maintain deep anaesthesia and neuromuscular blockade (NMB) to prevent inadvertent movement of the patient. Titrate NMB using Train of four monitoring to ensure adequate NM recovery at extubation at TOF ratio > 0.9.

- *Monitoring:* ECG, $EtCO_2$, Pulseoximetry, Temperature, Urine output and intraoperative Serum sodium. Patient with extensive resection of pituitary stalk may develop DI on table.

  Invasive blood pressure monitoring is mandatory. Allen's test should be performed prior to radial artery cannulation in view of high incidence of associated carpel tunnel syndrome especially in acormealy.

- Sphenoid bone fracture is performed to get access to pituitary. It is a is a painful stimulus and triggers severe sympathetic response. This can be attenuated by dexmedetomidine infusion or propofol bolus.

- *Complications:* Vascular damage, cranial nerve injury, cerebral ischaemia, and stroke as aresult of vasospasm. ICA injury is a catastrophic complication as controlling bleeding endoscopically is very difficult. In event of ICA injury, initially attempts are made to control bleeding by tamponed followed by cerebral angiography in radiology suite. Aggressive volume resuscitation by intravenous fluids and blood and blood products is essential to maintain haemodynamic stability and sustain intra-operative shifting for intervention procedure.

- *Emergence from anaesthesia:* Ensure smooth emergence from anaesthesia to prevent formation of haematoma in the surgical bed as well as to prevent dislodgement of the fat graft. Vigorous coughing could predispose the patient to Cerebro spinal fluid leak. Prevent hypertension and coughing or 'bucking' on the endotracheal tube[10].

53

- *Airway concerns at extubation:* Nasal packing, H/O difficult intubation, patient with OSA, obesity makes it difficult extubation. Nasal airway cannot be inserted. Continuous positive airway pressure (CPAP) should be avoided postoperatively to avoid potential graft dislodgment. These patients have some blood trickling in oral cavity in postoperative period. Fast track recovery from opioids and NMB is mandatory to ensure good cough reflex, to avoid postoperative respiratory depression, to prevent aspiration of blood, tongue fall and airway obstruction.

- *Postoperative analgesia:* Nonopioid analgesics are the choice to avoid opiod induced respiratory depression because patient may have postoperative nasal blood trickle in transphenoid approach. Also they may have sleep apnoea. Postoperatively, 24 hrs ICU monitoring is needed. Fentanyl-Patient-controlled analgesia (PCA) in monitored environment like ICU can be used.

Postoperative management

Patients require careful monitoring for potential neurologic or ophthalmologic deterioration.

Complications

Serious complications are relatively uncommon with experienced neurosurgical team[11]

- Endocrine related complications:

  Abnormalities of antidiuretic hormone (ADH) secretion

  - Diabetes Insipidus (DI)

  - Syndrome of inappropriate ADH secretion (SIADH)

- Endocrine related complications:

  - Visual loss/other cranial neuropathies

  - CSF leakage/meningitis

  - Stroke or other neurologic abnormalities

Incidence of meningitis, diabetes insipidus, cerebrospinal fluid leak, epistaxis or hypopituitarism is not significantly different between endoscopic and microscopic approach[12].

Abnormalities of ADH and Electrolyte imbalance

- Postoperative course is known to be variable due to unpredictable response to ADH[13]. Immediate postoperative DI is the most common finding seen in 31% of and prolonged DI in 10% of patients followed by Delayed hyponatraemia (SIADH) in 2.4%, biphasic response of DI followed by SIADH in 3.4% and triphasic pattern of DI-SIADH-DI in 1.1% of patients. Some patients (2.6%) have immediate postoperative SIADH without DI. Unfortunately, there is no way to predict the pattern prospectively. Therefore, frequent monitoring of sodium levels and serum and urine osmolarity is very important.

- **Diabetes Insipidus**

  Hallmark of DI is failure of kidneys to conserve water in face of increasing serum osmolarity.

  Patients can initially develop DI in the first 24 to 48 hours followed by transient SIADH developing 4 to 10 days postoperatively, followed by the return of DI in a matter of weeks.

  When DI returns as the third phase, this disturbance can be permanent. Fortunately, permanent DI occurs in only approximately 2% of patients.

  Permanent DI occurs when there is loss of 80% or more of the posterior pituitary neurons. The closer the surgical injury is to the hypothalamus, the more likely neuronal degeneration and cell death will arise[14].

Diagnostic criteria of DI[14]

Polyuria is hallmark of DI. In the literature different authors have described different thresholds of elevated urine output. Commonly used cutoff are > 250-500 ml/h (or > 4ml/kg/hour in children) for 2-3 consecutive hours or 2.5-18L/day. Other causes of polyuria like hyperglycemia, diuretic administration (including mannitol) and postoperative mobilization of excess fluid from the soft tissues in acromegalic patients should be excluded before treatment of DI is initiated.

Following laboratory parameters in presence of polyurea suggest diagnosis of DI, 1) hypernatrenmia, and 2) inability of kidneys to conserve water indicated by very low urinary specific gravity and low Urine osmolality in presence of increasing serum osmolality.

Parameters suggesting DI

- Urine output > 250-500 ml/h for 2-3 consecutive hours

- Urine specific gravity < 1.005

- Urine osmolality < 300 mOsm/kg and serum osmolality > 300 mOsm/kg

- Serum sodium > 140-145 mEq/L

Treatment of postoperative DI[14]: Aims at restoration of osmotic equilibrium and it should be individualized for every patient. Large fluctuations in sodium level should be avoided. Rapid rise of sodium level risks patient to irreversible brain damage due to osmotic demyelination syndromes like central pontine and extra pontine myelinolysis. Rapid fall of sodium level risks patient to cerebral edema and worsening of neurologic status.

- *Free water:* Patient is encouraged to drink water. In an awake patient with intact thirst mechanism, patient generally consumes a sufficient amount of water to maintain normal serum sodium and osmolality and no other treatment required especially when DI is transient.

- *Desmopressin:* It is synthetic analog of Arginine Vasopressin (AVP). It offers prolonged antidiuretic action with minimal vasopressor activity. Even though its plasma half-life is just about 3 hours, its antidiuretic effects can last up to 10 hours.

  - It is indicated if the polyuric patient with rise in serum sodium and osmolality if patient is unable to drink an adequate amount of fluids. Other causes of polyuria like hyperglycemia, or diuretic administration should be excluded before administration of desmopresin as it can cause severe and prolonged hyponatramia in absence of DI.

  - Route of Administration: orally, intranasally, subcutaneously, or intravenously. Intranasal desmopressin should be avoided in cases where nasal packing is placed during surgery.

  - Dose:

    - Oral: 100-800 mcg in two or three divided doses

    - Intranasal (10 mcg per spray): up to 40 mcg in two doses.

    - Intravenous: 2-4 mcg in two divided doses per day.

  - After administration of desmopressin and normalization of urine output, further free water administration should be done carefully to avoid rapid and severe hyponatremia.

- *Other Drugs.* Carbamazepine and chlorpropamide increase the sensitivity of renal collecting ducts to circulating AVP and potentiate its action. Thiazide diuretics crease sodium, and water absorption in the proximal tubules[15].

Non-endocrine related Complications

- Postoperative hematoma at surgical site[16]: It is rare but potentially lethal complication, typically seen within 24-48 hours of surgery. Reported incidence is 6-10%, and is often associated with headache, diplopia, visual loss, and also cerebrospinal fluid (CSF) leak. Small hematomas at operative site are more common and generally have no clinical manifestations. Large hematomas interfere with pituitary function by creating a mass effect and can also cause cranial nerve palsies, headaches and visual disturbances. Large hematomas with pituitary gland dysfunction is associated with acute onset of hypopituitarism characterized by a drastic reduction in the secretion of ACTH and ACTH-dependent steroids and simultaneous rise in serum prolactin levels.

  Treatment: Small hematomas generally require only observation. Hematomas with acute onset of hypopituitarism can be managed conservatively with immediate intravenous glucocorticoid administration. Recovery of pituitary function occurs in most of patients within 24 hours. Approximately one in six patients ultimately needs re-exploration for non-resolution of symptoms in 48 hours[17]. Very severe hematomas may require reintubation and mechanical ventilation and are associated with serious morbidity and mortality if not managed in timely.

- *Postoperative Visual loss.* Vision loss can occur due to various mechanisms like direct injury or devascularization of the optic apparatus, fracture of the orbit, postoperative hematoma, cerebral vasospasm, and prolapse of the optic chiasm into an empty sella. Incidence is 0.5% to 2.4%. The incidence is highest in apoplexy and lowest in prolactinoma patient[16]. Presence of a pituitary macroadenoma, previous visual impairment, a "bottleneck" or dumbbell-shaped tumor, previous surgery and/or radiation therapy, use of a lumbar subarachnoid catheter during operation are known to increase the risk of visual complications. Treatment is immediate glucocorticoid administration and early re-exploration may help in visual loss due to postoperative hematoma.

- Other neurologic abnormalities:

  1) Cranial neuropathies,

  2) Stroke due to Vasospasm, or cerebral ischaemia

- *CSF leakage and Meningitis:* Incidence of post-operative CSF leak after trans-sphenoidal surgery varies from 0.5 to 15% in various series. Large or recurrent adenomas, suprasellar extension, previous radiation, inexperienced surgeon, presence of preoperative leak and aggressive resection of the layer of the tumor adherent to the diaphragm sella increase incidence of intra-operative leak[18]. Macroadenomas particularly with suprasellar extension have four times higher incidence of postoperative CSF leak, than microadenomas. Coughing and bucking of patient during emergence of anesthesia can contribute to postoperative continuation of leak[3,10].

- *Management of post trans-sphenoid pituitary surgery CSF leak:* Use of external lumbar drain in postoperative persistence of CSF leak is controversial. Lumbar drain diverts CSF flow away from the sellar defect allowing healing of the reconstructed skull-base reducing the likelihood of recurrent CSF fistula. Some authors recommend conservative approach with trial of lumbar drainage for three or more days. Few authors prefer addressing the route cause and feel that immediate re-exploration with repacking is easier and more efficacious treatment.

The use of preoperative lumbar drain increases the risk of the intraoperative leak and probably delays recognition of the CSF leak.

Evidence supporting use of Lumbar drainage (LD) for treating CSF leaks is lacking.

Problems associated with lumbar drains:

- Headache and discomfort.

- Occasionally LD catheter can get fractured during removal especially in difficult placement requiring multiple punctures. Patient needs to be monitored for neurological deficit and informed regarding the fractured LD catheter, and managed conservatively in absence of pain or neurological deficits.

- Accidental over drainage. Considering normal adult CSF production of approximately 20 ml/h, some authors recommend limiting the rate of drainage to 5-10 ml/hour. Requirement of frequent opening and closing drain to control hourly drainage has potential of causing error. Over drainage with head elevation has potential of creating negative pressure gradient siphoning air into the intracranial space through the fistula. This may lead to pneumocephalus, subdural hemorrhage, neurological decline, or uncal herniation. Choice between re-exploration with repacking and Lumbar drainage is based on individual preference and practice varies from center to center.

Patients with CSF leak commonly receive prophylactic third-generation cephalosporin till nasal pack is removed to prevent meningitis however; there is no robust evidence to support this practice[19].

- *Hydrocephalus.* Preoperatively hydrocephalus occurs due to suprasellar extension of tumor leading to obstruction of third ventricle. Post-opetatively, intraventricular bleeding can cause hydrocephalus in early course and meningitis in later course.

CONCLUSION

Pituitary surgeries demand simultaneous intraoperative management of neuroanaesthesia and endocrine management. A good perioperative teamwork of endocrinologist, neurosurgeons, anaesthesiologist and intensivist is mandatory for a good outcome.

REFERENCES

1. Bithal PK. Neuroendocrine Lesions. Essentials of neuroanaesthesia 1st edition, Himanshu Prabhakar. Elsevier 2017: 376-89. ISBN: 978-0-12-805299-0.

2. Menon R, Murphy PG, LindleAM. Anaesthesia and pituitary disease. Continuing Education in Anaesthesia, Critical Care & Pain. 2011;11(4):133-37.

3. Abraham M. Perioperative management of patients with pituitary tumors. J Neuroanaesthesiol Crit Care 2016; 3:211-8.

4. Nemergut EC, Dumont A S, Barry UT, Laws E R. Perioperative Management of Patients Undergoing Trans sphenoidal Pituitary Surgery. Anesth Analg 2005; 101:1170 –81.

5. Bajwa SS, Bajwa SK. Anesthesia and Intensive care implications for pituitary surgery: Recent trends and advancements. Indian J Endocr Metab 2011; 15:224-32.

6. Herrmann BL, Bruch C, Saller B, Bartel T, Ferdin S, Erbel R, et al. Acromegaly: Evidence for a direct relation between diseaseactivity and cardiac dysfunction in patients without ventricular hypertrophy. Clin Endocrinol (Oxf) 2002; 56:595602.

7. Little AS, White WL. Prophylactic antibiotic trends in trans sphenoidal surgery for pituitary lesions. Pituitary. 2010;14(2):99-104.

8. Zada G, Du R, Laws ER Jr. Defining the "edge of the envelope": patient selection in treating complex Sella based neoplasms via trans sphenoidal versus open craniotomy Neurosurg. 2011; 114:286-300.

9. Ammirati M, Wei L, Ciric I. Short term outcome of endoscopic versus microscopic pituitary adenoma surgery: a systematic review and meta-analysis. J Neurol Neurosurg Psychiatr 2013; 84:843–9.

10. Anesthetic Considerations in Endoscopic Skull Base Surgeryhttp://www.springer.com/978-1-58829-814-0.

11. Woodmansee WW, Carmichael J, Kelly D, Katznelson L. American Association of Clinical Endocrinologists and American College of Endocrinology Disease State Clinical Review: Postoperative Management Following Pituitary Surgery. Endocrine Practice. 2015;21(7):832–8.

12. Gao Y, ZhongC, Wang Y, Xu S, Guo Y, Dai C, et al. Endoscopic versus microscopic trans sphenoidal pituitary adenoma surgery: a meta-analysis. World Journal of Surgical Oncology 2014, 12:94.

13. Hensen J, Henig A, Fahlbusch R et al. Prevalence, predictors and patterns of postoperative polyuria and hyponatremia in the immediate course after trans sphenoidal surgery for pituitary adenomas. Clin Endocrinol (Oxf) 1999; 50: 431–439.

14. Schreckinger M, Szerlip N, Mittal S. Diabetes insipidus following resection of pituitary tumors. Clinical Neurology and Neurosurgery. 2013;115(2):121–6.

15. Loffing J. Paradoxical Antidiuretic Effect of Thiazides in Diabetes Insipidus: Another Piece in the Puzzle. Journal of the American Society of Nephrology. 2004Jan;15(11):2948–50.

16. Chowdhury T, Prabhakar H, Bithal P, Schaller B, Dash H. Immediate postoperative complications in trans sphenoidal pituitary surgery: A prospective study. Saudi Journal of Anaesthesia. 2014;8(3):335.

17. El-Asmar N, El-Sibai K, Al-Aridi R, Selman WR, Arafah BM. Postoperative sellar hematoma after pituitary surgery: clinical and biochemical characteristics. European Journal of Endocrinology. 2016May;174(5):573–82.

18. Mansy A, Kersh A, Eissa E. Role of the External Lumbar Drain in Management of CSFLeak during or after Trans sphenoidalSurgery. Egypt J Neurol Psychiat Neurosurg2010;47(1):483-88.

19. Hadad G, Bassagasteguy L, Carrau RL, Mataza JC, Kassam A, Snyderman CH, et al. A Novel Reconstructive Technique After Endoscopic Expanded Endonasal Approaches: Vascular Pedicle Nasoseptal Flap. The Laryngoscope. 2006;116(10):1882–6.

MULTIPLE CHOICE QUESTIONS

1. **Which of the following is not a diagnostic criteria of DI**
   a. Urine output >250-500 ml/h for 2-3 consecutive hours
   b. Urine specific gravity >1.005
   c. serum osmolality >300 mOsm/kg
   d. Serum sodium >140-145 mEq/L

2. **Which of the following is correct dose of desmopresin**
   a. Oral 10 to 80 mcg
   b. Intranasal 2 mcg to 8 mcg
   c. Intravenous 2-4 mcg
   d. Oral 1 mg to 8 mg

3. **Triphasic pattern of DI- SIADH-DI is seen in _____ % of patients**
   a. Less than 2%
   b. More than 80%
   c. 10-20%
   d. 30-60%

4. **Which of the following is true regarding pituitary?**
   a. Posterior pituitary synthesizes oxytocin
   b. Anterior pituitary develops from neural crest cells
   c. Anterior lobe forms 30% of the pituitary
   d. Posterior pituitary develops from neural crest cells

5. **Which of the following statement regarding neurosurgical anatomy isnot correct?**
   a. Third ventricle is superior to pituitary
   b. Sphenoid bone is anterior to pituitary
   c. Internal carotid is at a distance of 2 cm from pituitary
   d. 3rd cranial nerve is lateral to pituitary

6. **Which of the following clinical manifestations can be seen in Acromegalic patient?**
   a. Recurrent laryngeal Nerve dysfunction
   b. Carpel tunnel syndrome
   c. Concentric LVH with diastolic dysfunction
   d. All of the above

7. **Which of the following statement regarding the Cushing's syndrome is not correct?**
   a. Patients may have myopathy
   b. LVH can be reversible if the pituitary lesion is treated
   c. Preoperative hydrocortisone administration affects postop serum cortisol assay
   d. Preoperative dexamethasone administration affects postop serum cortisol assay

8. **Which of the following statements regarding airway are true in Acromegaly patient?**
   a. Vocal cord palsy may be present preoperatively
   b. Mallampati score does not predict the difficulty in intubation
   c. Restrictive lung disease is the main feature
   d. All of the above

9. **Which surgical step is not a part of Transphenoidal endoscopic pituitary resection?**
   a. Durotomy
   b. Nasal Septal puncture
   c. Fracture of sphenoid bone
   d. Sublabial incision

10. **Which of the following statements are true regarding postoperative CSF leak after pituitary surgeries?**
    a. Lumbar drain is the gold standard therapy for this complication
    b. Uncle herniation is a possible complication
    c. Stormy emergence increases the possibility of postop CSF rhinorrhea
    d. All of the above

AWAKE CRANIOTOMY

Varun Jain, Falguni Shah

Introduction

Awake craniotomy, as the name suggests, are those neurosurgical procedures which are done while the patient is awake and alert. The reason for such complex and difficult surgeries to be carried out in awake state is because a conscious, oriented patient offers the advantage of helping in intraoperative neurological assessment which an otherwise sedated or anaesthetized patient will not be able to, thus optimizing the extent of successful resection.[1] Successful and smooth conduct of the procedure requires a good understanding and rapport between the patient and neuro-operative team, and attentive and involved neuroanaesthesiologist who knows the anticipated problems and their management.

Indications:

1. Deep Brain Stimulation surgery (DBS)

This is one of the fastest growing indication for awake craniotomy.[1] Idiopathic essential tremors, Parkinson's disease and primary dystonia are the common pathologies amenable to treatment by deep brain stimulation in refractory cases and all are FDA approved.

DBS implantation is a two-stage procedure. During the first stage, while the patient is awake, micro electrodes are placed at the desired intracerebral nuclei, e.g. subthalamic nuclei (STN), Globus pallidus internus (GPi) where maximal functional improvement is observed. This is followed by battery placement and tunnelling its connection to the microelectrodes under general anaesthesia.

2. Epilepsy surgery

Approximately 0.8-1.7% of world's population has epilepsy.[2] 30-40% of these people have epilepsy despite maximal medical treatment and may benefit from surgical resection of epileptic foci. Those foci near the eloquent cortex need intraoperative brain mapping or electrophysiological monitoring (such as electrocorticography) to achieve maximal resection while avoiding any permanent deficit. In general,

anaesthetic agents abolish the epileptic spikes and therefore an awake patient is preferred for such monitoring.

The procedure is usually preferred to be done in two stages although can be done in one stage. During the first stage subdural grid electrodes are placed under general anaesthesia and patient is latter monitored for few days to exactly localize the seizure focus. This is followed by second surgery to remove the grid electrodes and resect the seizure foci. The second procedure is usually performed while patient is awake and unlike DBS surgery which can be done with small burrholes, epilepsy surgery needs larger craniotomies.

3. For Tumours / Lesions near Eloquent Cortex

The eloquent cortex is one which has primary motor (pre-central gyri), sensory, memory, vision or speech (Broca's area in frontal lobe, Wernike's area in temporal lobe) centre located at it. Because of wide inter individual variability of eloquent cortex thorough precision is needed when removing a space-occupying lesion in these locations, so that maximum resection with minimal post-operative deficit is possible. Besides, cerebral cortex topography may itself be altered because of radiotherapy, or previous surgeries.

Intraoperatively, surgeon first stimulates the desired area to be resected and corresponding response is noted by a neuroanaesthesiologist, neurologist or neurophysiologist. In case of any abnormal motor or sensory response, further resection is averted.

4. To Enhance Perioperative Recovery

The length of ICU / hospital stay can be shortened by avoiding general anaesthesia, in patient with several comorbidities e.g. subdural hematoma evacuation by burr holes, stereotactic brain biopsy.

Advantages[3,4,5]

1. Higher gross total resection of the lesion

2. Lesser morbidity & therefore better preservation of speech and motor function

3. Avoidance of side-effects

4. Lesser resource utilisation leading to decreased procedure costs

5. Shorter ICU stay, faster recovery

Contraindications

Absolute contraindication is patient refusal.

Relative contraindications are:

1. Anticipated difficult airway - morbidly obese, history of OSA.

2. Anxiety disorder.

3. Claustrophobia.

4. Extreme age groups. Children less than 10 years may become uncooperative during prolonged procedures and elderly may develop delirium.

5. Drug abuse.

6. Low pain threshold or chronic pain syndrome.

7. Surgeries where higher blood loss is expected e.g. vascular lesion or lesions in vicinity of venous sinuses.

8. Uncontrolled hypertension.

Pre-operative Assessment & Patient Preparation

The responsibility of anaesthesiologist is to select and prepare the patient for the procedure in the best possible way. Earning patient's confidence is the first step towards this process. An understanding, motivated & cooperative personality is the most important trait in a patient to decide if he will be able to undergo prolonged procedure while awake. The steps of procedure, possible side-effects and complications, necessary intraoperative tests (like hand movement, speaking, visual assessment) should be explained and rehearsed with the patient to gain and boost patient's confidence about the surgery. Patient should be reassured that anaesthesiologist is prepared to handle all consequences and make a comfortable and safe environment for the patient.

Thorough airway assessment is most essential, as options to secure an airway are limited. A plan for emergency securement of airway must be available and practised. Predictors of difficult mask ventilation and intubation like high Mallampati score, history of difficult mask ventilation and intubation, obesity etc. must be thoroughly cross-checked.

Premedication

The preoperative anti-epileptics and benzodiazepines are usually omitted if patient is planned for intraoperative electro corticography (ECoG) monitoring. Injection Glycopyrrolate is to be avoided as a dry mouth may make the patient uncomfortable. Similarly, metoclopramide is also not recommended because of potential adverse effects of hastened peristalsis.[6]

Intraoperative Course

Monitoring

- ECG

- Pulse oximetry

- Non-invasive blood pressure monitoring

- End-tidal carbon dioxide monitoring by side-sampling method from nasal cannula or mask

- Arterial line: Preferred in cases where Asleep-Awake-Asleep (AAA) anaesthesia technique is planned, venous air embolism risk/ expected blood loss is high. As definite levels of $PaCO2$ cannot be correctly estimated by capnography (due to dilution by air/ oxygen when patient is on mask), arterial blood gas sampling may be required in some cases.

- Processed EEG monitoring (e.g. Bispectral index or Entropy) is helpful to regulate the dose of sedatives at various stages of procedure.

- Urine output monitoring: Condom catheter or Foley's is usually inserted when procedure is expected to last more than 3 hours and/or anti-oedema measures (mannitol, furosemide) are being used.

Positioning

The position is usually supine, semi-sitting or lateral as per surgical requirement and head is usually fixed on 3 pin Mayfield clamp or sometimes kept on horse-shoe. The operative field must be draped such that patient's visual field is clear and they don't feel claustrophobic (Fig. 1). Patient should be made as comfortable as possible. All pressure points must be adequately padded. The operating room (OR) temperature must be 20-22 degree Celsius and patient must be kept adequately warm to prevent shivering and noise levels in OR must be kept to minimum & sudden loud noises must be absolutely avoided.

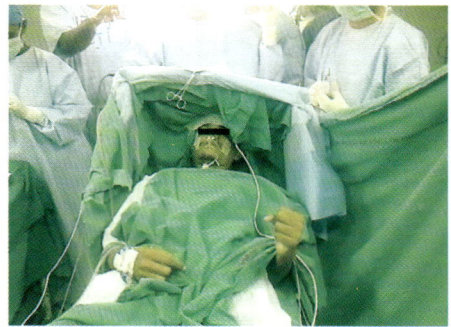

Fig. 1 : Positioning and draping

Various Anaesthesia Techniques

1. Exclusive Local Anaesthesia -

   Usually possible for small craniotomies like stereotactic biopsy, burr-holes or deep brain stimulation surgery, where procedure time is short. Patient is clear headed for the intraoperative testing with no residual effect of sedatives. Local anaesthesia at pin insertion site or incision site along with scalp block adequately alleviates the procedure pain.

2. Conscious Sedation -

   During conscious sedation, patient is moderately sedated so that the airway and breathing is not compromised, and patient is awake to follow purposeful commands for intraoperative testing.

   Sedatives can be given by intermittent boluses, continuous infusion or as target controlled infusion. Preferred agents for conscious sedation are dexmedetomidine, propofol, midazolam or fentanyl infusion. Dexmedetomidine, a highly selective alpha-2 agonist (loading 1 mcg/kg over 10-15 min followed by 0.2-1.0 mcg/kg/hr), is commonly preferred now because it does not compromise respiration and decreases opioid requirement. It also does not affect electrocorticography reading.

   Propofol (50-150 mcg/kg/min) is also widely used because of rapid onset and offset and antiemetic effect. Propofol must however be stopped 20-30 minutes before ECoG recordings as it also has anti-epileptic effect.[7] Remifentanil (0.03-0.09 mcg/kg/min, still not available in India) is most commonly preferred opioid in West because of its potent analgesia with ultrashort half-life. It however causes severe hypopnoea in spontaneously breathing patients and has risk of emergence excitement and hyperalgesia.[8]

   A nasal airway is a very useful adjuvant to keep airway patent during moderate sedation. Care must be taken to prevent an oxygen rich environment (from face mask) developing near the surgical site as it can precipitate surgical site fire while using cautery. The BIS, EtCO$_2$ and RR monitoring also aids to prevent over-sedation and respiratory depression. The scalp block and local anaesthesia is usually also given.

3. Asleep Awake Asleep anaesthesia (AAA):

   For AAA technique, patient is given general anaesthesia for first part of procedure i.e. head frame fixation, positioning, skin incision, craniotomy and dura opening. Supraglottic airway device or endotracheal tube is used to secure the airway. Some centres provide deep sedation with spontaneous respiration and nasopharyngeal airway in-situ. The patient is then gradually awakened, endotracheal tube or supraglottic

device removed and brain mapping or ECoG or sensory-motor testing performed. Once the lesion is resected, patient is again put to sleep and airway re-secured till the completion of surgery.[9]

There are two challenging situations for the anaesthesiologist during this technique one is when awakening the patient for neurological testing and second while re-establishing the airway for closure at later stage. The coughing, bucking, desaturation, head movement on pins and patient becoming restless will lead to cerebral oedema. A supraglottic airway devices are preferred for securing the airway, as lesser depth of anaesthesia is needed for their placement, muscle-relaxants can be avoided (therefore no reversal agent needed) and less chances of airway complications like laryngospasm. For re-securing the airway the tube exchanger and flexible fibreoptic scope are useful aids. Many anaesthesiologists modify the technique by using mild to moderate sedation during closure. The airway patency is maintained by means of nasal airway in such a scenario.

Intravenous and inhalational agents have all been tried for inducing and maintaining general anaesthesia. However, most of the regimens have preferred propofol and remifentanil because of smooth, predictable and rapid onset and awakening.

Scalp Block[10]

To alleviate pain for pin insertion and skin incision regional field block is effective. It must be considered in all types of anaesthesia plan for awake craniotomy as it decreases the opioid consumption, sedative requirement, minimizes hemodynamic disturbances and decreases post-operative analgesic requirement.

A complete scalp block requires anaesthetising six nerves bilaterally (Fig 2). However, this increases the risk of local anaesthetic toxicity because of large volume needed to block these nerves and the ample vascularity of scalp. Therefore, the nerves to be blocked must be carefully selected as per the surgical incision site and long-acting local anaesthetics (like bupivacaine, levo-bupivacaine or ropivacaine) along with 1:200000 Adrenaline must be used to prolong duration of block and decrease the systemic absorption.

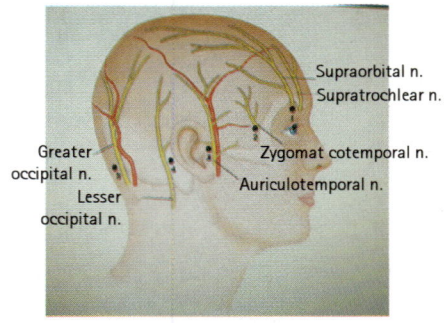

Fig. 2 : Nerve supply of the scalp

The maximum permissible amount to be infiltrated must be calculated (usually 0.2% bupivacaine max 2.5 mg/kg or 0.2% ropivacaine max 3.5 mg/kg)[11] and shared among the anaesthesiologist (for scalp block) and neurosurgeon (for incision site and pin site insertion).

The nerves to be anaesthetized are[10] (Fig. 3 & 4)

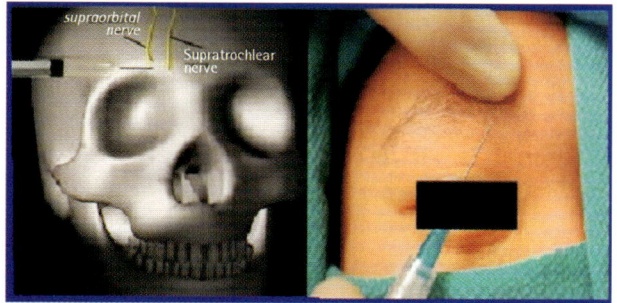

Fig. 3 : Supratrochlear & supraorbital nerve block

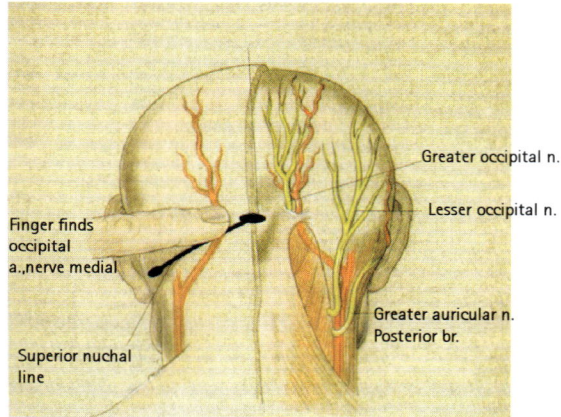

Fig. 4 : Scalp block – posterior landmarks

1. Supraorbital and Supratrochlear nerves -

    These are the branches of ophthalmic division of trigeminal nerve and gives sensory supply to forehead and upper eyelid. The nerve arises from the supraorbital notch which is in medial third of supraorbital ridge.

    A smaller gauge needle (25-26G) must be inserted perpendicular to skin till bone is contacted at 0.5-1.0 cm depth and slightly withdrawn. 2-3 ml of LA is infiltrated after negative aspiration for blood. The needle is then redirected 1- 1.5 cm medially and again 2-3 ml of LA is infiltrated to block supratrochlear nerve.

2. Auriculotemporal nerve-

    This is a branch of mandibular division of trigeminal nerve and supplies area in front of and above the ear. Chances of blocking the facial nerve are high while anaesthetizing this nerve. To block auriculotemporal nerve, palpate the temporal artery in front of the tragus. Enter the needle perpendicular to skin, just posterior to temporal artery. Inject 2-3 ml of LA at 0.5-1cm depth below and above the temporalis fascia.

3. Zygomaticotemporal nerve-

    This is a branch of the maxillary division of the trigeminal nerve and supplies the temple region of scalp. It is located at the frontotemporal suture line posterolateral to the lateral orbital rim. As this nerve branches extensively, both superficial and deep infiltration must be done. About 2-3 ml is usually effective. Effective blockade of this nerve obtunds the pain due to dissection and retraction of temporalis muscle.

4. Greater occipital nerve-

    This is a branch of C2 and supplies the posterior region of scalp. It lies medial to the occipital artery. Occipital artery can be palpated midway between the occipital protuberance and mastoid process. 3-4 ml of LA must be injected here.

5. Lesser occipital nerve-

    This nerve is a branch of C2 and C3 and supplies the postero-superior region of ear. It is blocked midway between the mastoid and occipital artery and about 3-4 ml is needed to block this nerve.

Complications[12]

1. Nausea and Vomiting -

    The nausea occurs in upto 4% of patients, however vomiting is rare could be due to anxiety, pain, opioids. The pain especially while resecting, the temporalis muscle and opening of dura and can induce nausea. It is advisable to infiltrate additional local anaesthetic over duramater before opening of dura to decrease the nociceptive response.

    Injection dexamethasone (as perioperative anti-oedema agent) and propofol (10-20 mg) are potent prophylactic anti-emetic agents. Injection ondansetrone (4 mg) is useful to prevent or control nausea and vomiting. A working suction must be readily available to clear the airway and prevent aspiration especially when the patient is sedated.

2. Airway obstruction or Loss of airway -

    Due to deep sedation, seizures, misplacement of airway can lead to hypoventilation, desaturation, CO_2 retention.

    The simple steps like jaw thrust, insertion of nasopharyngeal airway can circumvent the problem. In extreme cases, insertion of LMA or endotracheal tube followed by intermittent positive pressure ventilation may be necessary. The following of respiratory rate and $EtCO_2$ trend provides useful prediction about failing respiration.

When performing stereotactic biopsy, instrument must be available to release the head from the Leksell frame, which has a horizontal bar in front of mouth and may interfere even with LMA insertion.

3. Brain bulge –

The hypoventilation leading to hypercarbia causes brain bulge. If patient is having airway secured then hyper ventilating is effective, otherwise depth of anaesthesia is decreased, and patient awakened and asked to breathe deeply. Injection mannitol or hypertonic saline may also be needed.

4. Seizures –

The incidence of seizure during awake craniotomy varies from 2-20%. The anti-epileptic is usually withheld on day of surgery to improve electrocorticography readings. This along with bipolarstimulation of cortex (by Ojemann stimulator) for mapping decreases the seizure threshold. The seizure may be focal or generalized. The generalized seizures must be controlled urgently as head may be fixed on pins (leading to patient injury) or airway compromise can occur. Instillation of cold saline in the surgical field usually calms the seizure foci but at times propofol (20-50mg) or benzodiazepine or anti-epileptics may be necessary.

5. Conversion to general anaesthesia –

The failure of awake craniotomy for any of the above mentioned, complications or due to patient becoming overtly anxious and restless, may require conversion of conscious sedation to general anaesthesia. This can occur in up to 6% of cases. The failed awake craniotomy has lower incidence of gross-total resection, increased postoperative speech deterioration and longer hospital stay.[13]

6. Hemodynamic changes–

The hypertension, hypotension and tachycardia are frequently observed although mostly not harmful. The hypertension must however be attended to urgently which is the only consistent sign of intracranial bleed.

7. Venous air embolism (VAE) –

The incidence of VAE in sitting or semi-sitting position, recorded by precordial Doppler, has been reported in up to 4.5%. Coughing in an otherwise stable patient is symptom of VAE. The techniques of bending the head forwards, raising legs and bending abdomen increases the jugular venous pressure and helps to decrease air entrapment while surgeon tries to flood the surgical field with saline and apply bone wax.[6]

Postoperative Care

The routine ICU admission is not necessary after awake craniotomy but must be considered for patients with co-existent morbidities, complicated intraoperative course or any inadvertent intraoperative neurosurgical complication. The patients with uneventful intraoperative course can be safely observed in postanaesthesia care unit and then sent to ward. They usually have a shorter hospital stay. Incidence of postoperative nausea vomiting has been shown to be significantly less for awake craniotomy then craniotomies performed under general anaesthesia.[14] The requirement of analgesia is similar as for other neurosurgical craniotomies.

In Parkinson's disease patient who undergo DBS placement are continued with their medication as battery is activated after a few days when effect of local inflammation due to electrode placement settles. Similarly, all the anti-epileptics of the seizure patients are continued and gradually tapered by the neurologist over weeks. In few patients of tumour resection there may be aggravation of symptoms in the postoperative period due to oedema and retraction, but they must be reassured that this is transient.

CONCLUSION

The awake craniotomy is an increasingly expanding aspect of neurosurgery. The success of the procedure depends on right patient selection, excellent communication between the patient and the entire team, a good regional anaesthesia, timely and promptly rectification of complications. The neuroanaesthesiologist must be aware of the pathology and surgical steps in detail. He is like a pilot whose responsibility is to make sure that the procedure is conducted smoothly, maximally and safely.

REFERENCES

1. Erickson KM, Cole DJ. Anesthetic considerations for awake craniotomy for epilepsy and functional neurosurgery. Anesthesiol Clin. 2012;30(2):241–68.

2. WHO | Neurological Disorders: Public Health Challenges. WHO. World Health Organization; 2012.

3. De Benedictis A, Moritz-Gasser S, Duffau H. Awake mapping optimizes the extent of resection for low-grade gliomas in eloquent areas. Neurosurgery. 2010;66(6):1074–84; discussion 1084.

4. Sanai N, Mirzadeh Z, Berger MS. Functional Outcome after Language Mapping for Glioma Resection. N Engl J Med. 2008;358(1):18–27.

5. Blanshard HJ, Chung F, Manninen PH, Taylor MD, Bernstein M. Awake craniotomy for removal of intracranial tumor: considerations for early discharge. Anesth Analg. 2001;92(1):89–94.

6. Kayama T, Guidelines committee of the Japan awake surgery conference. The guidelines for awake craniotomy guidelines committee of the Japan awake surgery conference. Neurol Med Chir (Tokyo). 2012;52(3):119–41.

7. Ebrahim ZY, Schubert A, Van Ness P, Wolgamuth B, Awad I. The effect of propofol on the electroencephalogram of patients with epilepsy. Anesth Analg. 1994;78(2):275–9.

8. Schubert A, Lotto M. Awake Craniotomy, Epilepsy, Minimally invasive, and Robotic Surgery. In: Cottrell and Young's Neuroanesthesia. 5th Editio. Philadelphia,PA: MOSBY ELSEVIER; 2010. p. 296–315.

9. Sarang A, Dinsmore J. Anaesthesia for awake craniotomy—evolution of a technique that facilitates awake neurological testing. Br J Anaesth. 2003;90(2):161–5.

10. Assistant AP, Smith T, Certified C, Gottschalk A. A review of scalp blockade for cranial surgery &. J Clin Anesth. 2017;25(2):150–9.

11. Costello TG, Cormack JR, Hoy C, Wyss A, Braniff V, Martin K, et al. Plasma ropivacaine levels following scalp block for awake craniotomy. J Neurosurg Anesthesiol. 2004;16(2):147–50.

12. Skucas AP, Artru AA. Anesthetic complications of awake craniotomies for epilepsy surgery. Anesth Analg. 2006;102(3):882–7.

13. Nossek E, Matot I, Shahar T, Barzilai O, Rapoport Y, Gonen T, et al. Failed awake craniotomy: a retrospective analysis in 424 patients undergoing craniotomy for brain tumor. J Neurosurg. 2013;118(2):243–9.

14. Manninen PH, Tan TK. Postoperative nausea and vomiting after craniotomy for tumor surgery: A comparison between awake craniotomy and general anesthesia. J Clin Anesth. 2002;14(4):279–83.

MULTIPLE CHOICE QUESTIONS

1. **Awake craniotomy is preferred for which procedure?**
   a. Microvascular decompression
   b. Brainstem glioma excision
   c. EDH evacuation
   d. Surgical treatment of idiopathic essential tremors

2. **Not a preferred agent for conscious sedation during awake craniotomy**
   a. Dexmedetomidine
   b. Ketamine
   c. Propofol
   d. Fentanyl

3. **Which nerve can be accidently and undesirably blocked while giving scalp block?**
   a. Supraorbital
   b. Zygomaticotemporal
   c. Lesser occipital
   d. Facial

4. **A patient develops seizure intraoperatively while undergoing electrocorticography in awake craniotomy. 1st step should be**
   a. Instillation of iced saline by the neurosurgeon
   b. IV Midazolam
   c. IV propofol
   d. IV Phenytoin

5. **How long should propofol infusion be stopped before doing ECoG intraoperatively?**
   a. 2 min
   b. 5 min
   c. 20 min
   d. 50 min

6. **Not a contraindication for awake craniotomy?**
   a. Essential tremors
   b. Severe back pain
   c. 9 year old child
   d. Severe coughing

7. **Premedication to be prescribed before awake craniotomy for epilepsy surgery?**
   a. Glycopyrrolate
   b. Midazolam
   c. Pantoprazole
   d. Pheytoin

8. **Intraoperatively during awake craniotomy, patient develops coughing followed by hypotension and decrease in capnography trace. Treatment would be?**
   a. Insertion of intercostal drain
   b. Sedating the patient
   c. Flooding of surgical field with sterile saline by neurosurgeon
   d. Insertion of central line

9. **While giving scalp block, a patient becomes agitated, has seizures and loses consciousness. First line of treatment would be?**
   a. Intralipid 20% 1.5 ml/Kg
   b. Midazolam 5 mg
   c. Adernaline 1mg bolus
   d. Establish airway and ventilation.

10. **Drugs to enhance EEG seizure activity are?**
    a. Methohexital
    b. Etomidate
    c. Ketamine
    d. All of the Above

ANAESTHESIA MANAGEMENT OF CAROTID ENDARTERECTOMY

Ranjana Das, Vikram Karmarkar

Introduction

The main cause of carotid artery occlusion is atherosclerosis at bifurcation of common carotid artery with frequent extension into ICA and ECA. It's wide spread in western countries with increasing prevalence in developing countries.

The clinical features result from embolization of plaque or narrowing of lumen of carotid artery causing hypo perfusion and cerebral infarcts. This leads to fatal or debilitating stroke, TIA, transient mono ocular blindness. However, some patients may remain asymptomatic.

The degree of cerebral injury depends on the plaque morphology, characteristics of embolus, duration of hypo perfusion, integrity of circle of Willis and cerebral collateral circulation.

The symptomatic carotid disease is defined as focal neurological symptoms that are sudden in onset, ipsilateral to significant carotid atherosclerotic disease. There can be one or more TIA characterised by focal neurological dysfunction or transient mono ocular blindness.

The stroke is the third leading cause of death and long-term disability in USA. They perform more than 1 lakh carotid endarterectomy every year[1]. The surgical treatment of acute ischaemic stroke is controversial.

The emergency angioplasty and stenting and mechanical extraction of thrombi are alternative interventions. The approved therapy is intravenous recombinant tissue plasminogen activator[2].

The first carotid endarterectomy was performed at St. Mary Hospital, London in 1954. The North American Symptomatic Carotid Endarterectomy Trial (NASCET) and the European Carotid Surgery Trial (ECST) are two major trials which have defined current indications for carotid endarterectomy[3]. The European Asymptomatic Carotid Surgery Trial states that patient with asymptomatic carotid stenosis treated with carotid endarterectomy with medical treatment have reduced a five-year risk of stroke when compared with medical therapy alone. However, carotid endarterectomy is a controversial indication in asymptomatic patients with 50-90% carotid stenosis. The benefits of carotid endarterectomy are also uncertain in symptomatic stenosis of 50-70%.

AIM

The carotid endarterectomy is performed to prevent and to the reduce future risk of embolic stroke in both symptomatic and non-symptomatic patients. This should be performed as soon as possible after a TIA stroke. In centers of excellence, it is a low risk procedure with excellent long term durabiltiy[4].

ANESTHESIA MANAGEMENT

Preanaesthetic evaluation

History

- History of risk factors - age, sedentary lifestyle, smoking, hypertension, diabetes, hyperlipidemia, significant family history.

- History of cardiovascular disease- severity of coronary and cerebral vascular disease must be evaluated and decision must be taken to perform either treatment for coronary artery disease first or combined treatment.

- History of other comorbidiy - COPD, PVD, renal insufficiency

- History of any movement disorders e.g. Parkinsonism which is contraindicated for carotid endarterectomy under LA

- History of any surgery e.g. thyroidectomy. Patient may have recurrent laryngeal nerve palsy.

- History of any preexisting neurological deficit.

PHYSICAL EXAMINATION

- General and systemic examination
- Series of blood pressure and heart rate measurements

Investigations

- Baseline - CBC, serum electrolyte, coagulation profile, INR, lipid profile, blood sugar, renal function test
- 12 lead ECG, X ray chest
- 2D echo

- Investigations - Cerebral angiography to identify high risk patient because of high grade contralateral carotid disease or poor collateral circulation

Preoperative preparations

- Continue all long term cardiac medications. Aspirin and clopidogrel therapy should be continued throughout perioperative period to reduce the risk of MI and TIA. Keep platelets ready for possible transfusion.

- Reassure patient to reduce anxiety

- Document any preexisting neurological deficit

- Good glycemic control. Hyperglycaemia may worsen neurological deficit

- Optimise blood pressure

- Premedictation with short acting Benzodizepin

Anaesthesia technique

Aim

- To maintain Cerebral Perfusion Pressure

- To have minimum hemodynamic fluctuations

- Must maintain normocapnia

- Avoid vasoconstriction with hypocapnia and

- Avoid Steal phenomenon with Hypercapnia

- Neuro protection

- Provide optimal operating condition

- Good glycemic control

- Have rapid emergence to allow early neurological assessment and detection of complications

Choice of anaesthesia technique

Regional versus General Anaesthesia depends on surgeon's preference, patients comfort and Anaesthesiologists skills[5].

Regional anaesthesia

Method: Cervical epidural and deep and superficial Cervical plexus block to produce Anaesthesia of C2 to C4 dermatomes in combination with local infiltration around Carotid sheath.

Advantages:

- Minimal hemodynamic fluctuations

- Better Neurological evaluation

- Earlier detection and treatment of complications

- Less chances of Shunt Insertions

- Shorter hospital stay

- Useful in patients where General Anaesthesia is undesirable

Disadvantages:

- Requires patients Cooperation

- Difficult to protect airway in case of emergency

- Absence of Cerebral Protection

Technique

Cervical epidural : The recommended dose is Inj. Bupivacaine 0.5% 10-15 ml with or without 50-100 mcg Fentanyl.

The expected complications are hypotension, bradycardia, breathing difficulty and accidental dural puncture. It is advisable to have resuscitative measures ready while performing cervical epidural.

Deep cervical plexus block : A line is drawn from mastoid process (C1) to Cricoid cartilage (C6), one cm posterior to Sternocleidomastoid muscle. Now Inj. of Xylocaine 1% 3-5 ml each injected (at the roots of cervical plexus, C2,3,4) at distance of 1.5 cm along the line with needle directed posteriorly and caudally.

Complications : Accidental intravascular or Subarachnoid injection of LA can lead to loss of consciousness, convulsions, CVS collapse, block of Phrenic nerve, recurrent laryngeal and glossopharyngeal nerve and sympathetic chain. The treatment includes intubation and resuscitation.

Superficial cervical Block : Subcutaneous infiltration of 10 to 15 ml of Inj. Xylocaine along Posterior border and midpoint of Sternocleidomastoid muscle.

Sedation – Light sedation for insertion of lines and giving blocks. The commonly be used drugs are Propofol, Dexmedetomidine, Fentanyl and Midazolam in appropriate doses. It is advisable to discontinue sedation before Carotid artery cross Clamping for neurological monitoring of contralateral motor function,speechand cognition.

In addition, following things are observed:

- Supplement Oxygen and ensure airway

- Heamodynamic monitoring

- Non-claustrophobic draping (Clear drapes, adequate light, above and away from nose and mouth) which will help to communicate with the patient to reassure him always.

General anaesthesia

Advantages:

- Comfortable for patient, surgeons and OT staff

- Safe control over ventilatory parameters
- Cerebral metabolism protected by control over desired levels of CO_2
- Cerebral protection
- Better management of complications

Disadvantages:

- Difficult neurological assessment, hence alternative methods of cerebral functions Monitoring required
- More hemodynamic fluctuations
- Chances of shunt insertions high
- Hospital stay longer, thus expensive
- Delayed Emergence may confuse immediate Postoperative evaluation.

Technique

Induction: Choice of agents is based on experience of Anaesthesiologist however the advisable drugs and dosage are as follows

- Fantanyl 2-5 mcg/kg,
- Sufentanyl 0.5-1 mcg/kg
- Remifentanyl 0.1-0.5 mcg/kg
- Propofol
- Non Depolarising Muscle relaxants for intubation

Maintenance:

- Volatile Agents along with Nitrous oxide
- Opioid and Propofol infusion for maintainance
- Superficial cervical plexus block reduces intraoperative opiate requirement and provides post operative analgesia.
- Brain protection : barbiturates, benzodiazepines, etomidate, propofol and inhalational isoflurane or sevoflurane are used as brain protective agents as they decrease cerebral metabolic rate and cerebral blood flow. It can be used as bolus or IV infusion.
- IV fluids : Glucose free Cryatalloids
- Blood loss is not expected Intraoperative as there is good control over major blood vessels.

Cross Clamping

During CEA, Carotid artery is clamped above and below the disease area.

- It is important to maintain mean arterial pressure at baseline or higher during cross clamping to increase collateral blood flow and prevent ischemia.

- IV heparin 3000-5000 Units given before cross clamping.
- There are chances of hypoperfusion and ischemic injury to ipsilateral cerebral hemisphere specially when cross flow through Circle of Willis is insufficient.
- Clamping is often associated with rise in Mean arterial pressure
- Bradycardia and hypotension may occur due to Surgical stimuluation of Carotid sinus, this can be avoided by local infiltration.
- Surgical shunt should be inserted for any neurological deficit immediately.
- Shunt is used in selective patients. Risks are Thromboembolism, vessel wall injury and clotting.

Extubation:

- Standard reversal, smooth extubation with hemodynamic stability. Any rise in BP is to be treated with short acting antihypertensives
- All patients to be shifted in ICU, for at least 12 hours after surgery with continued hemodynamic and neurological monitoring.

In ICU

- Pain relief
- Blood pressure control below preoperative level to avoid hyper perfusion syndrome.
- Important to control stress response to pain, anemia, hypothermia, hemodynamic extremes and ventilatory insufficiency.

Intraoperative monitoring

Aim : To detect cerebral ischemia and prevent intraoperative stroke.

Routine

- 5 Lead ECG to detect ischemia
- Invasive Arterial Blood pressure in other arm. Minimum mean arterial pressure target should be at patient's preoperative value and or should not exceed 20% of it.

Hypotension and bradycardia may occur due to surgical interference with carotid sinus, treated by local infiltration around this area. Extremes of blood pressure changes are managed pharmacologically.

- End tidal CO_2 - Maintain normocapnea
- Pulse Oximetry
- Blood sugar - Maintain blood sugar level < 200 mg%.

Special neurological monitoring

- *Carotid artery stump pressure:* It represents the back pressure resulting from the collateral flow through Circle of Willis. Stump Pressure < 50 mmhg indicates Hypoperfusion.

- *TCD (MCA Blood flow):* Indicates continuous measurement of Mean Blood flow velocity and detects microemboli in MCA, and gives information about Carotid Shunt function.

- *EEG:* Detects early cerebral ischemia during Carotid Clamping, especially in patients with contralateral Carotid disease and if there is ischemia due to Hypotension, shunt malfunction or cerebral embolism. EEG does not detect subcortical ischemia[6].

- *SSEP:* Detects subcortical ischemia. Sensory cortex is at risk during carotid artery clamping. The decrease in amplitude and increase in latency occurs in ischemia, and waves are abolished when the flow is < 12 ml/min/ 100gm brain tissue[7].

- Cerebral oximetry: Jugular bulb venous oxygen saturation done from ipsilateral surgical site.

The near infrared Spectro photometry is non-invasive through scalp on ipsilateral side, which gives a continuous regional cerebral oxygen saturation monitoring.

The above special neurological monitoring has limitations as they get affected by anaesthetic depth, change in temperature and blood pressure.

Expected complications in postoperative period - Most neurological complications after Carotid Endarterectomy occur due to Intraoperative embolization, hypotension, thrombosis, Intracerebral hemorrhage and Cerebral hyperperfusion[8].

- Any Neurological defects requires prompt assessment of carotid artery patency by Carotid artery, duplex scanning or cerebral Angiography. If Occlusion is detected, then Surgical re-exploration to be done without delay.

- Wound hematoma : Expanding hematoma requires prompt evaluation exploration and evacuation especially when airway is getting compressed.

- Intracerebral hemorrhage : Excessive rise in blood pressure and CPP may cause cerebral hemorrhage or edema in areas of brain that have lost ability to autoregulate. Mostly it occurs 1-5 days after Endarterectomy, which has a significant morbidity and mortality.

- Hypertension may be due to Surgical denervation of carotid sinus baro receptors, to be treated by antihypertensives.

- Hypotension,could be because of regional anaesthesia or carotid sinus baroreceptors hyperactivity, treated by IV fluids and Vasopressors.

- *Myocardial infarction* : Responsible for 50% mortality.

- *Cerebral hyperperfusion syndrome :* Is an abrupt rise in blood flow in the surgically reperfusion brain having loss of autoregulation. It manifests as headache, seizures, brain oedema and focal neurological defecits this is more prone in severe stenosis and postoperative hypertension

- *Cranial and cervical nerve dysfunction :* Mostly these injuries are transient. Patient should be examined for injury to recurrent laryngeal, superior laryngeal, hypoglossal nerves immediately after extubation. Injury to unilateral recurrent laryngeal nerve may result in vocal cords palsy, hoarseness of voice and impaired cough. Bilateral recurrent laryngeal nerve injury can lead to upper airway obstruction[9].

- Carotid body dysfunction may occur after carotid endarterectomy. Unilateral injuryresults inimpaired ventilatory response to mild hypoxemia. Bilateral carotid endarterectomy may cause loss of Normal ventilatory response to acute hypoxia. Thus causes raised arterial $PaCO_2$.

- Coagulopathy due to residual heparin or massive blood transfusion.

CONCLUSION

The carotid endarterectomy continues to challenge the anesthesiologist as it is generally performed on a relatively elderly patient with high incidence of coexisting diseases.

Following may reduce the morbidity and give better overall outcome.

- Preoperative assessment and optimisation of cardiac risk

- Appropriate selection of cases

- Preference and experience of surgical and anaesthetist team

- Choice and implications of better anesthesia techniques

The early diagnosis, prevention and treatment of postoperative complication reduce morbidity and better overall outcome.

The medical management (of hypertension, diabetes, hyperlipidemia and smoking) and percutaneous carotid angioplasty and stenting are proposed alternatives and remain challenge to surgical vascularisation techniques.

REFERENCES

1. MoraschMD, Parker MA, FeinglassJ, et al: Carotid endarterectomy:Characterisation of recent increase in procedure rates. J Vascular Surg 31:901-909,2000.

2. Alberta MJ: Hyperacute strike therapy with tissue plasminogen activator. Am J Cardiology 80:29D, discussion 35D -39D, 1997.

3. Findlay JM, Tucker WAS, Ferguson GG, et Al: Guidelines for the use of carotid endarterectomy: Current recommendations from the Canadian Neurosurgical Society. CMAJ 157:653-659,1997.

4. EcherRD, Pichelmann MA, Meissner I, Meyer FB: Durability of carotid endarterectomy. Stroke 34:2941-2944,2003.

5. General anesthesia Vs local anesthesia for carotid surgery (GALA), a multi centre randomised controlled trial, The Lancet volume 372, issue 9656,2132-2142.

6. PlestisKA, LoubserP, MizrahiEM, et al: Continuous EEG monitoring and selective shunting reduces neurologic morbidity rates in CEA. J Vasc. Surgery 25:620-628,1997.

7. De Vleeschauwer P, Horsham S, Mamamoros R: Monitoring of somatosensory evoked potentials in carotid surgery: Results, usefulness and limitations of the method. Ann Vasc Surf 2:63-68, 1998.

8. KrulJM, van Gijn J, AckerstaffRG, et Al: Site and pathogenesis of infarcts associated with carotid endarterectomy. Stroke 20:324-328, 1989.

9. Schubert MD, Fontanelle LJ, Solomon JW, Hanson TL: Cranial/ cervical nerve dysfunction after carotid endarterectomy. J Vasc Surf 25: 481-487,1997.

MULTIPLE CHOICE QUESTIONS

1. **The commonest cause of chronic Internal Carotid Artery stenosis is**
   a. Embolus from heart
   b. Atherosclerosis
   c. Malignancy
   d. Vasculitis

2. **Clinical presentation commonly includes (more than 1 choice)**
   a. TIA
   b. Established stroke
   c. Transient monocular blindness
   d. Fever
   e. Convulsions

3. **Methods of treatment include (>1 answer)**
   a. Carotid endarterectomy
   b. Carotid stenting
   c. Medical management
   d. Chelation therapy
   e. Meditation

4. **The aim of carotid endarterectomy is,**
   a. Improve effort tolerance
   b. Prevent stroke on ipsilateral side
   c. Reverse effects of hyperlipidemia
   d. Treatment of brain infarction

5. **Specific investigations needed for decision making for surgery are**
   a. Digital subtraction angiography
   b. MRI brain
   c. HbA1c
   d. Cardiac stress test
   e. Colour doppler of neck vessels

6. **Goals of anaesthesia include,**
   a. Prevent hypocapnia
   b. Glycemic control
   c. Brain protection
   d. Maintain normal brain perfusion pressure

7. **Advantages of regional anaesthesia are,**
   a. Ability to monitor neurological functions
   b. Minimize hemodynamic fluctuations
   c. High risk for GA
   d. District hospital setting

8. **Brain protection agents include,**
   a. Propofol
   b. Barbiturates
   c. Ceftriaxone
   d. Sevoflurane
   e. Ketotifens

9. **Heparin dose used during cross clamping is**
   a. 100-500 u
   b. 10000- 12000 u
   c. 3000-5000u
   d. not required

10. **Complications of the procedure include**
    a. Neck hematoma
    b. Cerebral hyperperfusion syndrome
    c. Cranial nerve dysfunction
    d. Myocardial infarction
    e. Stroke

11. **Which nerve can possibly get injured during carotid endarterectomy?**
    a. Recurrent laryngeal
    b. Superior laryngeal
    c. Hypoglossal
    d. Phrenic

12. **Which monitoring technique helps to detect micro emboli?**
    a. TCD
    b. EEG
    c. SSEP
    d. Cerebral oximetry

CHAPTER 9

ANAESTHESIA FOR DEEP BRAIN STIMULATION (DBS)

Rajshree Deopujari, Vaibhavi Baxi

What is DBS

DBS (Deep Brain Stimulation) is a minimally invasive neurosurgical procedure used for the treatment of movement and neuropsychiatric disorders with alteration in function but not associated with much structural or anatomical changes. It involves implantation of a medical device called a neurostimulator (brain pacemaker), which sends high frequency electrical impulses, through implanted electrodes, to specific targets in the brain (brain nuclei). DBS has proved an extremely effective approach towards movement disorders like essential tremors, dystonia and parkinsons disease. Most of successful effects have been achieved using DBS in the vicinity of the subthalamic nucleus (STN), a small but integral part of the basal ganglia, which collectively control complex movements. The aim of this procedure is to improve the quality of life of the patient.

History

In the past for functional neurologic disorders invasive and more radical surgeries were performed for e.g. thalamotomy, pallidotomy, cingulotomy etc. Surgical removal of these deep brain structures was irreversible and left permanent side effects. As an alternative to theses ablative surgeries Thalamic deep brain stimulation was first developed for tremor control in the 1980. Later on, sub-thalamic nucleus (STN) and internal globus pallidus (GPi) stimulation were also investigated. Targeting the STN in 1987 resulted in improvement in a wide range of parkinsonian symptoms. After the initial success in parkinson's patient, its applications were extended for other functional disorders like dyskinesias, dystonia, epilepsy, chronic pain and alzheimer disease[1,2].

How does DBS Work

Tremor (14.5%), Parkinson disease (7%), and dystonia (1.8%) are three of the most common movement disorders[3]. These disorders eventually become refractory to medications and cause significant disability affecting the lifestyle of the suffering individual. These disorders can be significantly ameliorated by electrical stimulation of specific deep brain structures specific to each disorder. The mechanism by which DBS modifies neuronal activity in not exactly known[4]. For each disorder there is a specific target site and neuronal effects of the stimulation at each site too varies. DBS does not damage healthy brain tissue by destroying (Table 1) nerve cells. Instead the procedure blocks electrical signals from targeted areas in the brain. The effects are also frequency dependent with greatest relief between 50-100 Hz.

Table 1. Target site of each disorder and neuronal effects of stimulation.

Indication	Target site	Effect of Stimulation
Idiopathic parkinsons disease	Subthalamic Nuclei (STN)	Hyperpolarization (neuronal jamming) → activity inhibited → Glutamate production decreases
Dystonia	Globus pallidus pars internal (GPi)	Activation of GABAergic axons → inhibition of GPi
Idiopathic essential tremor (Vim)nucleus of	Ventralis intermedius thalamic nuclei thalamus	Activates reticular nucleus → inhibition of

Indications for DBS Surgery[5]

DBS implantation is an elective surgery to improve the quality of life in movement disorders no longer responsive to medical therapy.

Established indications include:

- Idiopathic parkinson's disease
- Idiopathic essential tremor
- Dystonia

Emerging indications include:

- Obsessive compulsive disorder
- Refractory epilepsy
- Tremor caused by multiple sclerosis
- Tourette syndrome
- Chronic pain
- Major Depression

Indications under experimental trial include:

- Other tremors like (kinetic, post-stroke, post-head injury)
- Alzheimer disease
- Minimally conscious vegetative state

Contraindications for DBS Surgery include

Coagulopathy, recent use of antiplatelet medications and uncontrolled hypertension as there is risk of intracranial haemorrhage.

Patients with ongoing electroconvulsive shock therapy or deep tissue heat treatment.

Procedures requiring electrocautery should be avoided if possible or use monopolar cautery with lowest energy and for shortest time; after DBS placement.

Surgical Technique

The DBS system consists of three components:

- Implanted pulse generator (IPG)
- Lead (micro-electrodes)
- An extension

The IPG is a battery-powered neurostimulator which sends electrical pulses to the brain that interferes with neural activity at the target site. The lead is a coiled insulated wire with four platinum-iridium micro-electrodes and is placed in one or two different nuclei of the brain. The extension is an insulated wire that connects the lead to the IPG. It runs subcutaneously, from the cranium, down the side of the neck, behind the ear to the IPG, which is placed subcutaneously below the clavicle or, in some cases, the abdomen. The IPG can be calibrated by a neurologist, nurse, or trained technician to optimize symptom suppression and control side-effects[6].

All three components are surgically implanted inside the body in a single operation or as a 2 stage procedure. The initial stage consists of micro-electrode implantation in the target area of the brain with internalization of the leads and subsequent implantation of programmable pulse generator which may be done immediately or after few days. One of the reasons to delay the IPG implantation is the 'microlesion' effect because of the edema around the freshly implanted electrode which impairs the ability to check for stimulation induced benefits[7].

The procedure in operating room begins with the placement of a rigid head frame to the patient's skull (Fig. 1). Magnetic resonance imaging of brain is then done to obtain reference of internal anatomy to external coordinates to plan a linear trajectory from parietal surface to the target deep brain structures avoiding the vasculature and ventricles. This allows accurate insertion of electrode into target area. After imaging, patient is positioned either in supine or semi-sitting position on the operating table with the stereotactic frame fixed to the table (Fig. 2). A bur hole is made in the cranium for electrode insertion. The electrode is inserted 10-15 mm above the target site and is advanced 0.5 to 1mm along its trajectory towards the target nuclei while spontaneous neuronal firing (microelectrode recordings, MER) is recorded by the neurophysiologist. The target nuclei in brain are localized by the neurophysiologist by using variations in spontaneous firing rates between specific nuclei and movement related changes in firing rate. Macrostimulation, which involves the clinical testing of the patient's movements, is then used to verify that the stimulation of the electrode at those nuclei will improve symptoms and not cause any side effects. The electrode is then secured and the lead is ready for tunnelled connection to the pulse generator.

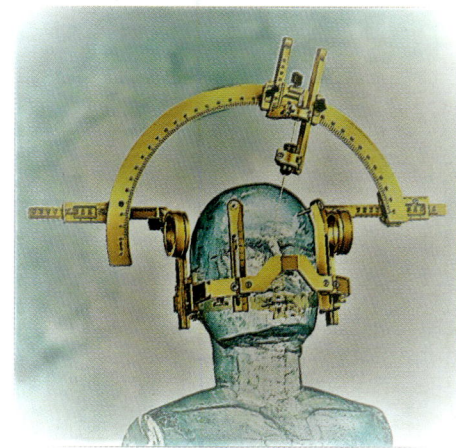

Fig. 1. Stereotactic Frame

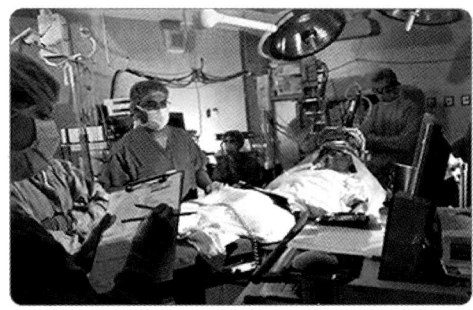

Fig. 2. Patient position during DBS surgery in OR

Anaesthetic Management

The anaesthetic technique varies depending upon the institution practices and has included monitored anaesthesia care (MAC), conscious sedation and general anaesthesia. Although none of them have been proven to be superior to other, due to need of intra-operative neurophysiologic mapping (microelectrode recordings-MER) and clinical testing of the patient, most of the DBS surgeries are preferred to be done under local anaesthesia and MAC. Conscious sedation may be given intermittently when testing is not being performed. General anaesthesia may be needed for paediatric patients and those with extreme anxiety for awake surgery and with chronic pain syndromes and severe 'off-medication' movement disorders/dystonia. Second stage of internalization is usually done under general anaesthesia.

Patient selection and preoperative evaluation

Careful patient selection is a major determinant of a successful postoperative outcome. The decision to operate is based on the risk to benefit assessment for the patient. For e.g. for parkinson's disease surgery is considered when patient develops moderate to severe motor fluctuation, medication induced dyskinesias, tremors refractory to medications or intolerance to medicines.

Patient is evaluated for general physical condition, psychiatric history, cognitive function, level of disability, general life expectancy and patient motivation. In awake technique patient's cooperation, communication, maturity and ability to cope in strange and stressful environment is crucial. Claustrophobia, anxiety disorder, psychiatric disorder and movement disorder may complicate positioning and compromise motionless surgical field. One case report does describe the role of regional block to eliminate involuntary movements in a patient with unilateral spontaneous movements[8].

Airway must be assessed for ease of mask ventilation, Mallampatti score, predictors of difficult airway and potential for airway obstruction. Obesity with obstructive sleep apnoea, wheezing, gastroesophageal reflux and chronic cough if severe may be a contraindication for awake

procedure. Others factors to be considered are type and frequency of seizures, haemorrhagic risk and haemodynamic instability.

Patient Preparation

The procedure is discussed with the patient and instructions are given about what to expect. Patient is reassured about his comfort as increased anxiety poses the risk of high blood pressure with intra cerebral bleed. Instructions regarding continuation or discontinuation of drugs are given too.

Positioning

Supine or semisitting position is used for DBS surgery. A soft mattress with padding of extremities and avoidance of extreme head rotation helps the patient to lie motionless for several hours on the operating table. The patient is surgically draped with sterile drapes such that patient doesn't feel claustrophobic and his facial expressions, speech, sight and motor movements of interest can be viewed. Some centres place a video to record patient's face which can be viewed by the surgical team[9].

Monitoring

Medical co-morbidities guide the monitoring needs in DBS surgery. Routine monitoring and a venous access depending upon the expectation of blood loss is usually sufficient. Exhaled carbon-di-oxide monitoring is essential for airway patency. Precordial Doppler is used for detection of any venous air embolism especially in patient in sitting position. Urinary catheterization may be done in some patients where surgery is expected to be prolonged so as to avoid discomfort of bladder distention.

Effect of anaesthetic drugs on MERs

Anaesthetics do not uniformly depress MERs but rather differ by disease as well as by deep brain stimuli. Hutchinson et al. have reported that the firing rates in the GPi nucleus were substantially decreased, and long pauses were present in patients with dystonia when given general anaesthesia with propofol compared to mapping under local anaesthesia[10]. Sanghera et al. studied the effect of general anaesthesia with desflurane in patients with dystonia and parkinson's disease. In dystonia group of patients there was no difference in the GPi nuclei firing rate in awake and anaesthetized patients; but there was a significant difference in GPi neuronal firing rate in the parkinson's group of patients[11].

The MER from STN nuclei have been successfully attained even under anaesthesia (TIVA/GA with ET).This is possibly due to higher GABA input in GPi neurons as compared to STN[12].

Role of Anaesthesiologist

In any kind of awake surgery the role anaesthetist broadens as he makes the patient comfortable, pain free, remains vigilant about patients rate and depth of breathing, communicates frequently with the patient giving reassurance and encouragement.

Premedication

Goals include anxiolysis, prevention of nausea, seizure, gastric reflux, pain and hemodynamic instability. For this midazolam, alprazolam, clonidine, metaclopramide, ondansetron, pantaprazole, ranitidine and antiepileptic medications are used. Dexamethasone for reducing intracranial pressure and acitoaminophen for mild analgesia may be given[13].

ANAESTHETIC TECHNIQUES

Monitored anaesthesia care

Local anaesthesia is used as subcutaneous infiltration at the pin sites, incision site and site of burr hole for electrode placement. Alternately scalp block by injecting local anaesthetic subcutaneously blocking supraorbital nerve, supratrochlear nerve, zygomaticotemporal nerve, auriculotemporal nerve, lesser and greater occipital nerve and greater auricular nerve; may be given. Local anaesthetics bupivacaine, ropivacaine and lignocaine are used with or without epinephrine.

Standard anaesthesia monitoring include electrocardiogram, pulse oximetry, end tidal CO_2 and non invasive blood pressure. Monitoring may be difficult in some patients with severe movement disorders and spasticity. Oxygen is supplemented through nasal prongs or oxygen mask. If the head frame is to be fixed then oxygen mask should be placed before the frame. Care should be taken to prevent an oxygen enriched environment to develop around the surgical site as electrocautery may cause fire.

Fluids should be administered to prevent hypovolaemia. Urinary catheter prevents discomfort of bladder distention. Position should be such that patient is comfortable for long hours and airway is accessible to secure in case of any emergency.

Conscious Sedation

Very often conscious sedation is used during opening and closing of the procedure. Drugs like midazolam, propofol, opioids and dexmedetomidine are used in small pulses or as infusions. Benzodiazepines may induce dyskinesias and may abolish MER; so its use is generally discouraged.

Propofol gives good patient satisfaction; is short acting, antiemetic and antiepileptic with predictable emergence. But it may cause oversedation, hypoventilation, may

attenuate tremors and MERs. Propofol is used in doses of 30 mic/kg/min to 180 mic/kg/min. Target controlled infusions devices are often used; but the pharmacokinetic behaviour in patients with parkinsons may vary from general population. Small doses of short acting opioids like fentanyl or remifentanil may be used in adjunct with propofol.

Dexmedetomidine from 0.2 mic/kg/hr to 0.8 mic/kg/hr preserves movement disorder symptom, MERs and does not ameliorate clinical signs of parkinson's disease. It also gives anxiolysis, analgesia and arousable sedation without respiratory depression. It is a good drug for neurological monitoring as it's action is non GABA mediated.

Depth of anaesthesia monitoring helps in titrating the drug doses and the state of arousal during DBS insertion. However its reliability during MER is questionable because the effects of anaesthetics are heterogenous across different regions of brain.

General Anaesthesia

Patient acceptance is higher for DBS surgery under general anaesthesia but the mapping and stimulation testing will be difficult. There are few reports of DBS insertion in general anaesthesia with limited electrophysiologic mapping and careful titration of anaesthetics.

Asleep–Awake–Asleep technique

The AAA technique in an interim technique with or without use of an airway. Patient is induced with popofol, short acting opioids and volatile anaesthetic is used during opening, closing and emergence of patients. LMA is the airway device most often used for the sleep portions due to ease of insertion, removal and re-insertion without changing the patient's head position.

Complications

Intraoperative complications are variable and needs vigilance for rapid detection and treatment. The incidence is variable due to differences in the practice, experience and duration of postoperative recording.

Airway complications include obstruction and de-saturation due to oversedation in patients with unprotected airway. This more often occurs in obese patient and few cases may also need intubation. Hence all appropriate airway instruments should be available all throughout the surgery, as handling the airway with the head fixed in the rigid frame can be difficult.

Hypertension may occur during the procedure due to patient's anxiety, agitation and discomfort in awake surgery. It needs to be controlled to systolic less than 140 mmof Hg, as it may cause intracerebral bleed. Frequently

Anaesthesia for deep brain stimulation (DBS)

used drugs include Labetalol, nitroglycerin, esmolol and nitroprusside. Hypotension may occur as a result of antiparkinson's drugs.

Venous air embolism may occur during DBS insertion in sitting/semi-sitting position especially in a hypovloaemic patient. Patient may vigorously cough with hypoxia and hypotension when there is a venous embolism. It can recorded by precordial Doppler. This needs to be communicated to the surgeon while maintain haemodynamic stability.

Seizures have been reported to occur in 0.8 to 4.5% of patients and often occur during stimulation testing[14]. Most seizures are focal and stop the moment surgeon stops his stimulation or pours ice cold saline directly on cortical surface. Seizures that do not stop simultaneously need to be treated with small dose of benzodiazepines, propofol or barbiturate. Risk factors for seizures include haemorrhage, age > 60 years, transventricular electrode trajectories and multiple sclerosis.

Haemorrhage is the most feared surgical complication during DBS implantation as functional structures are at risk and it may need an open craniotomy to control. Hypertension, age, number of microelectrode passes and transventricular lead trajectories are important risk factors for bleed.

Stroke, other neurologic deficit and death are rare events during DBS surgery. Tension pneumocephalus has been reported during DBS surgery. Complications are best managed when anticipated and prevented through proper patient selection, preparation and with appropriate care and medication.

CONCLUSION

With increasing elderly population, DBS will continue to increase in popularity for treatment of functional disorders with new indications emerging with time. The role of anaesthetist is also evolving in this kind of surgery with better drugs that do not interfere with the MER and lesser complications. The neuro-anaesthetist has to be aware of the unique requirements of his each patient with respect to his particular disease with its medications and severity of disorder and accordingly plan the awake or asleep technique for the surgery.

REFERENCES

1. Pereira EA, Green AL, Nandi D. Deep brain Stimulation: indications and evidence. Expert Rev Med Devices 2007;4:591-603.

2. Halpern C, Hurtig H, Jaggi J, Grossman M, Won M, Baltuch G. Deep brain stimulation in neurologic disorders. Parkinsonism Relat Disord 2007;13:1-16.

3. Wenning GK, Kiechl S, Seppi K. Prevalence of movement disorders in men and women aged 50-89 years (Bruneck Study Cohort): a population based study. Lancet Neurol 2005;4(12):815-20.

4. Dostrovsky JO,Lozano AM. Mechanisms of deep brain stimulation. Mov Disord 2002;17(3):S63-8.

5. Kirstin ME, Daniel JC. Anaesthetic considerations for epilepsy and functional neurosurgery. Anaesthesiology Clin 2012;30:241-268.

6. Volkmann J, Herzog J, Kopper F, Deuschl G. "Introduction to the programming of deep brain stimulators". Mov Disord 2002;17: S181-187.

7. Rezai AR,Kopell BH, Gross RE,Vitek J L,Sharan AD, Limousin P, Benabid A. Deep brain stimulation for Parkinson's disease:surgical issues. Mov Disord 2006;21:S197-218.

8. Kwan P, Brodie MJ. Early identification of refractory epilepsy. N Engl J Med 2000;342(5):314-9.

9. Costello TG, Cormack JR. Anaesthesia for awake craniotomy: a modern approach. J Clin Neurosci 2004;11(1):16-9.

10. Hutchinson WD, Lang AE, Dostrovsky JO, Lozano AM. Pallidal neuronal activity: implications for model of dystonia. Ann Neurol 2003;53:480-8.

11. Sanghera MK, Grossman RG, Kalhorn CG, Hamilton WJ, Ondo WJ, Jankovick J. Basal Ganglia neuronal discharge in primary and secondary dystonia in patients undergoing pallidotomy. Neurosurgery 2003;52;1358-73.

12. Benarroch EE. Subthalamic nucleus and its connections: anatomic substrate for the network effects of deep brain stimulation. Neurology 2008;70:1991-5.

13. Whittle IR, Midgley S, Georges H. Patient perceptions of "awake" brain tumour surgery. Acta Neurochir (Wien) 2005;147(3):275-7.

14. Khatib R, Ebrahim Z, Rezai A et al. Perioperative events during deep brain stimulation:the experience at Cleveland clinic. J Neurosurg Anesthesiol 2002;14(3):209-12.

MULTIPLE CHOICE QUESTIONS

1. **Deep Brain Stimulation is a minimally invasive neurosurgical procedure used for the treatment of the following except:**
   a. Essential tremors
   b. Parkinson's disease
   c. Dystonia
   d. Subarachnoid Haemorrhage

2. **True or False**
   a. Movement disorders can be significantly ameliorated by electrical stimulation of specific deep brain structures specific to each disorder
   b. DBS does not damage healthy brain tissue by destroying nerve cells
   c. DBS procedure blocks electrical signals from targeted areas in the brain with greatest relief between 50-100 Hz
   d. The target site for idiopathic parkinson's disease is Globus pallidus pars internal (GPi)

3. **Contra-indications for DBS surgery include**
   a. Tremor caused by multiple sclerosis
   b. Coagulopathy
   c. Refractory Epilepsy
   d. Idiopathic essential tremor

4. **The DBS system consists of the following components except**
   a. Implanted pulse generator (IPG)
   b. Lead (micro-electrodes)
   c. An extension (insulated wire)
   d. Electrocautery

5. **True or False**
   a. MRI of brain is done to obtain reference of internal anatomy to external coordinates to plan a linear trajectory from parietal surface to the target deep brain structures
   b. Patient is positioned either in supine or semi-sitting position on the operating table with the stereotactic frame (a rigid head frame to the patient's skull)
   c. A bur hole is made in the cranium for electrode insertion
   d. DBS surgeries are preferred to be done under General anaesthesia with controlled ventilation for all patients

6. **The following conditions are relative contraindications for Awake technique except:**
   a. Chronic Cough
   b. Obesity with severe OSA
   c. Mild anxiety
   d. Wheezing with gastroesophageal reflux.

7. **Following monitoring is essential for DBS procedures except**
   a. Pulse oximetry
   b. Exhaled CO2 monitoring
   c. ECG
   d. Rectal (core) Temperature monitoring

8. **The following nerves are blocked in Scalp block except**
   a. Infra and supra scapular nerve
   b. Supraorbital nerve and supratrochlear nerve
   c. Zygomaticotemporal nerve and auriculo-temporal nerve
   d. Lesser and greater occipital nerve and greater auricular nerve

9. **With respect to effect of anaesthetics on microelectrode recordings (MERs) state if True or False**
   a. Due to need of intra-operative neurophysiologic mapping (MER) and clinical testing of the patient, most of the DBS surgeries are preferred to be done under local anaesthesia and MAC
   b. Anaesthetics do not uniformly depress MERs but rather differ by disease as well as by deep brain stimuli
   c. All anaesthetics uniformly depress MERs
   d. The firing rates in the GPi nucleus is decreased with long pause in patients with dystonia when given general anaesthesia with propofol compared to mapping under local anaesthesia.

10. **Following anaesthetic drugs are used for conscious sedation during DBS surgery except:**
    a. Dexmedetomidine
    b. Propofol
    c. Atracurium
    d. Opioids

CHAPTER 10

ANAESTHESIA IMPLICATIONS IN EPILEPSY

Vidhu Bhatnagar, Rajshree Deopujari

Introduction

Epilepsy is a chronic neurological disorder, which leads to cognitive impairment, and progressively increases in frequency and severity of critical events characterized by recurrent seizures. Seizures can be explained as "a transient occurrence of signs and/or symptoms due to an abnormal excessive or synchronous neuronal activity in the brain." In simpler terms, a huge number of brain cells get activated abnormally, at the same time, behaving like an 'electrical storm' in the brain, during a seizure.

There are many factors which affect the nature, or the type of the seizure experienced by an individual:

(a) Patient's age

(b) Any prior injuries to the brain

(c) Congenital/genetic bearing

(d) Concurrent medications

(e) Sleep wake cycle disturbances and many others.

Classifying the seizures helps in treatment, management, prognosis, communication between clinicians, research etc.

History – Epilepsy was first described about 3,000 years ago in Akkadian, Mesopotamia (Iraq). The seizures were then attributed to the God of the Moon. William Gilbert, in the early 17th century, described the electrical phenomena responsible for epilepsy for the first time and rejected the supernatural theory. The word epilepsy is derived from the Greek verb "ëpilamvanein" which means attack or seizure.

Partial seizures start in one area or side of the brain and may or may not be associated with loss of awareness. Simple partial seizures are, when the patient is aware of the surroundings during the episode of seizure whereas complex partial seizure is denoted by some impaired awareness during the seizure. The patients may be confused, partially aware, or not aware of anything during the event of seizure episode. Generalized seizures commence simultaneously in both sides of the brain and usually have concomitant loss of awareness[1].

A revised basic classification (Fig. 1) was put forward in 2017 by International League against Epilepsy (ILAE) largely based upon the existing classification formulated in 1981.[2,3]

ILAE 2017 Classification of Seizure Types Expanded Version[1]

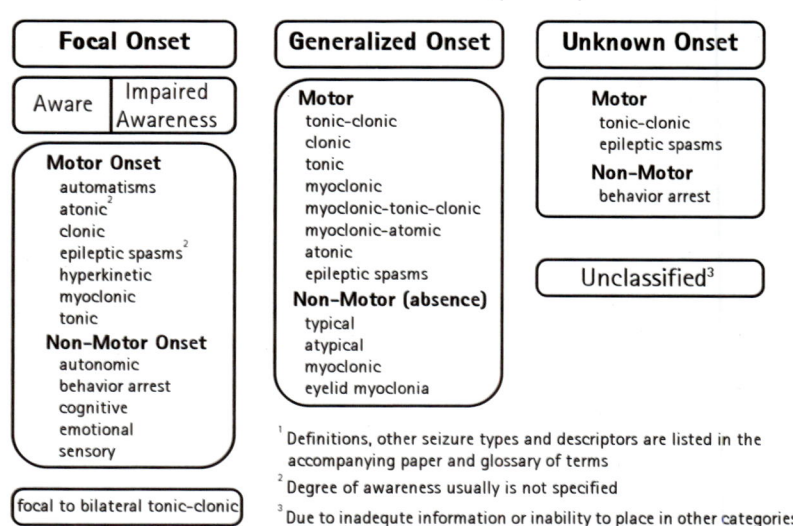

Fig. 1 : The New Basic Classification: 2017 Revised Classification of Seizures

Based on three key features so as to simplify the process of classifying seizures.
1. Where seizures begin in the brain 2. Level of awareness during a seizure 3. Other features of seizures

Epilepsy: Medical Management

Pathophysiology – The synchronous neuronal discharges which characterize the epileptic phenomenon, originate from one point of cerebral hemisphere (Focal seizures) and/ or may move to involve both hemispheres with loss of awareness (Generalized seizures). These synchronous and excessive neuronal impulses are triggered by excitatory stimuli (mediated by the major excitatory neurotransmitter, glutamate) or because of the deficiency of inhibitory neurotransmitter, GABA (gamma aminobutyric acid). The damage due to the generalized seizures is therefore because of influx of calcium ions during the depolarization and activation of excitatory amino acid receptors leading to acute cell necrosis leading to apoptosis in the long term.

Diagnosis: Based on:

(i) Clinical history: description of seizure activity by witnesses,

(ii) Physical examination: between seizures shows no abnormality but in the immediate postictal period, extensor plantar response may be observed.

(iii) Encephalographic findings

Triggers: Occasionally, there could be triggering factors like lack of sleep, poor diet, strong light or noise, stress of any kind, ingestion or withdrawal of alcohol or drugs etc. The differential diagnosis for seizures is given in Table 1. The diagnostic tests required for reaching a diagnosis are given in Table 2. The commonly used antiepileptic drugs for medical management of Epilepsy are discussed in Table 3.

Table 1: Differential diagnosis of epilepsy

Differential Diagnosis	Partial seizures	Generalized seizures
1	Transient ischemic attack	Syncope
2	aggressiveness attacks	Cardiac arrhythmias
3	Panic attacks	Brainstem ischemia

Table 2: Diagnostic Tests to diagnose Epilepsy

Diagnostic Tests	Neuroimaging Evaluation	Epileptiform EEG changes	Other tests
	CT scan	EEG	positron emission tomography (PET)
	MRI	Video EEG	single photon emission computed tomography (SPECT).
		functional magnetic resonance imaging (fMRI)	

Table 3: Medical Management: Commonly used Antiepileptic Drugs (AEDs)[4]

AED	Mechanism of Action	Side effects
Phenobarbital: long-term effect, barbiturate, effective against all types of epilepsy	1. Modulates the postsynaptic action of GABA 2. Blocks postsynaptic excitatory effect induced by glutamate receptors. 3. The GABAergic action increases duration of chloride channels opening thereby stimulating neuronal hyperpolarization, thus increasing the seizure threshold.	sedation, depression, hyperactivity (in children), confusion (in elderly), skin changes, megaloblastic anaemia, osteomalacia, nystagmus, ataxia, may precipitate attacks of porphyria. Not safe for pregnant women or neonates.
Valproic acid: It is effective in all generalized primary epilepsy and all convulsive epilepsy types.	It is a weak inhibitor of two enzymatic systems that inactivate GABA: the GABA trans- aminase and succinate semialdehyde dehydrogenase. It may potentiate the action of GABA by a postsynaptic action.	Tremors, weight gain, dyspepsia, nausea, vomiting, alopecia, hepatotoxicity encephalopathy teratogenicity, agranulocytosis, aplastic anaemia, Stevens-Johnson syndrome

Phenytoin: Effective in the treatment of partial and generalized epilepsies. It has a high therapeutic index. **Phosphofenitoin:** A prodrug of phenytoin	Regulates neuronal excitability, limits the spread of seizure activity from the seizure focus by blocking voltage-dependent sodium channels. It also acts on the second messenger systems as calmodulin and cyclic nucleotides	Nystagmus, Diplopia, Vestibular cerebellar dysfunction, nausea and vomiting, gingival hyperplasia, megaloblastic anaemia, agranulocytosis, aplastic anaemia, Stevens-Johnson syndrome, teratogenicity. It can cause congenital malformations if administered during pregnancy.
Carbamazepine: treatment of convulsive and non-convulsive partial epilepsy.	It changes the ionic conductance to sodium with a membrane stabilizing effect.	Sedation, diplopia, dizziness, neutropenia, nausea, drowsiness, diarrhoea, jaundice, oliguria, agranulo-cytosis, aplastic anaemia, allergic dermatitis, Stevens-Johnson syndrome.
Levetiracetam: Treatment of partial seizures as adjunctive or monotherapy	unclear, drug binds to protein A2, related to the release of glutamate in the synaptic vesicle	Drowsiness, weakness, dizziness, ataxia, amnesia, depression, anxiety, anorexia, diarrhoea, dyspepsia, skin changes and pancytopenia

Drug interactions: Interaction due to hepatic microsomal enzyme induction by Phenobarbital, Phenytoin, Carbamazepine. It exacerbates the hepatic metabolism of many liposoluble drugs: OCPs, beta-blockers, digoxin, anticoagulants, corticosteroids, other AEDs. The Valproic acid is an enzyme inhibitor, leading to a decrease in metabolic rate of phenytoin. On its chronic use the plasma concentration of phenobarbital increases by approximately 50%, probably due to inhibition of liver microsomal enzymes[5].

Limitations of medical therapy for epilepsy

The probability of achieving one-year freedom from seizures is between 63% and 79%, after regular administration of two to three drugs. Around 68% of patients with focal epilepsy are resistant to even multiple drug therapy. The resistance to drug therapy means that adequate trials of medical therapy with two "tolerated, appropriately chosen and used antiepileptic drug schedules have failed to achieve sustained seizure freedom"[6]. In view of these problems patients can be chosen for surgical management.

Epilepsy: Surgical Management

Preoperative assessment

1. Patient's history and physical examination findings,

2. Social circumstances, seizure syndrome and severity,

3. Diagnostic testing: basal investigations and disease specific evaluation.

Modalities used for evaluation of seizures:

A) Neuroimaging: Skull radiography, CT, MRI, PET CT, SPECT, Magnetoencephalography/magnetic source imaging (MEG/MSI)

B) Electroencephalography, video EEG

C) Neurocognitive/neuropsychological testing

D) Intracarotid amobarbital (Wada) test

E) Invasive intracranial monitoring e.g., intracranial EEG recording, or chronic electrocorticography [ECoG].

Surgical Plan

A surgical plan is established at a multidisciplinary team conference, to tailor the surgical approach according to the patient's disease.

(i) Definitive surgery – Aims to yield complete, or maximum improvement in seizures by physically removing seizure-producing cortex from the brain[7].

(ii) Palliative surgery – Aims to reduce seizure frequency whereas seizure freedom seems rare by disrupting pathways involved in seizure production and propagation[7].

Surgical techniques[7]

i) Anteromedial temporal resection (AMTR) – Most patients who get referred for AMTR have had epilepsy for approximately 20 years. This is most commonly performed procedure, with the best results and clearest indications:

   a) Complex partial seizures with semiology typical of mesial temporal lobe epilepsy

   b) Long standing complex partial and generalized tonic-clonic seizures.

ii) Corpus Callosotomy – This is a palliative procedure which aims to disrupt one or more major central nervous system (CNS) pathways used in seizure generalization, thereby decreasing the frequency and severity of primary or secondary generalized seizures. Indications: Not clearly defined

a) Performed to decrease the frequency of primarily and secondarily generalized seizures (i.e., tonic, clonic, tonic-clonic, and atonic seizures).

b) Callosotomy improves atonic seizures, but having atonic seizures does not guarantee that a patient will benefit from surgery.

c) Complex partial seizures may improve.

d) Aim to reduce seizure frequency and associated morbidity.

iii) Multiple subpial transection (MST) – This non-resective procedure aims to eradicate epileptiform discharges and correlative seizures from epileptogenic cortex by interrupting intracortical synchronization and thus attenuating or eliminating the epileptogenic potential of the seizure focus.

Indications:

a) Partial (focal) seizures

b) Seizures from chronic (Rasmussen) encephalitis that affects the speech-dominant hemisphere; however, results in these cases have not been good

c) Bilateral seizure foci in very difficult cases which are otherwise not considered for surgical intervention

iv) Functional hemispherectomy – The cortex is disconnected from all subcortical structures, and the interhemispheric commissures are divided. The goal of surgery is to isolate the affected brain from the healthier hemisphere thereby allowing the latter to function without the burden of seizures or interictal discharges.

Indications:

a) Injury and seizures limited to 1 hemisphere of the brain. The frequent seizures interfere with cognition and impair quality of life.

b) Rasmussen encephalitis

c) Sturge-Weber syndrome,

d) Cortical dysplasia,

e) Tuberous sclerosis

v) Ablative Procedures: Minimally invasive surgical procedures like radiofrequency ablation of the seizure producing focus by utilizing stereotactic probes implanted in brain have been undertaken with variable results. Minimally invasive (usually through a burr hole), probes are stereo tactically implanted in the brain for delivery of highly focused radiation, precise targeting of the well delineated lesion, minimum disruption of healthy brain tissue. Delayed benefits from surgery (after an interval of 10 to 12 months post-surgery) is main disadvantage.

Indication:

a) Well delineated lesion causing epilepsy

b) Some reports for being utilized in Mesial Temporal Lobe epilepsy

vi) Therapeutic devices: Electrical stimulation of vagus nerve, stimulation of deep brain cortex or deep brain nuclei have also been undertaken for treatment of epilepsy.

Therapeutic devices:

A. Vagal Nerve Stimulation[8]

Indication

i) Patients who have seizures refractory to medical management and who can't undergo respective surgery.

Procedure: A generator is placed subcutaneously, usually in the left chest area, and an electrode is placed with the end wrapping around the ipsilateral vagus nerve, connecting to the generator. The treating physician programs intermittent periods of stimulation into the generator. Voltage and timing of the stimulation can be altered using a wand device connected to a hand-held computer system to optimize individual devices. Thus, there is placement of helical electrodes on the left cervical vagus nerve, with intermittent stimulation which is provided by a small neurocybernetic prosthesis implanted subcutaneously in the upper chest. Most patients are stimulated using 20-30 Hz, a stimulation cycle of 30 seconds on, and 5 minutes off.

Mechanism of Action: Several theories exist regarding the therapeutic mechanisms of VNS, but it is certain that activation of vagal afferents through electrical stimulation influences seizure-related circuitry within the brain. This device increases the release of noradrenaline in the locus coeruleus,

Side Effects: voice changes (decreased volume or hoarseness), cough, and headache. Electromagnetic interference with the use of electrocautery and external defibrillator may take place, these devices can damage the electrodes and the generator of the vagus nerve stimulator. Similar care should be taken with patients with cardiac pacemakers.

B. Deep Brain Stimulation (DBS)[9]

Indications:

Medically refractory epilepsy

Procedure: Minimally invasive (through burr hole), stereo tactically implanted probes in brain for stimulation of anterior thalamus directly affects the ipsilateral hippocampus and/or mesial temporal lobe. Stimulation of one minute "on" with five minutes "off" mode or non-stimulation mode. (SANTE trial: Stimulation of Anterior Nucleus of the Thalamus in Epilepsy trial)

More studies required. Other areas of interest for DBS are cerebellum and subthalamic nuclei.

Anesthetic Management

Preoperative assessment and premedication

History: H/o an adequate control of the disease, a careful review of medical history, especially about the evolution of the disease, factors triggering the seizures (fasting, stress, sleep deprivation, alcohol and drugs), and comorbidities and their treatment. AEDs to continue till morning of surgery. Review the adverse effects and drug interactions of AEDs.

Induction: Thiopental, Benzodiazepines and, Propofol despite its pro-and anticonvulsant effects are commonly used. The use of ketamine and etomidate should be avoided. Isoflurane has the most potent anticonvulsant effect and Sevoflurane less than 1.5 MAC also seems safe in the epileptic patient. Though, Halothane and desflurane may be used safely but the use of nitrous oxide is controversial, and enflurane is contraindicated in those patients.

Meperidine can cause seizures through its metabolite normeperidine, and should be avoided. In the intraoperative period avoid changes that decrease the seizure threshold, such as hypoxia, hypotension, hypocapnia, and hyponatremia. The regional anesthesia techniques can be used safely in the epileptic patient. However, coagulation changes that may occur with the administration of most antiepileptic drugs should be evaluated[10,11].

Epilepsy surgery: Anaesthetic technique chosen is General anesthesia with airway secured endotracheally.

Sometimes, extra-operative mapping indicates that the ictal onset zone is close to or overlies critical motor or speech areas. On such occasions, using the advantages of awake operative language mapping (Awake craniotomy) may be helpful for resection of the epileptic focus. The utilization of Wada test intraoperatively is controversial but need for intraoperative electrocorticogram arises and resective surgery is performed, with the neurophysiologist present in the OR as necessary.

Premedication is with short acting opioids like Fentanyl (Remifentanil infusion if available)

Induction with Propofol and maintenance with inhalational agent (with a Minimum Alveolar Concentration of 0.5 to 0.6). Infusion of Propofol (50microgram/kg/min to 100 microgram/kg/min) for supplementing depth can be utilized.

Monitoring: consists of Heart Rate, ECG, Arterial Blood Pressure, temperature, capnography. The somatosensory evoked potentials (SSEPs) can be used during acute recording in the OR, using subdural strip electrodes to identify primary motor cortex.

Intraoperative Complications:

1. excessive bleeding from the superior sagittal sinus,
2. frontal lobe cerebral oedema,
3. venous infarction from sacrificing major bridging veins.
4. air embolism

At the end of surgery, patients can be reversed and woken up on table.

Postoperative Management

Re-start AEDs as soon as possible after surgery, according to the time of fasting. After surgery, whenever possible, the monitoring of plasma levels of antiepileptic drugs for at least 48 hours should be performed because there are significant variations in the apparent volume of distribution, linked to plasma proteins, hepatic metabolism and renal elimination[12].

Perioperative Seizures in Epileptic Patients

Seizures can happen up to 72 hours after surgery.

The risk is higher in patients with multiple AEDs or who had refractory seizures and in those patients who are administered GA. If the seizures get prolonged there could be brain damage from hypoxia, apnoea, prolonged postoperative mechanical ventilation, and delayed awakening from anesthesia. The seizure activity may even impair the physiological regulation of cardiac and respiratory activities and may lead to tachy-brady arrhythmias, apnoea, autonomic instability, pulmonary oedema and even sudden death.

Management: Maintain a patent airway and adequate ventilation and protect the patient from injuries resulting from seizures. Continuous monitoring is to be performed. If seizures last more than five minutes intravenous benzodiazepine (Lorazepam) should be given. Phenytoin (18 to 20 mg/kg given over 30 minutes) may be used.

Other drugs which can be used are:

1. Phenobarbital (15 mg/kg).
2. Midazolam (0.1-0.3 mg/kg in 2 to 5 minutes, followed by infusion of 0.05 to 0.4 mg.kg- per hr).
3. Propofol (1-2 mg/kg, followed infusion of 2-10 mg/kg/hour).
4. Thiopental (5-10 mg/kg in 10 minutes).
5. Lidocaine (1.5-2 mg/kg in 2-5 minutes, followed by infusion of 2-3mg/kg/hour for 12 hours).

Postoperative Complications

a)   hemogenic meningitis,

b)   ventriculitis,

c)   CSF leakage,

d)   hydrocephalus,

e)   Less common: stroke, infection, coma, or postoperative haemorrhage.

CONCLUSION

Epilepsy, as a chronic illness, has a huge impact on the life of the patient, creating hurdles in activities like sleep, safety while crossing roads, driving and swimming. It may also contribute to mood changes and have a bearing on relationships. Anything that disrupts the normal brain network of neuronal activity, which could be ranging from disease process to brain injury to abnormal development of brain may lead to this crippling illness. Well-designed imaging studies help us in localizing lesions and diagnosis. Medical management may give adequate control in some patients and the rest with intractable epilepsy may resort to surgical techniques for relief. The best advice is prompt diagnosis and early institution of management.

REFERENCES

1.   Berg AT, Berkovic SF, Brodie MJ, et al. Revised terminology and concepts for organization of seizures and epilepsies: report of the ILAE Commission on Classification and Terminology, 2005–2009, Epilepsia 2010;51: 676-85.

2.   Operational Classification of Seizure Types by the International League Against Epilepsy. 2017.

3.   Proposal for revised clinical and electroencephalographic classification of epileptic seizures. From the Commission on Classification and Terminology of the International League Against Epilepsy. Epilepsia1981; 22:489-501.

4.   Anderson J, Moor CC. Antiepileptic drugs: a guide for the non-neurologist, Clin Med 2010;10:54-8.

5.   Johannessen Landmark C, Patsalos PN. Drug interactions involving the new second- and third-generation antiepileptic drugs, Expert Rev Neurother, 2010;10:119-40.

6.   Kwan P, Arzimanoglou A, Berg AT, et al. Definition of drug resistant epilepsy: consensus proposal by the ad hoc Task Force of the ILAE Commission on Therapeutic Strategies. Epilepsia2010; 51:1069– 77.

7.   Wiebe S, Jette N. Epilepsy surgery utilization: Who, when, where, and why? CurrOpinNeurol2012; 25:187–93.

8.   Tecoma ES, Iragui VJ. Vagus nerve stimulation use and effect in epilepsy: What have we learned? Epilepsy Behav2006; 8:127–36.

9.   Quigg M, Rolston J, Barbaro NM. Radiosurgery for epilepsy: clinical experience and potential antiepileptic mechanisms. Epilepsia2012; 53:7–15.

10. Kofke WA. Anesthetic management of the patient with epilepsy or prior seizures, Curr Opin Anesthesiol 2010;23:391-9.

11. Maranhao MV, Gomes EA, Carvalho PE. Epilepsy and Anesthesia. Rev Bras Anestesiol. 2011; 61:232-41.

12. Téllez-Zenteno JF, Hernández Ronquillo L, Moien-Afshari F, et al. Surgical outcomes in lesional and non-lesional epilepsy: a systematic review and meta-analysis. Epilepsy Res 2010; 89:310-8.

MULTIPLE CHOICE QUESTIONS

1. **The new basic classification (2017 Revised Classification of Seizures) is based on one of these key features so as to simplify the process of classifying seizures**
   a. Synchronous neuronal discharges
   b. Level of awareness during a seizure
   c. Sleep wake cycle disturbances
   d. Any prior injuries to the brain

2. **The synchronous and excessive neuronal impulses are triggered by**
   a. Excitatory stimuli (mediated by the major excitatory neurotransmitter, glutamate)
   b. Excessive inhibitory neurotransmitter
   c. Excessive concentration of GABA
   d. None of the above

3. **Differential Diagnosis of Seizures are**
   a. Transient ischemic attack
   b. Diabetes Mellitus
   c. Alcohol Withdrawal
   d. Persistent hypertension

4. **Diagnostic Tests for Epilepsy is**
   a. Functional Magnetic Resonance Imaging
   b. Ultrasonography
   c. Biochemical profile
   d. X-ray

5. **Various surgical techniques utilized for epilepsy are**
   a. Multiple subpial transactions
   b. Functional hemisperectomy
   c. None of the above
   d. Both a and b

6. **In Vagal Nerve Stimulation procedure for epilepsy**
   a. there is placement of helical electrodes on the left cervical vagus nerve, with persistent stimulation
   b. there is placement of helical electrodes on the right cervical vagus nerve, with intermittent stimulation
   c. There is placement of helical electrodes on the left cervical vagus nerve, with intermittent stimulation
   d. None of the above

7. **Anesthetic agents which can be utilized for epileptic patients are**
   a. Ketamine
   b. Enflurane
   c. Meperidine
   d. Thiopentone

8. **Intraoperative seizure activity may lead to**
   a. Delayed awakening
   b. Cardiac arrhythmias
   c. Apnea
   d. All of the above

9. **Postoperative complications in epilepsy surgery could be**
   a. Hydrocephalus
   b. Respiratory depression
   c. Hypothermia
   d. Hypotension

10. **What is true for Corpus Callosotomy?**
   a. This is a definitive procedure
   b. This aims to disrupt one or more major central nervous system pathways used in seizure generalization
   c. The cortex is disconnected from all subcortical structures
   d. The goal of surgery is to isolate the affected brain from the healthier hemisphere.

CHAPTER 11

MANAGEMENT OF CEREBRAL ANEURYSMS AND ARTERIOVENOUS MALFORMATIONS

Pratima Kothare, Smita Sharma

Introduction

Aneurysm:

A Cerebral **aneurysm** is an excessive localized enlargement of a brain **artery** caused by weakness in the arterial wall. It can be congenital or acquired secondary to degenerative changes in muscular and elastic component of vessel wall occurring at branching points of major cerebral vessels where there is a turbulent flow[1].

Aneurysms can be classified both by size and by shape:

According to size:	According to the shape:
Small < 12 mm diameter	Fusiform
Large 12 to 25 mm diameter	Saccular (Berry)
Giant 25 to 50 mm diameter	

Subarachnoid hemorrhage:

Aneurysm rupture is one of the commonest causes of Subarachnoid hemorrhage. The other common cause is traumatic injury.

AVM (Arterio-venous malformation):

An AVM is a tangle of abnormal and poorly formed blood vessels (arteries and veins) generally congenital, manifesting before 40 years of age. A cerebral AVM is of concern because of the damage they cause when they bleed.

ANEURYSM

LOCATION (Fig. 1 & 2)

1) 40% in the region of Anterior Cerebral artery

2) 55% in the Middle Cerebral artery origin or bifurcation

3) 4% at origin of Posterior Communicating artery

4) 0.5 to 1% in the Basilar artery

5) A small number at the internal Carotid artery bifurcation

There can be multiple aneurysms and a patient can have both aneurysm and AVM as well.

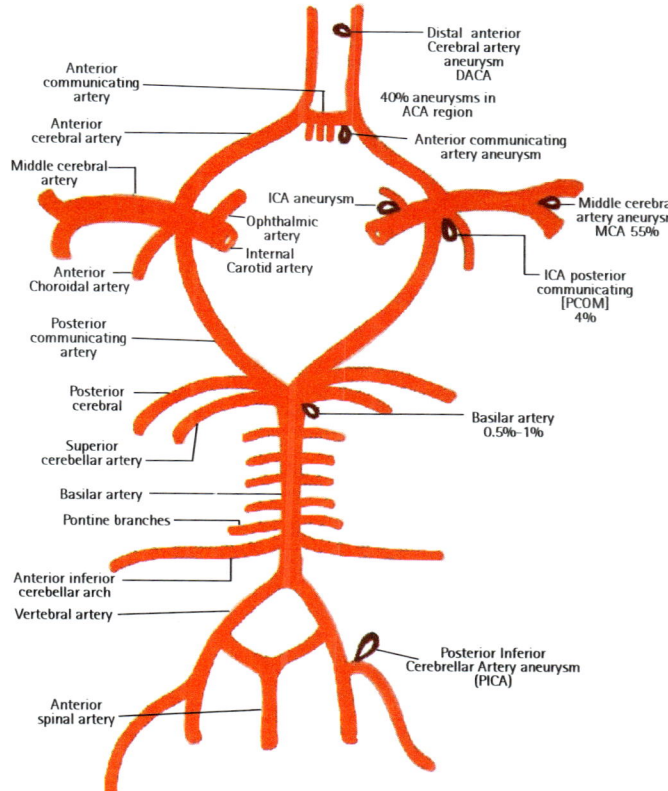

Fig. 1. *Circle of Willis* (Symbolic Line Diagram)

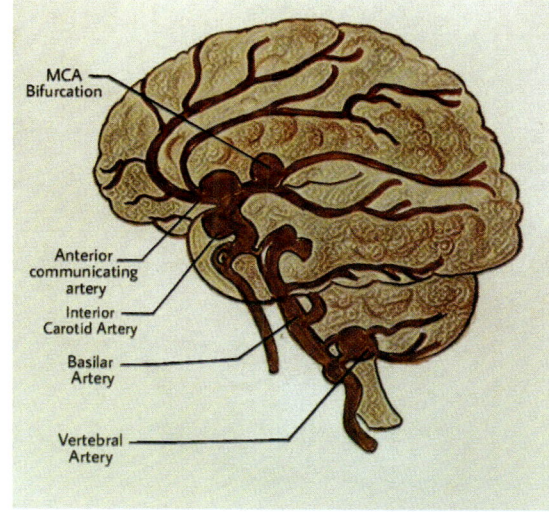

Fig. 2. Location of Aneurysms *(Symbolic Line Diagram)*

Why should an aneurysm be treated?

Both ruptured and unruptured aneurysms should be treated by clipping or coiling. Unruptured aneurysms have a 1-2% risk of Hemorrhage. There is a significant risk of disability/ death if the aneurysm ruptures. The rupture will lead to subarachnoid hemorrhage. The overall morbidity and mortality following subarachnoid hemorrhage is significantly high. 30-day morbidity is 30% and mortality is about 50%[2]. Hence both rupture and unrupture aneurysm should be treated by clipping or coiling. In the case of ruptured aneurysms, the chances of re-bleed are about 50%.

Causes of severe disability / death after aneurysm rupture are:

a) Extreme neuronal injury after initial bleeding

b) Re-bleeding

c) Vasospasm leading to profound Cerebral ischemia and hence infarction.

Subarachnoid haemorrhage

Ruptured Aneurysms lead to subarachnoid hemorrhage. A patient with SAH may be classified or graded according to the well documented grading systems. These systems can be clinical or radiological.

Clinical grading systems:

Hunt and Hess (1968)

I – Asymptomatic or mild headache

II – Moderate-severe headache, meningism and no weakness

III – Mild alteration in mental status

IV – Depressed level of consciousness and/or hemiparesis

V – Posturing or comatose

It is subjective and helps to evaluate surgical risk. If there is a serious systemic disease or severe vasospasm on angiography the grade increases by 1[3].

Hunt and Kosnick modification (1974) :

0 – Unruptured Aneurysm

1 – Ruptured aneurysm with minimal headache

1a – Grade for a fixed neurological deficit in the absence of other signs of SAH

2 – Moderate to severe headache no deficit other than cranial nerve palsy

3 – Drowsiness /confusion or mild focal deficit

4 – Stupor, significant hemiparesis, early decerebration, vegetative disturbances

5 – Deep coma, decerebrate rigidity, moribund

WFNS (1998)[4]

I   – GCS 15, no motor deficit

II – GCS 13-14, no motor deficit

III – GCS 13-14, motor deficit

IV – GCS 7-12 +/- motor deficit

V   – GCS 3-6 +/- motor deficit

It is more objective, but reliant on accurate GCS

Radiological grading systems[5]

Fisher (1980)

I   – No blood

II – Diffuse deposition of SAH without clots or layers of blood >1mm

III – Localized clots and/or vertical layers of blood 1mm or > thickness

IV – Diffuse or no subarachnoid blood but intracerebral or intraventricular clots

It is a useful scale to predict likelihood of vasospasm.

Hess and Hunt prognosis prediction[6]

Grade	Mortality%	Morbidity%
0	0-2	0-2
1	2-5	2
2	5-10	7
3	5-10	25
4	25-30	25
5	40-50	35-40

Once a subarachnoid bleed is detected the investigation should proceed towards detecting/ruling out an aneurysm or AVM.

Diagnosis

- CT scan
- MRI
- MR Angiography
- DSA-gold standard

DEFINITIVE TREATMENT OF CEREBRAL ANEURYSMS

- Surgical Clipping
- Endovascular Coiling
- SAH-Evacuation of hematoma

Clipping of Aneurysm

The goal of surgical clipping is to isolate an aneurysm from the normal circulation without blocking any small perforating arteries nearby.

A small titanium clip is placed across the base or neck of the aneurysm to block its blood supply. The aneurysm should be totally isolated from the circulation. These clips are MRI compatible.

Endovascular Coiling

80% of aneurysms can be treated by platinum coils. It may be the treatment of choice in unruptured aneurysm. It is done in the in the DSA suite using fluoroscopy. Being noninvasive it is more suitable option for the elderly and for the patients with co-morbidities.

It is best suited for posterior circulation aneurysms particularly the basilar aneurysm.

The procedure is done under general anaesthesia and the considerations for anaesthesia remain the same as clipping. The safety of anaesthesia is somewhat compromised when done in the DSA suite as it may not have all the facilities and monitoring as the operation theatre.

The short-term disadvantage is the need for a repeat procedure if the neck is not adequately plugged. In the long-term, there is a high possibility of recurrence of aneurysm.

TIMING OF SURGERY AFTER SAH[7]

EARLY OPERATION: Within 48 hours

- Prevents complications of re-bleeding
- Decreases risk of Vasospasm by evacuating all blood

INTERMEDIATE PERIOD: 7–10 days

- Maximum risk of Re-bleeding and Vasospasm
- Worst surgical outcomes

LATE OPERATION: 11–14 days

- Brain edema is resolved by treatment so better dissection
- Stabilized aneurysmal clot
- Adjuvant medical conditions treated
- Hence good surgical outcomes

Surgeon's requirements for Clipping of Aneurysm

- Steroids -Dexamethasone 4 – 10 mg
- Lumbar drain to facilitate brain relaxation
- Anticonvulsants
- Good brain relaxation

- Monitoring temporary Clipping time and reperfusion time before re clipping
- Brain protection measures
- Intraoperative Indocyanine dye
- Adenosine if indicated
- SSEP monitoring

ANAESTHESIA CONSIDERATIONS IN ANEURYSM SURGERY

Anaesthesia for aneurysm clipping is a challenging clinical scenario. It calls for very precise and tight control of hemodynamic and brain management with a narrow margin of safety and error.

Preoperative understanding of relevant systems affected

This is very important to conduct a smooth and safe anesthetic.

CNS

(a) Intracranial pressure correlates with clinical grades. Only the patients of Grade I and II have normal ICP. Grade III onward the ICP is raised

Causes of raised ICP in Cerebral Aneurysms

- Increase in Blood Pressure.
- SAH
- Formation of Blood clot causing a space occupying effect
- Intracerebral and intraventricular hematoma
- Hydrocephalous
- Vasospasm decreases the CBF so exacerbates ICP
- Hypovolemia
- Compensatory vasodilatation in distal vessels

It is essential not to normalize the ICP too rapidly as it may increase the transmural pressure gradient (TMP) across the aneurysm wall and may cause it to rupture. CPP of 60-80 mmhg is a reasonable goal.

(b) Autoregulation

It is the ability of the blood vessels to maintain CBF at a relatively constant level by altering cerebrovascular resistance (CVR) despite wide fluctuations in cerebral perfusion pressure (CPP). SAH disturbs this autoregulatory mechanism. The degree of impairment of the autoregulatory capacity increased significantly with the severity of the SAH. It would be ideal to monitor autoregulation[8].

In absence of monitoring this impaired autoregulation should be kept in mind throughout the operation starting from induction. This is done by keeping a keen attention to the blood pressure and cerebral perfusion pressure levels which are to be kept in a very tight range as close to the pre-induction state as possible. The cerebrovascular response to hyperventilation is generally preserved after SAH and patients can tolerate hyperventilation upto a PCO_2 of 25 mm Hg[9].

(c) Intravascular volume and electrolyte status

The degree of hypovolemia correlates with grades of SAH and this hypovolemia increases risk of vasospasm. Hyponatremia may also trigger vasospasm. Hence a low sodium may be used for the prediction of an impending vasospasm[10]. Patients should be given normal saline as IV infusion. There can also be hypokalemia and hypocalcemia.

(d) CVS

SAH causes sympathetic hyperactivity leading to increased norepinephrine levels. ECG changes in SAH are mostly of neurogenic origin. An echocardiogram and cardiac enzyme testing can be done to rule out a cardiogenic cause. There can be a variety of ECG changes and they primarily reflect repolarization abnormalities involving the ST segment, T wave, U wave, and QTc interval. Patients can also be at a high risk for malignant ventricular arrhythmias, including ventricular tachycardia, and ventricular fibrillation, particularly if the QT interval is prolonged.

(e) Respiratory system

Respiratory disturbances are not common but there should be high index of suspicion for Neurogenic pulmonary edema and Aspiration Pneumonia. It is important to distinguish between the two as treatment approach is very different.

Preoperative evaluation and preparation

A thorough medical examination to understand the above mentioned systemic involvement is necessary. All the relevant investigations should be sent out immediately. As the surgical decisions are being planned the hemodynamic, physiological and biochemical optimization should be done.

Surgical preparation includes the clinical grading of SAH and CT scan and DSA to understand the underlying pathology.

Communication and planning with the neurosurgeon: This is a very important part of aneurysm surgery.

- Position of the patient
- Use of clamps
- Need for neuronavigation

- Plan of temporary clipping and permissible clip time
- Need to use ICG dye
- Use of adenosine
- Post-operative plan to extubate or ventilate

Anaesthetic goals

- Prevention of rupture of aneurysm during induction. This is done avoiding increase in Transmural pressure gradient. Maintain adequate CPP and cerebral oxygenation (TMP and CPP are determined by same equation MAP- ICP)
- To keep the brain slack
- Brain protection when indicated
- Prompt awakening and assessment in SAH I, II, III

Induction of anaesthesia

Premedication must be given judiciously so that patient is calm and sedated while taking the arterial line. Fentanyl and midazolam can be used. Glycopyrrolate should be avoided. Remifentanyl or sufentanyl can be used if available.

Dexamethasone to be given to reduce brain edema.

Arterial cannulation and display of arterial BP during induction would be recommended in most cases.

Induction can be done with propofol or thiopentone or etomidate. Etomidate should be an option only when it hemodynamic benefits justify its use.

Intubation is to be done with a non-depolarizing agent- vecuronium, rocuronium atracurium or cisatracurium. It is very important to ensure that the BP does not deviate much from baseline. Xylocard and xyclocaine topical spray may be used to attenuate the sympathetic response to intubation. If needed, esmolol or labetolol can be used to control BP.

If there is a strong reason to use succinylcholine it is safe to use in acute SAH but to be avoided in sub-acute stages with motor deficits and raised ICP. If using succinylcholine, it is prudent to precede it with defasciculating dose of a nondepolarizing agent.

- Endotracheal tube: It may be plain cuffed or flexometalic depending on position of neck & need to ventilate post operatively
- Vascular access
- Two peripheral veins 20/18/16 gauge
- Central access with Triple Lumen Internal Jugular or Subclavian.
- A Lumbar drain may be inserted if needed keeping a strict watch on hemodynamics during the process

Care during positioning :

During neck positioning special attention should be given to airway pressure and venous engorgement. A flexometalic tube to be used when indicated.

Monitoring

Routine	Optional Monitoring	Advanced monitoring
ECG	BIS	Transcranial doppler
Arterial BP	TOF	SSEP
SaO_2		Jugular venous oximetry
$EtCO_2$		Cerebral oximetry
U/O		
CVP		
Core temperature		

Maintenance of anaesthesia

$N_2O + O_2$ or air $+ O_2$ remains a topic of debate and the anaesthetist can make a choice depending on other factors. The vasodilator effects of N_2O must be kept in mind. Balanced general anaesthesia should be used with following options.

IV agents	Inhalational agents
Propofol	Isoflurane
Fentanyl	Sevoflurane
Dexmedetomidine	Desflurane
Muscle relaxant	

If additional BP control is needed labetolol or esmolol can be used. Nitroglycerine to be avoided.

Mannitol, furesamide and lumbar drainage may be used to give a slack brain.

Controlled Hyperventilation used to decrease CBV, Mild Hypocapnia 30-35mm Hg before Dura is open, Moderate Hypocapnia 25-30 mm Hg after Dura is open & Normocapnia 35 mm Hg after Clipping is complete. $EtCO_2$ values should be continuously and vigilantly monitored

IV fluids

Crystalloid fluids are routinely used. Normovolemia is to be maintained even if induced hypotension is planned to maintain CPP. No glucose containing solutions to be infused as hyperglycemia aggravates both local and global transient cerebral ischemia[11] Colloid of preference should be 5% Albumin, HES fluids should be used with caution as they interfere with coagulation.

Clipping of aneurysm:

These are critical and crucial minutes of the surgery. Clipping of aneurysm can be a direct clipping after dissection or may involve the process of temporary clipping (temporary arterial occlusion).

Measures to be taken during temporary clipping:

Note the exact ischaemia time and inform the surgeon every 3 minutes or as per discussion with surgeon. Blood pressure should be kept on the higher side during this period. Pharmacoprotection with thiopentone 1 to 2mg/kg, Propofol 1 to 2 mg/kg or Etomidate 0.5 mg/kg with a constant infusion of 12 mg/min Dexamethasone may be repeated.

Thiopentone is the gold standard but causes delayed recovery.

Some studies are emerging supporting the role of etomidate but the disadvantages should be kept in mind.

While the advantages of hypothermia are debatable the patient should be allowed to spontaneously reach a temperature of 34 to 35 degress[13].

It is always a good idea to discuss with the surgeon what is the clip time that is permissible for that case and how he should be cautioned.

Additional considerations:

SSEP:

SSEP monitoring whenever available helps to guide the surgeon for impending ischaemia.

Indocyanine dye:

Use of Indocyanine green dye after clipping is done where the facilities are available. This helps to verify that the aneurysm is completely clipped and the rest of the circulation and perfusion is not disturbed in any way. The dye is safe. It must be given in the central venous line preferably dedicated for this. 5 cc of the dye is given at a time. The dye should be flushed slowly with distilled water. Too fast an injection will make the dye disappear quickly. It can be repeated 2 to 3 times.

Adenosine

Adenosine induced asystole for cerebral aneurysm was first described by Groff et al in 1999 in posterior circulation aneurysms. This is used for transient circulatory arrest before dissection and clipping of giant or complex aneurysms[14]:

- Adenosine has a very short half-life of < 10 seconds
- Dose upto 0.3-0.4mg/kg is safe
- After IV injection, effect on heart rate is seen within 10 to 20 seconds

Management of cerebral aneurysms and arteriovenous malformations

- Asystole occurs after 30 seconds and reaches a plateau between 40-60 seconds

- Hypotension for one minute

- Multiple doses may be required

- Repeat only after 3 to 10 minutes

- Recovery to Sinus rhythm is spontaneous

- Some may develop atrial fibrillation and may require Amiodarone treatment

Advantages of adenosine

A 30-60 seconds of controlled hypotension which gives a bloodless field of 360^0 manipulation of giant / difficult location aneurysm and briefly reduces the CPP and turgor of the aneurysm, hence chances of bursting are reduced. Useful if there is a rupture and surgeon can get a bloodless field for a minute.

Disadvantages of adenosine:

Dysrhythmia and coronary insufficiency- it may cause a rise in Troponin T levels and may have persistent hypotension due to systemic vasodilation, can cause bronchoconstriction and hence contraindicated in COPD and asthma.

Precautions: External defibrillator pads to be applied to all patients for cardioversion.

Management of intraoperative aneurysm rupture

The management of rupture on the operation table needs fine balance between maintaining cerebral perfusion and giving the surgeon a relatively bloodless field to complete the clipping.

- Transient induction of hypotension but maintaining volume (CVP and CPP)

- Use of IV fluids and blood transfusion. Colloids if needed

- Brain protection

- Steroids to control edema

- Communication with the surgeon

- Consider the use of adenosine in experienced hands[15]

An aneurysm is not expected to rupture during coiling most of the time. The incidence of rupture is 2 to 4 %. This has come down due to the use of balloon remodeling technique. Haemostasis can be done with the balloon. Heparin which is routinely used is reversed. The bleeding does not cause haemodynamic instability.

Giant aneurysms

Aneurysms > 2.5 cms, lack of anatomical neck, with atheromatous changes and perforators originating from neck come under this catergory.

If these are to be operated then the use proximal and distal temporary occlusion to collapse the sac is done. Transient circulatory arrest using adenosine or profound hypothermia is also considered for these[16].

These procedures had a high morbidity and mortality. Fortunately, today most of these patients have better outcomes due to coiling treatment. Another option is trapping of the aneurysm. Trapping can also be done if there is an inability to clip after a rupture.

Reversal of anaesthesia and extubation

- Grade I and II with Uneventful Surgical Clipping should be extubated

- Grade III SAH with difficult surgery to be decided on clinical picture

- Grade IV and V SAH should be ventilated

- Intra operative rupture may require ventilation

- Vertebrobasilar aneurysms are slow to recover therefore prudent to ventilate.

- Prevention of coughing during extubation with lidocaine 1.5mg/kg

- Hypertension should also be controlled beyond 180mm Hg. It is better to monitor arterial BP and use short acting drug such as esmolol.

Post-operative care

- Avoid hypotension. BP should be maintained around 160 mm Hg systolic to prevent vasospasm. Hypertension < 180mm can be accepted, BP > 200 mm must be treated as it may cause Hemorrhage or edema.

- Nimodipine to be given orally by Ryle's tube 60 mg 4 times a day. Nimodipine should not be omitted if BP drops. Instead BP should be maintained using noradrenalin

- Arterial BP to be displayed for 48 hours

- CVP should be maintained at a minimum of 10 cms H_2O

Triple H (Hypertension, Hypervolumia and Haemodilution) is now replaced with the Hypertension and Euvolemia[17]. All these measures are implemented for prevention of vasospasm.

Vasospasm

Clinically Vasospasm occurs after about 4 to 9 days of SAH, It does not occur later than two weeks after aneurysmal rupture.

Symptoms are diminution of level of consciousness or development of focal deficits. There should be a high index of suspicion to pick up vasospasm and do an immediate DSA. Intra-arterial Nimodipine is injected during DSA. The additional measures are aggressively continued.

Arteriovenous malformations

AVM is an abnormal collection of dysplastic vessels, 75% of which are supratemporal. There is a central nidus surrounded by dilated draining veins. In the nidus, the blood flows from dilated arteries directly to veins with no capillary bed or neural parenchyma. 10 % have associated Aneurysms.

They present with headache, seizures, focal deficits and raised ICP.

Diagnosis: MRI, DSA.

Treatment:

- Surgical excision

- Endovascular Onyx embolization

- Stereotactic radiosurgery

Principles of Anaesthesia for AVM resection are same as in SAH / Aneurysms Clipping. Embolisation also requires General Aneasthesia.

Expected Intra-operative Complications:

- Severe bleeding

- Slow insidious bleeding-blood should be given

- Venous Hemorrhage

- Cerebral edema

- Hypertension

- Seizures

Normal pressure breakthrough perfusion (NPBP)

This is a dreaded complication that can occur after an uneventful surgery. It presents as cerebral edema and hemorrhage in the adjacent brain tissue. The hemodynamic basis for this phenomenon is disordered autoregulation causing NPBP and obstruction of venous drainage leading to occlusive hyperemia[18]. NPBP occurs both after excision of AVM and embolization.

Treatment is supportive with controlled hyperventilation, steroids, and osmotic dehydrating agents to control raised ICP. Blood pressure reduction to the lower levels of the normal cerebral perfusion curve and the use of barbiturates is advocated. Once the storm is controlled the patient is taken up for hematoma evacuation. Prognosis is guarded with improvement seen in some patients.

CONCLUSION

Aneurysm and AVM surgery are one of the most challenging clinical situations in neuroanaesthesia. It requires a deep understanding of the underlying pathology and multisystemic implications. It also involves a very committed participation by the anaesthetist in the operation theatre and for a few days post operatively. Vasospasm is a dreaded complication of an otherwise successful surgery and all measures for its prevention and early detection should be taken. Neuroradiological treatment is on the rise and these procedures require high level of expertise as a neuroanaesthetist. Thus, it is important to be updated with the recent advances in aneurysm and AVM surgery that have taken place in the last decade to have a successful outcome in our patients.

REFERENCES

1) Stehbens WE. Etiology of intracranial berry aneurysms. J Neurosurg. 1989 Jun;70(6):823-31.

2) Mark J Kotapka, Eugene S Flamm. Editors James E Cottrell, David Smith. Anaesthesia and Neurosurgery 3rd Ed 1994.

3) Hunt WE, Hess RM. Surgical risk as related to time of intervention in the repair of intracranial aneurysms. J Neurosurg 1968; 28:14–20.

4) Drake CG. Report of World Federation of Neurological Surgeons Committee. on a universal subarachnoid hemorrhage scale. J Neurosurg 1988; 68:985-6.

5) Fisher C M, Kistler J P, Davis J M; Relation of Cerebral Vasospasm to subarachnoid hemorrhage visualizes by Computerized tomographic scanning. Neurosurgery 6:1, 1980.

6) Hunt WE, Hess RM. Surgical risk as related to time of intervention in the repair of intracranial aneurysms. J Neurosurg 1968; 28:14–20.

7) Kassell N F, Toner J C, Jane J et al the International Co Operative study on the timing of aneurysm surgery. part 2 Surgical results J Neurosurgery 73:37-47 1990.

8) Schmieder K, Möller F, Engelhardt M, Scholz M, Schregel W, Christmann A, Harders A. Dynamic cerebral autoregulation in patients with ruptured and unruptured aneurysms after induction of general anesthesia. ZentralblNeurochir. 2006 May;67(2):81-7.

9) Dernbach PD, Little JR, Jones SC, Ebrahim ZY. Altered cerebral autoregulation and CO_2 reactivity after aneurysmal subarachnoid hemorrhage. Neurosurgery. 1988 May;22(5):822-6.

10) Chandy D, Sy R, Aronow WS, Lee WN, Maguire G, Murali R. Hyponatremia and cerebrovascular spasm in aneurysmal subarachnoid hemorrhage. Neurol India. 2006; 54:273–5.

11) Lam Am, Winner, Cullen BF, et al: Hyperglycemia and neurological outcome in patients with head injury, J Neurosurgery 75 :545,1991.

12) Rosenwasser RH, Jimenez DF, Wending WW, Carlsson C: Routine use of etomidate and temporary vessel occlusion during aneurysm surgery. Neurol Res 13:224–228, 1991.

13) Pong RP, Lam AM. Anesthetic management of cerebral aneurysm surgery, editors. Cottrell's and Young's Neuroanesthesia. 5th ed. Philadelphia: Mosby Elsevier; 2010. pp. 218–46.

14) Guinn NR, McDonagh DL, Borel CO, et al. Adenosine-induced transient asystole for intracranial aneurysm surgery: a retrospective review. *J NeurosurgAnesthesiol*. 2011 Jan;23(1):35–40.

15) Luostarinen T1, Takala RS, Niemi TT, Katila AJ, Niemelä M, Hernesniemi J, Randell. T. Adenosine-induced cardiac arrest during intraoperative cerebral aneurysm rupture.

World Neurosurg. 2010 Feb;73(2):79-83;

16) Botterell EH, Lougheed WM, Scott JW, Vandewater SL. Hypothermia, and interruption of carotid, or carotid and vertebral circulation, in the surgical management of intracranial aneurysms. J Neurosurg. 1956 Jan;13(1):1-42.

17) Treggiari MM1; Participants in the International Multi-disciplinary Consensus Conference on the Critical Care Management of Subarachnoid Hemorrhage. Hemodynamic management of subarachnoid hemorrhage. Neurocrit Care. 2011 Sep;15(2):329-35.

18) Kumar S, Kato Y, Sano H, Imizu S, Nagahisa S, Kanno T. Normal perfusion pressure breakthrough in arteriovenous malformation surgery: The concept revisited with a case report. Neurol India 2004; 52:111-5.

MULTIPLE CHOICE QUESTIONS

1. Aneurysm clip is made of
   a. Gold
   b. Silver
   c. Titanium
   d. Platinum

2) The following treatment is not useful in providing brain relaxation in aneurysm surgery
   a. Steroids
   b. Lumbar drain
   c. Balanced anaesthesia
   d. Anti convulsants

3) The following drug should not be used to control hypertension in aneursym surgery
   a. Esmolol
   b. Nitroglycerine
   c. Labetolol
   d. Dexmedetomidine

4) The following drug is used to cause transient cardiac standstill for clipping of giant aneursym
   a. Atenolol
   b. Adenosine
   c. Verampil
   d. Xylocard

5) How many days after subarachnoid heamorrhage does vasospasm commonly occur
   a. within 48 hours
   b. 2 to 7 days
   c. 4 to 9 days
   d. after 1 month

6) The following IV fluid should not be used in aneursym surgery
   a. Lactated ringer
   b. Normal saline
   c. Colloids
   d. Glucose containing fluid

7) The following drug is used to as study the vasculature after clippping of aneurysm
   a. Thiopentone
   b. Remifentanyl
   c. Iohexol
   d. Indocyanine

8) The following is not a treatment for AVM
   a. Clipping
   b. Surgical excision
   c. Endovasular coiling
   d. Radiosurgery

9) The following is a common but dreaded complication in spite of a successful aneurysm clipping
   a. Hypertension
   b. Vasospasm
   c. Cardiac arrhythmias
   d. Normal pressure breakthrough perfusion

10) The following drug is used to treat vasospasm
    a. Nimodipine
    b. Atenolol
    c. Propofol
    d. Dexamethosone

CHAPTER 12

AIRWAY IN NEUROSURGICAL PATIENTS

Tasneem Dhansura, Nitin Bhorkar

Introduction

The demands for airway management in neuroanaesthesia require expertise in the various modes of securing the airway while considering the patient's physiological requirements as well as the unique surgical demands. The primary goal during induction is a smooth transition to anesthesia while maintaining hemodynamic stability. Even brief episodes of hypoxia and hypercapnia cause cerebral vasodilation and are especially deleterious in the neurosurgical patient.

Hemodynamics, Hypoxia and Airway-why is it relevant in neuroanaesthesia?

ICP, mean arterial pressure (MAP) and cerebral perfusion pressure are interrelated by an equation [1]:

Cerebral perfusion pressure CPP = MAP - ICP. Factors which affect any of these will lead to deleterious effects.

CNS requires a constant blood supply as it lacks substrate reserve and even brief episodes of hypoxia can lead to cerebral vasodilation which can prove to be deleterious in neurosurgical patients.

On the other hand, the hyperventilation may cause vasoconstriction and worsen cerebral ischemia.

In addition, hypoxemia may lead to secondary brain injury and increase morbidity and mortality. The CBF is normally 50 mL/100 g tissue/min and bood flow of less than 15 mL/100 g/min will eventually lead to cell death.

The laryngoscopy and intubation, if improperly performed, may severely compromise intracranial dynamics and increase morbidity, especially, in patients with decreased spatial compensatory capabilities, and cerebral edema with cerebral ischemia. Both preoperative history and physical examination and computed tomography or magnetic resonance imaging scans give valuable information into the possibility of increased ICP (>10 mm midline shift and/or brain edema indicate markedly increased ICP) [1].

An increase in ICP during intubation can occur due to a reflex sympathetic response to laryngoscopy, resulting in an increase in catecholamines. This in turn increases the heart rate and blood pressure causing intracranial hypertension with the loss of cerebral autoregulation. Another reason for raised ICP would be a direct cough reflex from airway manipulation.

The routine use of lignocaine pre-treatment to prevent, these reflexes remains controversial. A recent review of the literature cited several studies in which the reflex sympathetic effects of endotracheal intubation were described [2]. Lignocaine prior to endotracheal intubation was associated with a significant reduction in catecholamine release; however, none of the studies specifically addressed ICP. The best available evidence suggests a treatment benefit for reduction of ICP during intubation with no clear evidence of harm, leading to a recommendation to routinely pre-treat prior to intubation [3].

In addition, the outcome is also related to the ventilation during the time the airway is secured, PaCO2 varies directly with CBF and CBV with the effect greatest for changes in PaCO2 in the physiologic range: CBF increases 1 to 2 mL/100 g/min for each 1 mm Hg increase in the PaCO2 and vice versa (especially in the PaCO2 range of 20 to 80 mmHg) and CBV increases 0.04 mL/100 g/rain for each 1 mm Hg increase in the PaCO2 and vice versa [1].

Positioning and the axis of intubation is very relevant especially in traumatic spines and traumatic brain injuries. All patients with severe trauma or head injury should be assumed to have cervcal spine injury until proven otherwise. The immobilization of the injured cervical spine is of utmost importance if a fracture is suspected, stabilization and early intubation is essential as these patients are prone to respiratory failure after acute cervical cord injury.

As compared to sniffing position decreases laryngoscopic view in 45% of the patients [4] and use of the gum elastic bougie should be encouraged. (Awake fiberoptic, videolaryngoscopy, direct laryngoscopy and use of supraglottic devices like laryngeal mask airways should all be available).

Airway Requirements Related To Surgical Demands

PITUITARY

In Acromegaly patients multiple airway anomalies have been described. Unanticipated difficulty with airway management is three times more common in acromegalic patients[5]. (Airway management may also be difficult in a patient with acromegaly due to hypertrophy of facial bones and mandible, large bulbous nose, thick tongue and lips can cause adifficult mask fit and hypertrophy of the nasal turbinates, soft palate, tonsils, epiglottis and larynx can lead to difficulty in ventilation and laryngeal visualization). Patients may have preoperative hoarseness and dyspnoea due to glottic stenosis due to tissue overgrowth leading to post-extubation oedema. Vocal cord paralysis may result from stretching of recurrent laryngeal nerve, impaired mobility of cricoarytenoid joints, or compression of recurrent laryngeal nerve by thyroid enlargement.There may be impaired mobility of the cervical spine and the cricoarytenoid joints.

Any history of stridor, difficult intubation, hoarseness, and obstructive sleep apnea suggests glottic or infraglottic involvement and therefore warrants smaller than usual ETT to be always available.

Patients undergoing Transsphenoidal Hypophysectomy in addition have the surgical approach involving incising the nasal septum and pharyngeal bleeding and a secure aiway to prevent aspiration is essential.

Intracranial space occupying lesions and endotracheal intubation for elective craniotomy

Choice of relaxant for intubation is controversial. Succinyl choline causes a transient increase in ICP by muscle fasciculation. Defasciculation with a small dose of nondepolariser muscle relaxant helps prevent an increase in ICP. Drugs such as thiopentone, propofol or lignocaine may help to reduce the effect of succinylcholine. Rocuronium, which has an onset of action that is close to that of succinylcholine can be an ideal nondepolariser muscle relaxant for rapid sequence intubation unfortunately its long duration of action makes it risky in patients with difficult airway. Inability to intubate rapidly or ventilate adequately after administration of the relaxant may aggravate the cerebral injury. Therefore despite its potential to increase ICP transiently, succinylcholine remains the relaxant of choice for rapid intubation and institution of mechanical ventilation in a head injury patient[6].

Surgical position and aggravation of intracranial hypertension due to airway manipulation are two major considerations in the airway management for an elective craniotomy.

Sterotactic neurosurgery

The areas of stereotactic surgery and its applications is increasing. The care of these patients will demand more of the anesthesiologist's participation in the future. Stereotactic neurosurgery can be conducted with conscious sedation, whereas others may require a general anesthetic and the airway can be secured prior to application of the head frame.Many centres may employ head frame devices that interfere less with air- way management and have crossbar equivalents that can be removed with ease and without distorting the head frame. Even in these cases, ,the amount of head frame behind the patient's head and neck may make proper positioning for airway management extremely difficult

Intraoperative neurologic events that require airway management one required in 16% of the patients.

When these do occur it is challenging due to position away from the anaesthesia provider in the MRI consoles and the presence of the headframe which though has a hinge anteriorly for access to the airway, the frame makes the head and neck immobile and changes the airway axis due to the sheer size of the frame. Laryngoscpy maybe rendered difficult and supraglottic airway devices should be at hand.

These patients are usually transported between the operating room and the MRI suite in the absence of hybrid OTs.

Hydrocephalus and other spinal cord anomalies

The presence of a large head circumference leads to positioning difficulties in aligning the airway axis for intubation (Fig. 1). Ensuring a preanaesthetic vist to assess the head circumference so that adequate arrangements can be made for creating a suitable pillow or an appropriate sized cushion can be designed from locally available material such that the head remains stable on a ring and the torso of the child is lifted to the appropriate height such that the airway axis are aligned (Fig. 2).

Similarly with the presence of a myelocoele (Fig. 3) or a meningomyelocoele either cervical or lumbar an adequate cushion will have to be designed so as to accommodate the lesion within it while the patient is positioned supine (Fig. 4).

These patients are usually of the pediatric age group, which adds to the level of difficulty of intubation.

Similarly these patients are also encountered in the remote locations for MRI scans where they are anaesthetised for the diagnostic procedure and management of the airway has to be dealt with using the same principles.

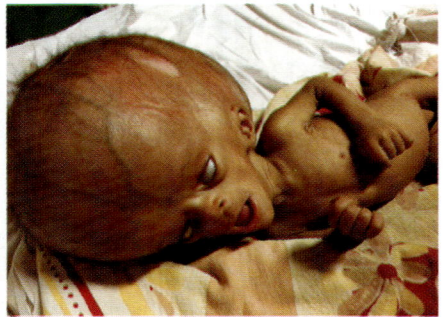

Fig. 1. Hydrocephalus

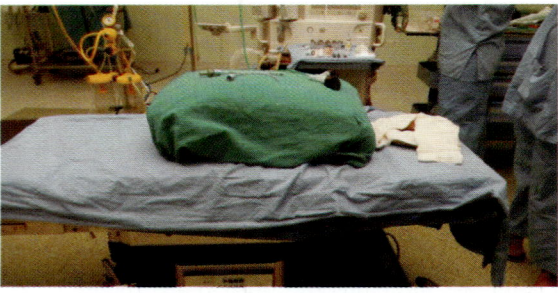

Fig. 2. Position for hydrocephalus

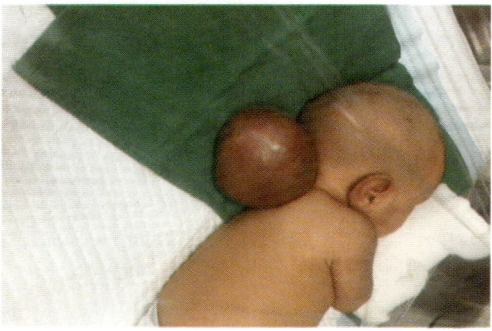

Fig. 3. Cervical myelocele

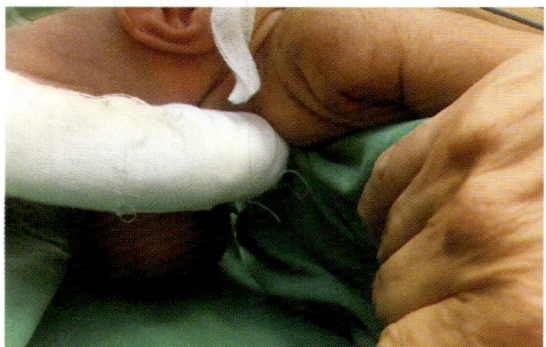

Fig. 4. Position of myelocele in doughnut

Traumatic brain injury

Patients with severe traumatic brain injury require endotracheal intubation in the emergency room.

Uncooperative head injury patients may require sedation for computed tomographic scanning and sedatives cannot be administered without an endotracheal tube in place and institution of controlled ventilation.The major goals during intubation of a brain injured patient are to prevent an increase in intracranial pressure (ICP), prevent pulmonary aspiration and avoid aggravation of a coexisting spinal injury.

A profound decrease in CPP caused by the anaesthetic agents may be more detrimental to cerebral oxygenation than a transient increase in ICP caused by intubation. It is very well established now that cerebral blood flow in a patient with traumatic brain injury is lowest during the first 24 hours after injury, which is precisely the time when he is most likely to require emergency endotracheal intubation[7].

Airway difculties occur with over 50–70% of head injuries which are associated facial injury[8]. Airway compromise can arise from associated soft tissue swelling, haemorrhage and secretions, and fractured teeth. Maxillary fractures lead to facial edema and pharyngeal blood, and disrupt the skeletal support of the oropharyngeal musculature causing reduced pharyngeal dimensions, and increased susceptibility to obstruction.

Focal neurological insults to the midbrain, cerebellum, or brain stem (injury, stroke, demyelination) can affect airway control centers.

More diffuse disease (injury, infection, inflamation, ischemia) can alter the consciousness with impairment of cough and swallowing reflux leading to a vicious cycle which can further propogate morbidity. A decreased level of consciousness can lead to a reduction in airway muscle tone which may lead to airway obstruction. Obstruction of the airway results in hypoxia, hypercarbia, and further diminishes airway control and finally increase in respiratory effort which generates negative intrathoracic pressure and further collapses the airways.

Complete neuromuscular blockade should be verified with a nerve stimulator before laryngoscopy to prevent cough and associated increases in ICP.

Management of the difficult airway in a patient with increased ICP should be approached in the same fashion as the mangement of the difficult airway in any patient.

The laryngeal mask airway (LMA) may provide an advantage for short neurosurgical procedures in patients with elevated ICP because its placement has less impact on haemodynamics (and therefore intracerebral dynamics) than endotracheal intubation. However, every patient with raised ICP is at increased risk for aspiration and almost always require positive pressure hyperventilation; both limitations with an LMA. In addition, most neurosurgical procedures make intraoperative access to the airway and readjustments of the LMA difficult.

Craniofacial anomalies

There are over 58 syndromes associated with craniofacial defects[9,10]. Airway management is often complicated by severly abnormal upper and lower airway anatomy, associated cardiopulmonary or neurological dysfunction, increased ICP, a history of sleep apnoea, and surgical requirements specific to each case. Micrognathia, retrognathia or mandibular hypoplasia, are common.

Laxity of transverse ligament is seen in 14-22% of children with 'Down's syndrome'[11]. Extension of the head may cause subluxation of atlas over axis with resultant compression of the spinal cord by the odontoid process. Rotatory subluxation of the atlanto-axial joint and posterior subluxation of the axis have been reported in the postoperative period in patients with Down's syndrome. Increased prevalence of lower cervical spondylosis and cervical myelopathy are known to occur in adults with Down's syndrome. Other spinal anomalies with specific relevance to airway management seen in patients with Down's syndrome include spina bifida of the atlas, vertebral occipitalisation, congenital nonunion of the odontoid process and Klippel-Feil syndrome. The importance of all the above anomalies lies in the fact that tracheal intubation may be difficult in these patients. Also, cervical spinal movements during intubation may worsen the spinal cord compression. Awake fibreoptic intubation under regional anaesthesia is preferred in these patients. Anaesthetic drugs should not be administered until the trachea is intubated, patient is positioned for surgery and neurological examination carried out.

Cervical spine injury

Our goal as clinicians encountering the patient, is to attempt to limit injury further than the primary insult and prevent damage by complicating factors as hypoxia, inadequate perfusion pressures, and increased ICP. Current research is being aimed at the better understanding of and limitation of secondary injury after the primary insult that occurred at the time of mechanical trauma. This secondary injury seems to be mediated by microvascular and subsequent biochemical forces set in motion by the primary injury.

Airway management is crucial in patients with cervical spine injury as airway management techniques may cause secondary neurologic injury. The objective during airway management of patient with cervical spine injury is to secure the airway rapidly and efficiently with minimal or no movement of the neck. Videofluoroscopic studies in anaesthetized patients and cadaver models of cervical spine injury have improved our understanding of the movement of spine during intubation in normal individuals and in patients with spinal cord injury[12].

Cervical spine immobilization should be the standard of care until exclusion of spinal injury. Cervical collars and manual in-line stabilization can be used for immobilization. Rigid collars are better.. While collars restrict the spinal motion they also limit mouth opening. During airway management, removal of the anterior portion of the collar and applying manual in-line stabilization should be practised[12].

Manual in-line stabilization (MILS): MILS is used during procedures like airway management where other stabilization techniques are not appropriate. For achieving this maneuver the provider stands at the side of the patient and grasps the mastoid and occiput of the patient with their hands. The aim of MILS is to apply opposite and equal forces to laryngoscope to fix the head and neck in a neutral position. MILS decreases laryngeal visualization and hinders intubation[12]. Nolan et al. 4 showed that MILS impairs glottic view in 45% of patients. However, glottic view is better with MILS when compared with collars. In addition to intubation techniques, mask ventilation can cause cervical motion. Direct Laryngoscopy (DL): DL has many advantages. It causes greatest cervical movement when MILS is applied glottic view is reduced. Gum elastic bougie is an important adjunct for direct laryngoscopic intubation. By using a bougie, the laryngoscopist tends to use less pressure, thus avoiding a displacement of the fractured spine. Video laryngoscopes we know, may improve glottic view and ease intubation but it is not certain that they decrease cervical spine motion. Cervical spine movement is least with fibreoptc intubation. It needs experience. Urgency of the procedure and experience of the anesthetist are the main determinants to decide which airway management should be used. Currently awake fiberoptic intubation is the recommended intubation technique. However, there is not enough evidence to reveal the ideal intubation technique with least neurologic adverse effects[12].

Effect of basic airway manoeuvers on cervical spine mobility Chin lift and jaw thrust in an adult cadaver model of C5-6 ligamentous injury causes a greater than 5 mm increase in the disc space.[13]. This widening is not prevented by a Philadelphia collar. Introduction of an oesophageal obturator airway causes a 3-4 mm increase in disc space. Anterior neck pressure to facilitate nasotracheal intubation causes a posterior subluxation of more than 5 mm. Head tilt, and insertion of an oropharyngal or nasopharyngeal airway are not associated with any significant displacement of the spinal segments[13]. Cricoid pressure should be applied during emergency[13].

Occipito-Atlanto-Axial Complex

Diseases of the OAA complex have comparatively more chances of affecting the airway management than those of lower levels. Difficult laryngoscopy rates in patients with cervical spine diseases when affecting OAA complex and below C3 level have been found to be 40% and 7% respectively[12,13].

Role of OAA complex in airway management

Head tilt achieved by extension at OAA complex is a basic requirement for face mask ventilation and direct laryngoscopy. However, cervical spine disease has not been found to be a risk factor for difficult face mask ventilation. Mouth opening is also dependent on OAA extension. Reduced inter-incisor distance or a Mallampati grade 3 should raise suspicion of poor OAA movement. Diseases associated with atlanto-axial instability include rheumatoid arthritis, Down's syndrome, mucopolysaccharidoses, infection and Klippel Feil deformity. However, a reliable and accurate non invasive clinical method of detecting significantly reduced OAA mobility is ambiguous [12,13].

Cervical stenosis and cervical instability

Cervical stenosis may result from encroachment on the vertebral canal by arthritic osteophytes or pannus, disc protrusion or thickening of ligaments, loss of ability, under normal physiological loads, to maintain relationship between vertebrae.

A particular, established method of airway management in unstable spine remains missing due to the multifactorial nature of neurological deterioration in cervical spine diseases The basic airway management techniques do carry a risk of displacement or angulation of cervical spine. Aiding intubation with devices such as Bullard, glidescope, Airtraq laryngoscopes, lightwand or Bonfil's endoscope offer better visualization of glottis with less cervical movement. The risk of further injury to cervical spine is minimum with use of flexible fibreoptic technique.

Criteria for stability after cervical trauma

In a conscious patient, alert, no distracting injuries, no midline pain, normal movement, no neurologic abnormalities.

In an unconscious patient the combination of plain films and computed tomography (CT) is adequate to diagnose bony and ligamentous instability. MRI is not required for exclusion of instability [12].

Approximately 5% of patients with traumatic cervical injury deteriorate neurologically, mostly early (within 24 hours). Some show delayed deterioration (1-7 days) and occasionally late (weeks) due to subacute post traumatic ascending myelopathy [12].

Currently, there is no clear evidence that airway management has any significant influence on neurological outcome, as there are many other factors involved [12].

The position of the patient in neuroanaesthesiology and the airway

Due to the surgical demands in neuroanaesthesiology the patient is placed in various positions which affect the maintenance of the airway intraoperatively.

In the sitting position, the extreme flexion and long duration of surgery can lead to obstruction of the venous and lymphatic drainage of the tongue leading to edema and macroglossia, edema of the pharyngeal structures and the use of transoesophageal echo probes add to the edema. This affects the extubation with the potential of airway obstruction at extubation.

The sitting, prone and lateral positions have the potential of accidental extubation if the endotracheal tube is not secured well.

CONCLUSION

The airway management in neuroanaesthesia is vast and encompasses a practical knowledge in use of a wide variety of devices to secure the airway. It also requires the operator to have a sound understanding of the physiology of the ccerebral circulation and control of cerebral blood flow alongwith the alterations in the airway anatomy that are widely encountered in the practice of neuroanaesthesia.

Acknowledgement:
Fig. 1 & 2 Dr Poonam Ghodki & Fig. 3 & 4 Dr Aslam Shaikh

REFERENCES

1. Iyer RR. Airway management in neurological emergencies and neuroanaesthesia. In:Seminars in Anesthesia, Perioperative Medicine and Pain. 2001 Sep 30 (Vol. 20, No, 3, pp 154-165). WB Saunders.

2. Robinson, N, Clancy, M. In patients with head injury undergoing rapid sequence intubation, does pretreatment with intravenous lignocaine/lidocaine lead to an improved neurological outcome? A review of literature. Emerg Med J. 2001 Nov;18(6): 453-457. (Review).

3. Wang Y.M, Chung K.C, Lu H.F, et al: Lidocaine: the optimal timing of intravenous administration in attenuation of increase of intraocular pressure during tracheal intubation. Acta Anaesthesiol Sin. 2003;41:71-75. (Prospective; 135 patients).

4. Goutcher CM, Lochhead V. Reduction in mouth opening with semi-rigid cervical collars. Br J Anaesth 2005 Sep; 95(3): 344-8.

5. Nemergut EC, Zuo Z. Airway management in patients with pituitary disease: a review of 746 patients. J Neurosurg Anesthesiol 2006 Jan; 18(1): 73-7.

6. Kovarik WD, Mayberg TS, Lam AM, et al. Succinylcholine does not change intracranial pressure, cerebral blood flow velocity, or the electroencephalogram in patients with neurologic injury. Anesth Analg 1994;78:469.

7. GS Umamaheshwara. Airway management in neurosurgical patients.Indian J. Anaesth. 2005; 49 (4) : 336 – 343.

8. Souter MJ. Airway management in the neurological and neurosurgical patient. Emergency Management in Neurocritical Care. 2012 Mar 20; 10:12

9. Broennle MA, Teller L. Anesthesia for craniofacial procedures. Clin Plast Surg 1987; 14: 17-26.

10. Posnick .IC. Craniofacial dysostosis. Staging of recon- struction and management of the midface deformity. Neurosurg Clin N Am 1991; 2: 683-702.

11. Peuschel SM, Scola FH. Atlantoaxial instability in individuals with Down's syndrome; epidemiologic, radiographic and clinical studies. Pediatrics 1987; 80: 555-560.

12. Erden A,Kanburolu Ç. Airway management in adults with cervical spine injury. Acta Medica 2015; 4: 3-4.

13. Aprahamian C, Thompson BM, Finger WA, Darin JC. Experimental cervical spine injury model; evaluation of airway management and splinting techniques. Ann Emerg Med. 1984; 13: 584-58.

MULTIPLE CHOICE QUESTIONS

1. **All are true about cerebral autoregulation except**
   a. It occurs between 50-150 mm Hg
   b. It is a Myogenic response
   c. Occurs immediately after the pressure change
   d. Range of autoregulation is shifted to a higher pressure in hypertensives
   e. Abolished by trauma, hypoxia, and inhalational anesthetics

2. **When the brain is stiff (low compliance) and enlarged, ICP**
   a. Rises only minimally when the patient coughs
   b. Rises significantly with a small increase in arterial CO_2
   c. Is unaffected by arterial desaturation (hypoxia)
   d. Falls if the patient is put in the head-down position
   e. Rises if the head is twisted to the left or right

3. **Following a severe head injury, ICP will rise to damaging levels if**
   a. The patient develops airway obstruction
   b. The patient becomes severely hypertensive
   c. The patient is allowed to breathe halothane spontaneously during an anaesthetic
   d. Arterial hypoxemia occurs
   e. The patient suffers severe pain from other injuries which is not treated

4. **Which of the following features does not increase the difficulty of direct laryngoscopy in Acromegaly?**
   a. Distorted facial anatomy
   b. Macroglossia
   c. Glottic stenosis
   d. Prognathic Mandible
   e. Arthritis of the neck

5. **What is the threshold value of decrease in Pao_2 that results in an exponential increase in CBF ?**
   a. 70mmHg
   b. 80mmHg
   c. 40 mmHg
   d. 50 mmHg

6. **The goal of induction in neuroanesthesia is (multiple answer)**
   a. to blunt the stimulation of direct laryngoscopy
   b. without compromising cerebral perfusion by increasing ICP
   c. without decreasing MAP
   d. attaining low PaCo2

7. **To attenuate the response to laryngoscopy, the drugs used are**
   a. lignocaine
   b. succinyl choline
   c. Propofol
   d. thiopentone

8. **Which of the following are indications of an unstable cervical spine**
   a. Blunt trauma
   b. Rheumatoid arthritis
   c. Head injury
   d. Diabetes mellitus

9. **These airway manoeuvres cause the maximum movement in the cervical spine**
   a. Mask ventilation
   b. Direct laryngoscopy
   c. Fibreoptic intubation
   d. Laryngeal mask airways

CHAPTER 13

NEUROMONITORING

Joanna S. Rodrigues, Shwetal U. Goraksha, Joseph N. Monteiro

Introduction

Intraoperative neurophysiological monitoring improves patient outcome by allowing early diagnosis of ischaemia or hypoxia before irreversible damage occurs, enabling surgeons to provide the optimal intervention required to preserve function.[1]

Key Principles

- Pathway at risk must be amenable to monitoring.
- Monitoring must provide reliable and reproducible data.
- If evidence of injury is detected, some intervention should be possible.
- If changes are detected and no intervention is possible it should be of prognostic value.

Brain can be monitored for (Table 1)
- Function
- Blood flow
- Metabolism

Table 1: Monitoing of function

1. **Monitoring function**
   - Electroencephalogram
     - Raw EEG
     - Computerised processed
       - Computerised special array
       - Density spectral array
       - Aperiodic analysis
   - Evoked potentials
     - Sensory evoked potentials
       - Somatosensory EP
       - Brain Stem auditory EP
       - Visual EP
     - Motor evoked potentials
       - Transcranial magnetic
       - Transcranial electric
       - Direct spinal cord stimulation

2. **Monitoring of function**
   - Cerebral blood flow
     - Nitrous oxide wash in
     - Radioactive Xenon clearance
     - Laser Doppler blood flow
     - Transcranial Doppler
   - Intracranial pressure
     - Non-invasive
       - Clinical examination
       - Imaging modalities
         - Non-contrast CT
         - MRI
         - TCD
         - Tympanic membrane displacement
         - Optic nerve sheath diameter
     - Invasive
       - Intraventricular devices
       - Subrachnoid devices
       - Epidural / subdural devices
       - Pneumatic sensor
       - Intraparenchymal devices
         - Fibreoptic devices
         - Implanted microchip transducers

3. **Monitoring of metabolism**
   - Invasive monitoring
     - Intracerebral PO_2 electrode
     - Cerebral micro dialysis
   - Non-invasive monitoring
     - Transcranial cerebral oximetry
     - Jugular venous oximetry

Fig. 1 & Table 2 : Electroencephalogram

EEG is a recording of spontaneous electrical activity of the brain. It is a summation of the excitatory postsynaptic potentials produced from the pyramidal cells of the cerebral cortex.[1]

- EEG is recorded from electrodes placed on the scalp.
- A pair of electrodes is called montage.
  - i) Bipolar montage: Both the electrodes are active.
  - ii) Referential montage: Only one electrode is the active recording electrode, the other is referential.
- Focal lesions are better picked up by the bipolar montage, and diffuse lesions by referential montage.
- Intraoperatively, a 2-4 channel EEG with computer processing is commonly used.
- Gold standard:16-channel recording (8 channels for each hemisphere) with electrodes placed according to the international 10-20 system.
  - 10% or 20% of the Nasion-inion, preaurical or hemi circumference line.
  - Midline electrodes are designated "z", while right side electrodes are even and left side are odd numbers.
  - According to position, they are designated as:
- Frontal prominence (Fp)
- Frontal (F)
- Central (C)
- Parietal (P)
- Occipital (O)

Normal EEG

- It is a plot of voltage versus time 1-35 Hz Frequency.
- Based on the frequency, waveforms are classified into different bands.

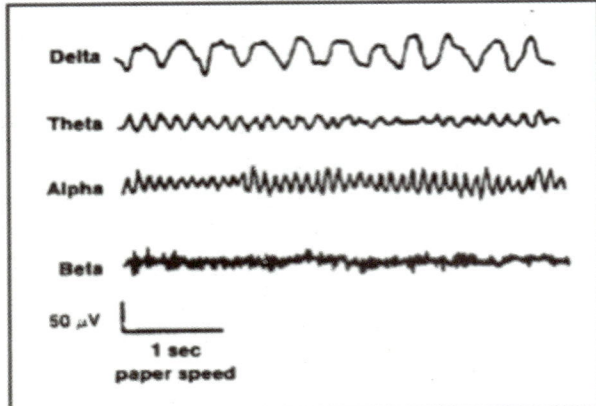

Fig 1: EEG waves

Table 2 : EEG Waves, frequency and amplitude.[2]

Waves	Frequency Hz	Amplitude mV	Characteristics
Beta	> 13	20	With mental activity, mainly frontal
Alpha	8-12.5	40-100	Adults with eyes closed mainly occipital
Theta	4-7.5	> 50	Sedation / Anaesthesia/ Sleep
Delta	0.5-3.5	> 50	Sedation / Anaesthesia/ sleep / Ischaemia

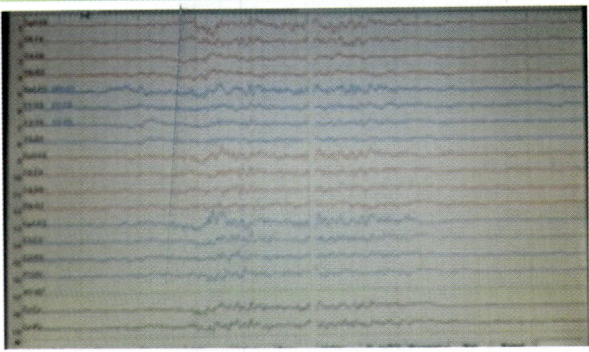

Fig. 2 : EEG recording

EEG analysed for frequency, amplitude, wave pattern, burst suppression, spikes and sleep spindles.[2]

Factors affecting EEG:

- Cerebral ischaemia
- Hypothermia
- Hypercarbia / Hypocarbia
- Hypoxia
- Hypotension

Electrocorticography (ECoG)

It is the recording of spontaneous electrical activity directly from the surface of the brain.

Wave forms are better localised and delineated.

It is recorded intraoperatively to delineate seizure focus and area of surgical resection.

Uses of EEG

- Reflects cortical neuronal function.
- To detect cerebral ischaemia before tissue damage occurs. EEG shows abnormal changes at Cerebral blood flow (CBF) < 20ml/100g/min much before the level at which cellular integrity is threatened (12ml/100g/min).
- To detect cerebral ischaemia during cross clamping in carotid end arterectomy.

- To detect cerebral ischaemia during temporary occlusion in aneurysm surgery.
- Seizures evaluation surgery - mapping and resection.
- Spine surgery – scoliosis, spinal cord decompression and resection of spinal cord tumours.
- Extracranial-Intracranial bypass.
- Thoracic aortic aneurysm repair.
- Cardiopulmonary bypass.
- ICU
  - Used to titrate sedation.
  - Detect subclinical seizures.
  - Monitor adequacy of metabolic suppression.
  - Assess the degree of anoxic damage.
  - Prognosticate ICU patients.

Fig. 3 & Table 3 : Bispectral index (BIS)

- Derived EEG parameter to monitor the degree of hypnosis and monitors the depth of anaesthesia.
- Based on power spectrum analysis and time domain analysis.[3]

Table 3 : BIS range

BIS	State
	Awake
100	Respond to commands
80	Respond to loud commands or mild prodding / shaking
60	GENERAL ANAETHESIA Low probability of recall Unresponsive to verbal commands
40	DEEP HYPNOTIC STATE
20	BURST SUPPRESSION
0	FLAT LINE

i) Uses a 4-electrode sensor placed on the patients forehead, and is less sensitive to development of regional ischaemia.

ii) It calculates the index of the state of sedation by an algorithm.

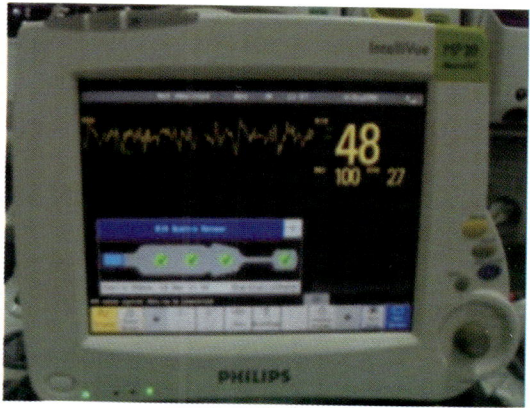

Fig 3 : BIS Bispectral Index

Entropy

- Entropy module monitors the depth of anaesthesia
- It describes the irregularity of the signal and not the predictability of the same.
- Uses frontal EMG and EEG.
  - i) Response entropy:
    - Fast reacting parameter.
    - Sensitive to facial muscle activation.
    - Early activation.
  - ii) State entropy:
    - Stable
    - Measures hypnotic effect of anaesthetic drugs.
- Scale 0-91: 0- no brain activity - 100-fully awake. Clinically relevant 40-60.

Uses of BIS and entropy[3]

- Helps identify patients at risk of awareness recall and pain under anaesthesia when patients are paralysed.
- Guides sedation and analgesia.
- Titrating sedation in ventilated and ICU patients.
- Titrate mediations used in inducing coma.

2. Evoked potential monitoring

- Recordings of electrical activity of specific neuronal pathways in response to external stimuli.
- When neural tissues are stimulated, the electrical activity ascends along specific neuronal pathways.
- Based on stimulation site and recording location, a characteristic waveform is obtained.
- Both sensory and motor.

1) Somato sensory evoked potential (SSEP)

EEG generated in response to electrical stimulation of a cranial or peripheral nerve. If peripheral nerve is stimulated it can record proximally along entire tract (peripheral nerve – spinal cord- brainstem-thalamus-cerebral cortex).[2]

- Time locked
- Event related
- Pathway specific
- Recorded plot of VOLTAGE VERSUS TIME has an initial artefact representing the stimulation of the tract followed by the neuronal response, recorded as a series of peaks and valleys.

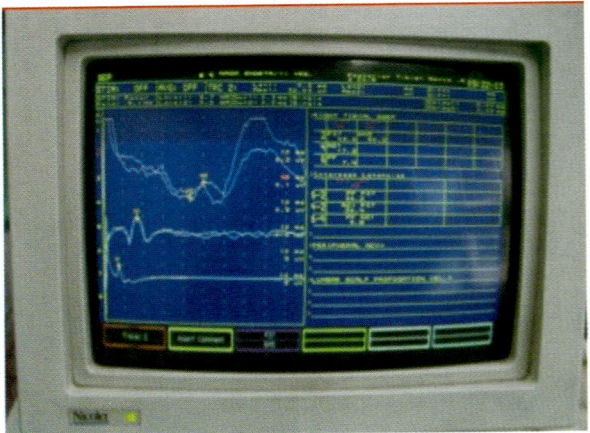

Fig 4 : SSEP Somatosensory Evoked Potential

Nerves monitored

- Median (C6-T1)
- Ulnar (C8-T1) } MCA and ICA territory
- Common peroneal (L4-S1)
- Posterior Tibial nerve(L4-S2) } ACA territory

Peripheral stimulation
↓
Electrical activity passes
↓
Posterior column and spinothalamic pathways (Supplied by posterior spinal artery)

Changes considered significant

- Latency prolongation ≥ 10%
- Amplitude decrease by ≥ 50%

Variables affecting SSEP:

1) Anaesthetic agents (Table 4):
2) Temperature: Hypothermia

Mild: ↑ Latency of cortical SSEP

Profound: Cortical potential disappear followed by ↑ latency and ↓ amplitude of sub cortical potentials.

Table 4: Effect of Anaesthetic agents on SSEP and MEP.

Anaesthetic agent	Somatosensory evoked	Motor evoked potential
Halothane (MAC 0.5-1)	↓ A ↑ L	++
Isoflurane (MAC 0.5-1)	↓ A ↑ L	++
Savoflurane (MAC 1.5)	↓ A ↑ L	++
Desflurane (MAC 1.5)	↓ A ↑ L	++
Nitrous Oxide (60-70%)	↓ A - L	++
Barbiturates	↓ A ↑ L	++
Propofol	↓ A	++
Ketamine	↓ A	+
Etomidate	↓ A	+
Opioids	↓ A ↑ L	-
Benzodiazopines	-	+++
Dexmedetomidine	-	+
Neuromuscular Blockade	-	+++

2) Temperature: Cortical potential disappear followed by ↑ latency and ↓ amplitude of sub cortical potentials.

3) Hemodynamics:
   - Ischaemia ↑ latency, ↓ amplitude.
   - Severe anaemia – affects cortical latency and amplitude.
   - ↑ ICP ↓ amplitude and ↑ latency of cortical SSEP.

4) Ventilation
   Severe hypoxemia changes amplitude.

Uses:

- For spinal procedures
  - Intramedullary tumours
  - Scoliosis surgery
  - Spine stabilization
- For cerebral vascular surgeries like intracranial aneurysm and CEA to check
  - For adequacy of collateral blood flow
  - Tolerance to temporary vessel clamping
  - Adequacy of systolic blood pressure in specific sensory cortex.

- To locate sensory and motor cortex.
- To identify procedure related nerve injury.
- During neuroradiological procedures- occlusion of vessels and thrombolysis of clots.
- Brain death: Used as a confirmatory test.

Limitations

- Does not monitor spinal cord supplied by anterior spinal artery.
- Normal intraoperative SSEP does not rule out occurrence of postoperative paraplegia.
- Artefacts by operating table, cautery machine, convection warmer, anaesthesia machine, drill, CUSA may pose problems in SSEP.

2) Brainstem Auditory Evoked Potential BAEP (Fig.5)

Recording of activities of neural generators involved in the auditory pathways following stimulation of cochlear nerve.

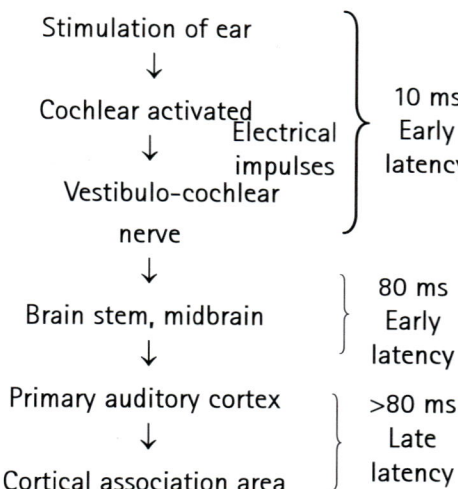

BAEPs produced by delivering repetitive clicks or tones through foam ear inserts attached to stimulus transducers. BAEP waveform consists of 7 short latency peaks.

- Interpretation involves measuring the absolute latency of the three most prominent vertex positive peaks I, III, and V
- Changes considered significant are
- V waveform latency prolongation >0.5 ms
- 50% decrease in amplitude
- Prolonged interpeak latency III-V
- I and V are preserved - hearing is preserved.

Factors affecting BAEP

1. Early latency is resistant and mid latency is sensitive to anaesthetic agents effects.
2. Use of drill can interfere with the recording.

Uses

- Monitoring during posterior fossa surgeries.
- Posterior circulation vascular surgeries.
- Microvascular decompression – Facial nerve monitoring.

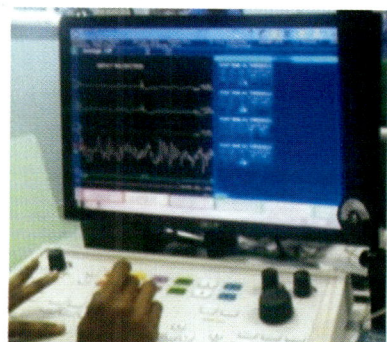

Fig 5 : BAEP Brainstem auditory evoked potential

3) Visual Evoked Potentials VEP

- Records electrical activity from neural generators along the visual pathways.
- Following light stimuli retinal receptors get activated.
- Electrical activity travels along optic nerve, optic chiasm, optic tracts, LGB and reach visual projection areas in occipital cortex.
- Responses recorded bilaterally in the visual cortex.
- High contrast checkerboard pattern of stimulation in awake patients and flash stimulation in anaesthetised patients.

Drawbacks

- Flash stimulation
- Large bulky goggles pose technical problems
- Bilateral nature of response may obscure some focal changes and anaesthetic sensitivity makes recording difficult.

Motor Evoked Potential:

Following stimulation of the motor cortex, electrical impulses travel along the cortical spinal tract crossing at the midline in lower lateral part of the brainstem, and travel down to the anterior ipsilateral funiculi of spinal cord and results in muscle activity.

- Types
  - Transcranial magnetic MEP
  - Transcranial electrical MEP
  - Direct spinal cord stimulation.
- MEP evaluates descending motor pathways (cerebral cortex→past the neuromuscular junction → to peripheral muscle groups).
- Changes considered significant:

i) Increased requirement of stimulus strength (>50 v) to produce same initial response.

ii) Increased number of stimuli to achieve same initial response.

iii) Decreased amplitude by more than 80%.

Uses

- For spinal procedures as a supplement to SSEP e.g.: scoliosis correction surgery, intramedullary tumours, spinal decompression.
- To map motor cortex during tumour resection.
- Vascular lesions: vasospasm, incorrect placement of aneurysm clip.

Complications

- Tongue injury.
- Bone fractures including mandible skull defects
- Patient fall from the table.

Contraindications:

- Patients with implantable DBS, clips.
- Epilepsy, cortex lesions, high ICP
- Recent craniotomy
- Cardiac pacemaker, implanted pumps.

3. ELECTROMYOGRAPHY (Fig. 6)

- Spontaneous or triggered.[4]

- Continuous recording of EMG activity in the muscle of regions innervated by nerve roots around which surgeons are working.
- Impingement on a nerve root by an instrument will cause immediate motor activity.
- Cranial nerves with motor components or peripheral nerves involved.
- To record muscle activity, needle pairs are placed near the muscles of interest and electrical activity recorded.
- Direct feedback to the surgeon can be achieved by playing of these responses through a loudspeaker.

Short bursts or blurps indicate nerve irritation, while continuous bursts indicate nerve damage.

Uses

- Warn the surgeon of impeding nerve damage.
- Help locate a nerve within the field for biopsy.
- Localise the level of any conduction block or delay.
- Release of tethered cord surgery- risk of damage to nerve roots of lower limbs, anal and urethral sphincters.

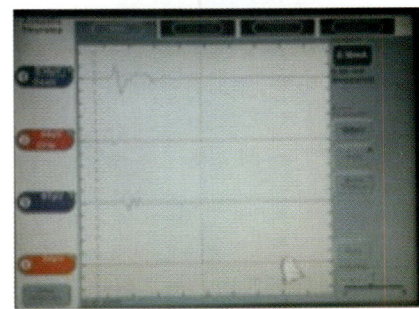

Fig 6: Facial nerve monitoring

Fig 7: Anaesthesia for SSEP, VEP, BAEP, MEP

Monitoring	Types of anaesthetic agent	Dose
Auditory evoked potential No limitations	-	-
Visual evoked potential Similar to SSEP	-	-
Somatosensory evoked potential (SSEP)	Volatile agent	0.5 - 1.0 MAC acceptable
	N 20	50-70% baseline SSEP not compromised
	IV anesthetics fentanyl	1-2 mcg / kg / hr
	Neuromuscular blockers	No limitations
Spinal cord stimulation Similar to SSEP	-	-
Motor evoked potential		
EMG	Volatile agent	No limitations
	N 20	No limitations
	IV anaesthetics	No limitations
	Neuromuscular blockers	Limited use ; try to avoid
Tc MEP and cMEP	Volatile agent	Limited use 0.3 MAC maximum
	N 20	50-70% acceptable
	IV anaesthetics propofol	50-300 mcg / kg / min
	Neuromuscular blockers	Very limited use

II. MONITORING OF FLOW/ PRESSURE

CEREBRAL BLOOD FLOW

1. Laser Doppler Flowmetry (Fig. 8)

- Basic principle: A laser beam is directed to an area of tissue. Upon contact with RBCs in target tissue, light waves are reflected and scattered, resulting in broadening of light wave frequency, which is detected and received by a photodetector.
- Parenchymal or surface Doppler probe which measures local CBF in a quantitative manner.
- Allows instantaneous, continuous and non-invasive measurement in a small tissue sample.

Limitation:

- Volume monitored is limited to 1 mm- Use limited.
- Requires a burr hole for insertion.

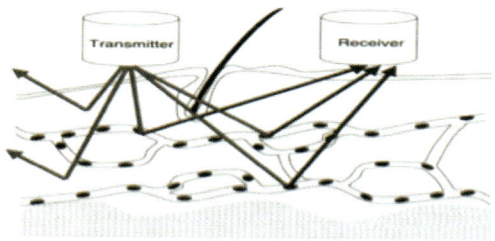

Fig. 8: Laser doppler flowmetry

Basic principle: A laser beam is directed to an area of tissue. Upon contact with RBCs in target tissue, light waves are reflected and scattered, rsulting in broadening of light wave frequency, which is detected and received by a photodetector.

2. TRANSCRANIAL DOPPLER[1,2]

- Non-invasive
- Cost effective bedside tool
- Provides realtime information of cerebral hemodynamics.
- Insonation: commonly defined acoustic windows
  - Temporal
  - Orbital
  - Sub occipital
  - Submandibular
- Doppler Principle: Doppler shift of the ultrasonic beam after its reflection on the moving blood column within the vessel is proportional to blood flow velocity.
- Reflection of ultrasound waves occurs at the interface between different tissue types and depends on the resistance to the ultrasound breakthrough or acoustic impedance.
- When reflected waves are sent back to the transducer the piezoelectric crystals convert mechanical energy into electrical energy which is processed by the ultrasound machine to produce two-dimensional grey scale image.

- During their travel into tissues, ultrasound waves are attenuated by
  - Attenuation coefficient of tissue
  - Travelled distance
  - Ultrasound frequency
- Low frequency transducer 2MHz is used.
- Flow within structures can be studied by using colour flow Doppler.
- To use TCD as an indirect measure of CBF, two main assumptions are:
  - Constant vessel diameter.
  - Unchanged angle of insonation.
- Measured velocity = Real velocity × cosine of angle of incidence.
- Pulsatility describes the shape of the maximal shift of the Doppler spectrum from peak systolic pressure to end-diastolic pressure with each cardiac cycle.
- In the absence of vessel stenosis or vasospasm, with constant pulsatility of ABP and during constant cerebral perfusion pressure (CPP), changes in pulsatility reflect the changes in cerebrovascular resistance.
- Factors affecting diameter of vessels.
  - $PaCO_2$
  - Blood pressure
  - Anaesethetic agents
  - Vasoactive drugs.

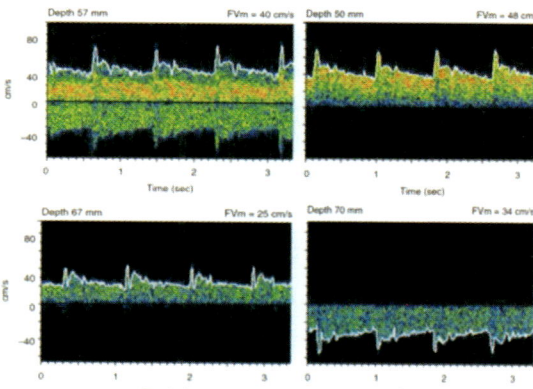

Fig. 9: TCD waveforms

Practical application

- Carotid Endarterectomy
  - Preoperative assessment of cerebrovascular reserve.
  - Determining the need for shunting by examination of CO_2 reactivity.
  - To detect shunt malfunction caused by kinking or thrombosis.
  - Testing the integrity of cerebral autoregulation.
  - Detection of preoperative and postoperative embolic phenomena.

- Detection of cerebral ischemia during cross-clamping of the carotid artery.
- Early detection of hyperperfusion syndrome
- Identification of spinal cord disease.
- Sub Arachnoid Haemorrhage
  - Valuable for diagnosing vasospasm noninvasively before the onset of clinical symptoms.
  - FVMCA > 120 cm/sec
  - 'Lindegaard Ratio'
  - FVMCA : FVICA > 3 } VASOSPASM
- Right to left shunt identification.
- Arteriovenous malformations.
- Estimating the completeness of resection and diagnosis and treatment of hyperperfusion syndrome.
- Diagnosis of cerebral circulatory arrest.
- Stroke
  - To identify cerebral arterial occlusion and recanalization.
  - To detect early (<2 hours) reocclusion following tPA.
- Head injury
  - Testing cerebrovascular reserve, autoregulation status
  - Post traumatic vasospasm.

Fig. 10 : Typical patterns for identification of arteries

Artery	Academic window	Probe angle	Depth	Flow Direction	Resistance	Adult MFV (cm/sec)
ECICA	Retromendibular	Superior-Medial	45-50	Away	Low	30 ± 9
MCA	Middle transtemporal	Straight/Anterior-Superior	30-65	Towards	Low	55 ± 12
ACA	Middle transtemporal	Straight/Anterior-Superior	60-75	Away	Low	50 ± 11
PCA - Segment 1	Posterior transtemporal	Straight/Posterior	60-70	Towards	Low	39 ± 10
PCA- Segment 2	Middle transtemporal	Straight/Posterior-Superior	60-70	Away	Low	40 ± 10
BA	Suboccipital	Superior	80-120	Away	Low	41 ± 10
VA	Suboccipital	Superior lateral	60-75	Away	Low	35 ± 10
OA	Transorbital	Staright	40-55	Towards	High	21 ± 5
Supradinold ICA	Transorbital	Superior	65-80	Away	Low	41 ± 11
Paraseller ICA	Transorbital	Inferior	65-80	Towards	Low	47 ± 14

Fig. 11: Degree of vasospasm measured by TCD

Degree of MCA or ICA	MFV (cm/sec)		I.R.
Mild (<25%)	120-149	A	3 - 6
Moderate (25-50%)	150-199	N	3 - 6
Severe (>50%)	>200%	D	>6

Degree of vasospasm	MFV (cm/s)		Modified I.R.
May represent vasospasm	70-85	A	2 - 2.49
Moderate (25-50%)	>85%	N	2.5 - 2.99
Severe (>50%)	>85%	D	>3

Intracranial Monitoring[5]

I. NON INVASIVE

- Tympanic Membrane Displacement.
    - CSF and perilymph communicate through cochlear aqueduct and increased ICP is directly transmitted to the footplate of stapes.
    - Inward displacement -normal or low ICP
- Optic Nerve Sheath Displacement (ONSD)
    - Optic nerve part of CNS and the space between optic nerve and sheath is continuation of subarachnoid space filled with CSF whose pressure is equal to the ICP.
    - In case of increased ICP, the diameter of the sheath increases and blood flow through the retinal vein is impeded.
    - ONSD > 5 mm → ↑ ICP

II. INVASIVE

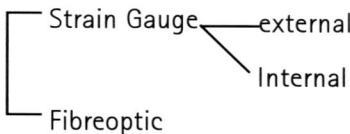

- **INTRAVENTRICULAR CATHETER**
    - External Ventricular Drain
    - Catheter is placed into one of the lateral ventricles through a burr hole.
    - Fluid coupled device connected to an external strain gauge.
    - Recalibrated in vivo against external reference – foramen of Monroe.

Advantages:
- Minimal expense.
- Maximum accuracy
- Therapeutic CSF drainage.
- Instillation of medication intrathecally.

Disadvantages:
- Most invasive.
- Infection.
- Difficult in young patients with slit like ventricles.

- **SUBARACHNOID DEVICES**
    - Subarachnoid bolt/Richmond screw is a hollow screw that goes into the skull abutting the dura.

- Dura is perforated to fill the bolt with CSF which is then connected to a fluid filled tubing and a pressure transducer.

Advantages:
- Devices easily and quickly placed without invading the brain.

Disadvantages:
- Prone to errors.
- ICP underestimation.
- Misplacement of screws.
- Occlusion by debris.

- **PNEUMATIC SENSOR**
    - Fluid filled catheter transducer system which uses a distal air filled balloon tipped catheter to measure ICP.
    - The monitor connects to an internal strain gauge transducer used to measure the internal balloon pressure.

Advantages:
- Capable of automatic zero drift correction.

Disadvantages:
- Limited bandwidth.

- **EPIDURAL/SUBDURAL DEVICES**
    - Least invasive.
    - Easily and quickly placed.

- **INTRAPARENCHYMAL DEVICES**

Group of devices that are non-fluid coupled devices and can be divided into
- Fibre optic devices.
- Strain gauge devices.

These ICP microtransducers can be used at any location.
- Intraventricular
- Intraparenchymal
- Epidural
- Sub dural

Advantages:
- Accurate
- Easily transported
- Recordings independent of patient positioning
- No measurement of artefact, dampening of waveform.
- Does not require irrigation
- Low risk of infection.

Disadvantage:

- Cannot be recalibrated.

Not reflective of global ICP

- Therapeutic CSF drainage not possible.

I. FIBREOPTIC CATHETER TIP TRANSDUCER.

- Transmits light via a fibreoptic cable towards a displaceable diaphragm.
- Light is reflected off the diaphragm and the change in light intensity interpreted in terms of pressure.
- Requires dedicated microprocessor.
- Costly
- Catheters cannot be recalibrated.
- Drift occurs if monitoring continued longer than 5 days.
- Catheters are fragile.

II. IMPLANTED MICROCHIP TRANSDUCER

- Miniature solid state pressure transducer mounted on a titanium case at the end of a 100cms flexible Nylon tube.
- Transducer tip contains a silicon microchip with diffuse piezoelectric strain gauges.
- Microsensor monitors ICP at the source.
- Information relayed electronically
- Accurate.
- Stable.
- Daily drift is 0.13–0.11 mmHg/day
- When this is incorporated into a ventricular system the system allows simultaneous drainage of CSF and ICP recording.
- Flexible and tunnelled beneath the scalp.
- Microsensor at the tip eliminates the need for constant realignment of transducer with the patient's head.

3. Monitoring of Metabolism

INVASIVE:

1. Brain tissue oxygen absorption

- Measures focal oxygen tension in the interstitial space of the brain.
- It represents oxygen available for mitochondrial oxidative phosphorylation.
- It is determined by CBF and the difference between arterial and venous oxygen tension.[1,2]

Technology

(1) Modified Clark Electrode (e.g., Licox, Neurovent-P)

(2) Optical fluorescence (e.g. Neurotrend, Codman)

Clarke's electrode

- A membrane surrounds an electrolyte layer and two electrodes made of a noble metal.
- Oxygen diffuses in to the membrane, electrochemically gets reduced and cases a voltage difference which is proportional to the oxygen tension.
- This process is temperature dependent, brain temperature must be simultaneously measured.

Optical Fluorescence Technology

- Sensors are coated with coloured markers that emit colour when in contact with oxygen.
- Intensity of colour depends upon the oxygen tension, detected by fluorescent sensors.
- Probe requires calibration with known oxygen concentration prior to insertion.
- Focal measurement
- In diffuse injury, values correlate with global monitors – jugular venous oximetry.
- Probe placement: $PbtO_2$ (Table 5) probes are fine catheters placed in white matter close to injured brain, preferably in the penumbral region. Position confirmed with CT.

Table 5: $PbtO_2$ values

Normal	20-35 mmHg
Compromised	20 mmHg
Brain hypoxia	< 15 mmHg

Uses

- Detection of cerebral hypoxia.
- Titrate individualised therapy-osmotherapy, hyperventilation, CPP, patient positioning and deciding timing on decompressive craniectomy.
- Identify delayed cerebral ischaemia in SAH before ICP use or clinical deterioration.
- $PbtO_2$ useful to determine transfusion trigger and blood product administration can be rationalised.

Limitations

- Regional differences in blood flow and metabolism.

2. CEREBRAL MICRODIALYSIS

It measures brains metabolic substrate both aerobic and anaerobic in the interstitial space.[1,2]

- Substances present in the area of higher concentration diffuse across a semipermeable membrane present in the tip of the microdialysis probe to an area of lower concentration.
- Probe consists of a coaxial double lumen tube (outer diameter 0.6 mm) covered by dialysis membrane in the distal 10mm and is continuously infused with an artificial CSF with known concentration.
- Depending on the concentration gradient and pore size of the membrane, metabolic substrates diffuse through the dialysis membrane into the probe and are collected in to the sample bottle.
- The sample is analysed for substrates using photometric enzyme kinetic analysis.
- Probe is placed either separately or with a triple bolt system into the white matter.
- Diffuse injury:
  - Non-dominant frontal cortex
  - Subcortical white matter
  - Values representative of global changes.
- Focal changes in penumbra
- Pericontusional area or in the vasospastic territory in SAH.

Table 6: Cerebral Micro dialysis analysis.

Conditions	Lactate	Pyruvate	LPR	Glutamate	Glycerol
Ischaemia	↑	↓	↑		
Hyperglycolysis	↑	↑	Normal		
Mitochondrial dysfunction	↑↑	Normal to↑	↑		
Excitotoxicity				↑	
Cell death					↑

Uses

- Monitoring substrates to detect neuronal ischaemia at a reversible stage.
- In SAH, metabolic changes occur before clinical manifestations of vasospasm.
- Glucose management in ICU.

Limitations

- Localised measurement
- Expensive
- Intermittent
- Invasive - prone to infection.

NON INVASIVE:

1. Near-Infra Sprectoscopy[2]

- NIRS measures near infrared light absorption by the superficial part of brain tissues.
- Optical Spectrophotometry: Light emitted through the skin and the skull enters the brain tissue to a depth of 1-2 cm. Absorption at different wavelength allows estimating the mixed capillary venous regional cerebral oxygen saturation ($rSCO_2$)
- $rSCO_2$ depends on the balance between local metabolism and oxygen delivery which in turn depends on
  - Regional cerebral blood flow
  - Blood oxygen content
- If metabolism is constant then $rSCO_2$ is regarded as a surrogate marker of regional CBF changes.
- Normal $rSCO_2$ values range from 62% in cardiac surgery to 11% in healthy young men.

Indications

- Aortic arch surgeries
- CEA

Limitations

- Contamination by blood originating from external carotid artery.
- Non-haem tissue chromophobes such as melanin or increased bilirubin can confound values.

Disadvantages

- Regional monitoring technique
- Impossible to detect changes in areas located distant from monitoring site.
- Potential for contamination of signal by extracranial tissue and ambient light.
- Wide intra and interindividual baseline variability.
- Best used as a trend monitor.

2. Jugular Venous Oximetry

The jugular bulb, a dilatation in the upper end of the IJV is the final common pathway for venous blood draining from the cerebral hemispheres, cerebellum and brainstem.

- It contains blood drained from both the sides of the brain, 70% from the same and 30% from opposite hemisphere.
- $SjVO_2$ reflects the balance between the brain supply and oxygen consumption.
- $SjVO_2$ accurately reflects global and hemispheric cerebral oxygenation when the dominant jugular bulb is cannulated.

Technique:

- Insertion at the junction between sternal and clavicular heads of the sternocleidomastoid with a 16-gauge catheter. With gentle aspiration, needle is passed 1-2 cm cranially at 15-20p angle in sagittal plane.[6]
- SjVO2: Normal Range: 55% to 75%
  - Levels < 55% suggest cerebral hypoperfusion with oxygen demand exceeding supply, an increase in oxygen extraction or a reduction in oxygen delivery which may be an early warning sign of ischaemia
  - Levels > 85% indicate relative hyperaemia or decreased oxygen supply (infarct)
- $SjVO_2$ depends on CBF, $CMRO_2$, CaO_2, Hemoglobin

Table 7: Jugular venous oxygen saturation (%). Many factors alter the relationship between cerebral oxygen consumption (CMRO2) and supply.

Desuturation	**SjVO$_2$ 55–75%**	**Luxuriant**
↑ ICP	↓ CMRO:Hypothermia, sedatives	
↓ $PaCO_2$	↑ CBF:Hyperemia	
↓ Systolic blood pressure	↓ Arterial O_2 content (CaO_2)	
↑ $CMRO_2$:Fever, seizures	A V communications	
Cerebral vasospasm	Brain Death	
Arterial hypoxia		

Clinical applications:

- Traumatic brain injury.
- Ischaemia detection due to systemic or intracranial causes.
- To help maintain the appropriate MAP and $PaCO_2$
- Intracranial aneurysm.
- $SjVO_2$ values are higher in the non-survivors than the survivors of cardiac arrest.

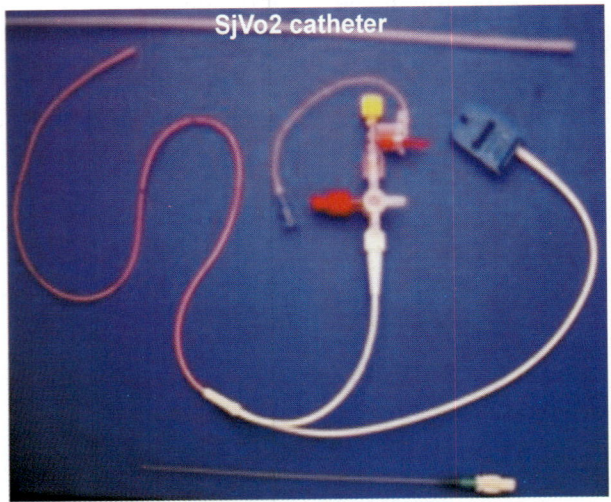

Fig. 12: $SjVO_2$ Catheter Normal range 55% to 75%

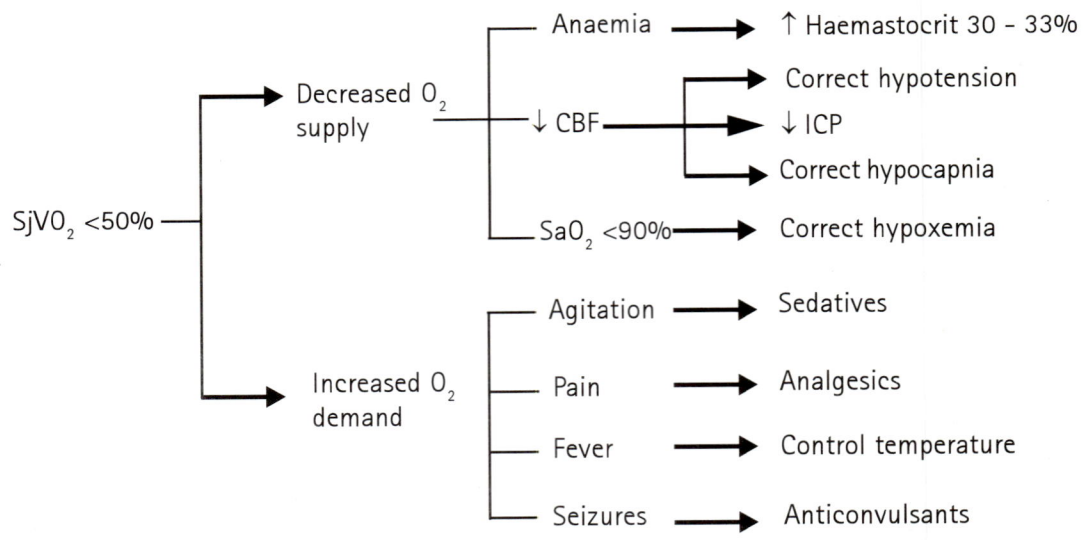

Fig .13: Management of Low $SjVO_2$

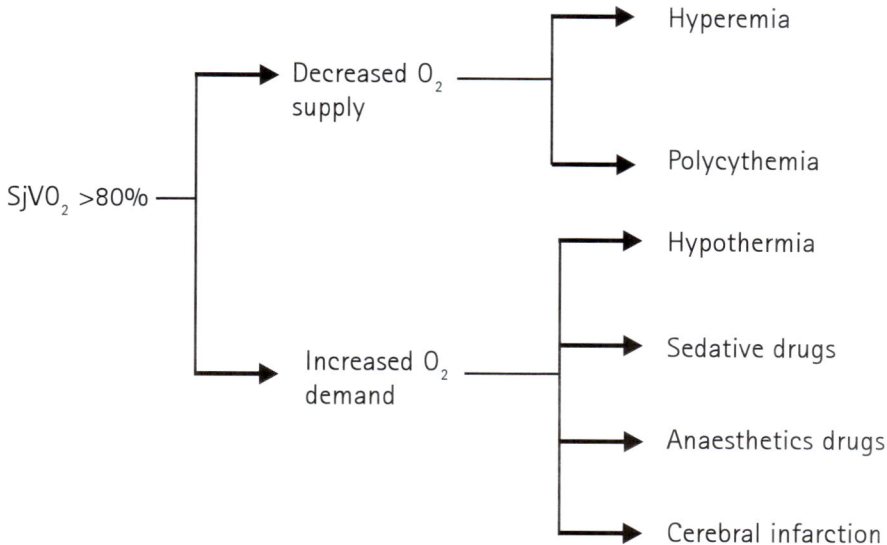

Fig. 14: Management of High SjVO$_2$

CONCLUSION

- Intraoperative Neuromonitoring (IONM) is useful in predicting intraoperative and postoperative nerve damage.

- **Multimodality monitoring**: Individually neuromonitoring techniques may have false-negative as well as false positive results, however their combined use, significantly improves their sensitivity and specificity hence gives greater versatility and power of diagnosis, and is preferred over any single monitoring technique.

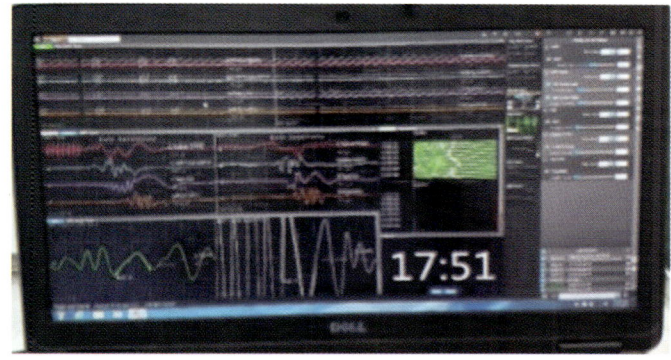

Fig. 15: Multimodality monitoring

REFERENCES

1. Cottrell JE, Young WL.Cottrell and Young's Neuroanesthesia, 5th ed. United States of America: ; 2010.

2. Hemanshu Prabhakar. Essentials of Neuroanesthesia: Elsevier Inc, San Francisco; 2017.

3. Gupta N, Singh GP. Electroencephalography based monitors. J Neuroanaesthesiol Crit Care 2015;2:168-78.

4. Ali Z, Bithal PK. Intra-operative neurophysiological monitoring. J Neuroanaesthesiol Crit Care 2015;2:179-92.

5. Abraham M, Singhal V. Intracranial pressure monitoring. J Neuroanaesthesiol Crit Care 2015;2:193-203.

6. Schell RM, Cole DJ. Cerebral Monitoring: Jugular Venous Oximetry. ANESTH ANALG 2000;90:559–66.

MULTIPLE CHOICE QUESTIONS

1. **24 year old man without significant past medical history posted for thoracolumber spine deformity correction. Planned neuromonitoring modalities are tcMEPS, SSEP and EMG. It is expected that most anaesthetic regimes will have a more pronounced effect on evoked potential latency than amplitude.**

   a. True

   b. False

2. **Rank the evoked potential modalities in order of decreasing sensitivity to anaesthetic agents**

   a. VEP, MEP, SSEP, BAEP

   b. MEP, VEP, SSEP, BAEP

   c. BAEP, SSEP, VEP, MEP

   d. BAEP, SSEP, MEP, VEP

3. **A young adult with a midthoracic fracture and uncleared cervical spine following a fall presented for spine stabilisation and fusion. What neuromonitoring modalities should be applied in this case**

   a. EMG triggered only

   b. SSEP

   c. EMG spontaneous only

   d. MEP

   e. SSEP, EMG triggered and MEP

4. **What intravenous anaesthetic agent can be added to maintenance regimen to increase evoked potential amplitude?**

   a. Dexmedetomidine

   b. Lignocaine

   c. Ketamine

5. **45 year old adult posted for left acoustic neuroma excision with BAEP monitoring. During resection of tumour, BAEP.**

   a. are robust and not affected by external stimuli such as drilling and extraneous noise

   b. are significantly altered by both intravenous and inhalation agents

   c. Waves I and V presence best correlates postoperative hearing preservation

   d. Provides realtime monitoring of 8th nerve and brainstem integrity

6. **EEG – following is true.**

   a. Generated by pyramidal cells of granular cortex

   b. Deep sleep and deep anaesthesia produce delta waves

   c. Theta waves are high frequency, low amplitude waves seen in awake adults

   d. Indicated intraoperatively in detection of cerebral ischemia, assessment of pharmacological interventions (burst suppression)and brain death, diagnosis and management of intractable epilepsy.

   e. Plot of voltage against time

7. **All the following are true about sensory evoked potentials except,**

   a. There are 3 modalities – SSEP, MEP, BAEP

   b. Individual peaks are described in terms of amplitude, latency and polarity

   c. For SSEP – 50% decrease in amplitude is clinically signifiant

   d. Evoked potentials of brainstem origin are more vulnerable to anaesthetic influence when compared to those of cortical origin

   e. Volatile agents cause dose dependent increase in latency and decrease in amplitude of cortical evoked potentials

8. **About Jugular venous oximetry, all are true except**

   a. Estimates balance betwenn cerebral oxygen demand and supply

   b. Normal $SjvO_2$ is 70–80%

   c. Change of oxygention of systemic blood influences $SjvO_2$

   d. $SjvO_2$ increases to > 75% during ischaemic injury

   e. It does not detect focal ischaemia

9. **Surgeries for which one would consider omitting an intermediate or long acting neuromuscular blockade at the time of induction and intubation include**

   a. Craniotomy for aneurysm clipping with EEG, MEP and SSEP monitoring planned

   b. Multilevel thoracolumber posterior spinal fusion without 'pre flip' baseline neuromonitoring signals planned

   c. Cervical posterior spinal fusion with 'pre flip' baseline SSEP amd MEP neuromonitoring signals requested

   d. Microvascular decompression for hemifacial spasm with neuromonitoring

11. **Transcranial Doppler: all are true except**

   a. Readings assume no change in diameter of MCA

   b. Anaemia may affect the readings

   c. Blood pressure is an important component of FV mean

   d) Lindegaard ratio of 6 implies hyperemia in a patient with SAH

   e) May be used to improve outcome in carotid surgery.

CHAPTER 14

ANAESTHETIC CONSIDERATIONS IN SPINE SURGERIES

Prerna Gomes, Aparna Budhakar

Introduction

The surgical procedures on the spine and spinal cord are common and performed for a variety of conditions. These surgeries can be elective or emergency. Both adults and paediatric patients present for surgery.

They mainly present with following pathologies: trauma, unstable vertebral fractures, vertebral abscess, vascular malformations, benign and malignant tumours (metastatic or primary diseases with spinal instability, pain and neurological compromise), congenital/ idiopathic scoliosis or degenerative disease.

Surgery may be required at any site in the spine from cervical to lumbosacral and ranges from minimally invasive micro discectomy to prolonged operations involving multiple spinal levels and significant blood loss. The stabilization of the spine involves instrumentation above and below the unstable spinal level especially in scoliotic surgeries. The approach for insertion of such devices may be through a posterior, anterior or a combined approach involving reposition of the patient half way through the procedure and with major blood loss.

The challenges to the Anaesthesiologist is to provide optimal surgical conditions. The pre-anaesthetic evaluation should be meticulous and complete. The main intraoperative concerns are related to the approach, positioning, blood loss and monitoring of neurologic functions of spinal cord. The anaesthetic technique should be tailored to best suit the type of intraoperative neurologic monitoring technique used.

The major concern is postoperative pain and is a challenging task for the anaesthesiologist and a multimodal approach of systemic analgesics in combination with regional techniques are helpful.

Preoperative assessment

Pre-anaesthetic evaluation of patients undergoing spinal surgery is most important and should involve assessment of airway, respiratory system, cardiovascular system and nervous system. There should be a thorough discussion with the surgeon about the type of spine surgery, position involved and the anticipated blood loss.

Airway assessment: Airway assessment is especially important in surgery of upper thoracic and cervical spine. A careful assessment of stability of cervical spine should be done. Apart from stability, other assessment tools like Mallampatti classification, mouth opening etc. should also be assessed.

Cardiovascular evaluation: Due to the pre-existing underlying cardiac disease or due to direct effect of the spinal deformity, long standing scoliosis may have corpulmonale secondary to the chronic hypoxia and pulmonary hypertension. The cardiac dysfunction may also result from the underlying systemic pathology like rheumatoid arthritis, muscular dystrophy etc. These patients should be evaluated preoperatively with electrocardiogram and echocardiogram to assess left ventricular function and severity of pulmonary hypertension.

Respiratory system assessment: Patients having high thoracic and cervical involvement, often have impaired pulmonary functions with repeated chest infections and many of them may be mechanically ventilated preoperatively. The patients having scoliosis have restricted pulmonary disease with reduced vital capacity and total lung capacity and the severity often depends upon the angle of Cobb, the number of vertebrae involved, the cephalad position of curve and loss of normal thoracic kyphosis.[1,2] The abnormality in arterial blood gas is usually reduced oxygen tension with normal carbon dioxide levels indicating a ventilation perfusion mismatch.

Preoperatively, all the reversible conditions should be corrected like control of chest infection by appropriate antibiotics and optimisation of chest conditions by use of chest physiotherapy and bronchodilators.

Neurological evaluation. The degree of neurologic impairment should be assessed thoroughly preoperatively and should appropriately documented. The knowledge of existing deficits is essential for accurate surveillance and diagnosis of new postoperative deficits[1].

Hematologic evaluation: This includes complete hemogram, serum electrolytes and renal function tests. These patients may be on chronic therapy with non-steroidal anti-inflammatory drugs (NSAID's) and thromboprophylaxis for deep vein thrombosis, so a coagulation profile is important preoperatively.

Premedication - It depends upon neurological deficit and hemodynamic stability of the patient. Preoperative bronchodilators and antibiotics are continued to optimise pulmonary status. The usual premedication drugs used in spine surgery are anti sialagogue's like glycopyrrolate and aspiration prophylaxis with proton pump inhibitors or histamine-2 receptor antagonists.

Intraoperative management

Anaesthesia induction : Most cases of spine surgeries require general anaesthesia, consisting of inducing agents, opioids, muscle relaxants and inhalational agents. Mandatory monitoring for all cases include electrocardiography, non-invasive blood pressure, pulse oximetry, capnography and temperature.

A large bore intravenous cannula should be inserted and secured to prevent dislodgement in prone position[3]. These surgeries have massive blood loss. The additional iv access is useful for potential multiple infusions. The decision to invasively monitor arterial pressure should be based on the planned operation, expected blood loss, patient co-morbidities, and a requirement for postoperative critical care management.[1] The threshold for arterial cannulation and monitoring should be low as haemodynamic instability secondary to patient position and blood loss is common. It also allows sequential intraoperative blood investigations. The use of a central venous cannula will depend upon haemodynamic. It provides an additional route for intravenous infusions. Nowadays minimally invasive monitors of cardiac output (CO) using arterial waveform pulse contour analysis or transoesophageal Doppler are widely used. The urinary catheterization and urine output monitoring is required for all major cases and those anticipated to last > 2 hrs. An enlarging bladder may cause increased intraoperative blood loss as pressure is transmitted to the valve less epidural veins. All patients with a spinal cord injury should have a urinary catheter inserted. Patients should be kept warm with appropriate warming devices.

Airway management

The decision for the method of intubation is made preoperatively by careful assessment of the patient's condition. The awake intubation is usually indicated in patients with documented unstable cervical spine and presence of neck stabilisation devices. The direct laryngoscopy with manual in line stabilization of spine may be an acceptable option if the intubation can be performed without significant neck flexion but in cases of fixed flexion deformity of cervical or upper thoracic spine, micrognathia, limited mouth opening and unstable cervical spine, the use of fibre optic laryngoscopy is preferable. The video laryngoscopeis an attractive alternative to the fibre optic bronchoscope especially if the availability is under question. The use of reinforced flexo-mettalic tube is recommended. A double lumen endobronchial tube may be required in surgery of thoracic spine when anterior approach is used to deflate one lung to facilitate the exposure of thoracic spine. It is important to fix the tube carefully to avoid dislodgement.

Positioning

The prone position is the most commonly used position for spine surgeries, other positions like lateral decubitus and sitting are also used. While positioning, special consideration should be given to the proper padding of pressure sensitive areas like bony prominences, eyes and peripheral nerves[4].

For safe prone positioning appropriate support should be selected. The foam bolsters are commonly used, one at the level of the chest below the axillae and the other at the level of the anterior superior iliac spines (Fig. 1).

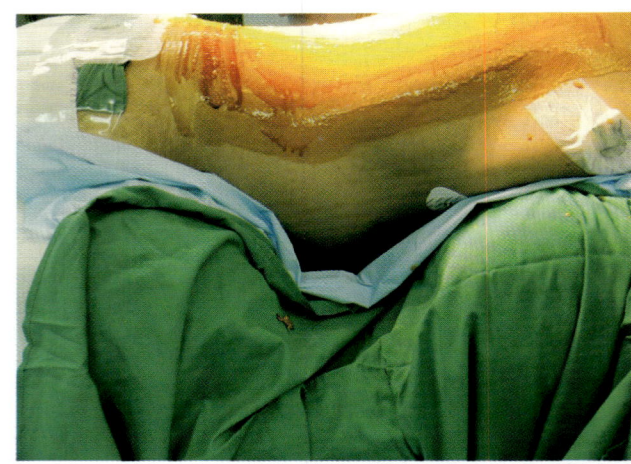

Fig. 1. Positioning of foam bolster in prone position

It is important to avoid pressure on abdomen as it will transmit to venous system leading to increase bleeding. Obstruction of inferior vena cava will lead to decrease venous return hence a decrease in CO and increased risk of lower limb thrombosis. The arms should be abducted to no more than 90° with slight internal rotation to avoid injury tobrachial plexus (Fig. 2).

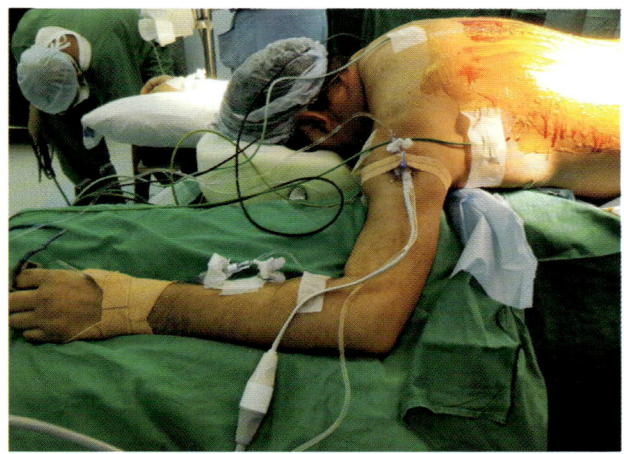

Fig. 2. Positioning of arms in prone position

The Ulnar nerve at the elbow is at high risk of pressure-related injury. The patient's arms are usually tucked at the sides for cervical procedures. After the arms are tucked, IV flow should be confirmed. Anterior cervical procedures are usually done with the patient's head on a padded head rest. For posterior cervical procedures or for procedures requiring intraoperative traction, the Mayfield device with skull pins is often used. The most commonly used specific devices are Andrews operating table, Jackson operating table and Wilson frame.

Patients are anesthetized on a stretcher and then turned prone onto the operating table. Prior to the turn the eyes are covered with clear plastic adhesive dressing, bite blocks are placed. Foam headrest is placed over the patient's face while supine, making sure that the eyes and nose are free. After turning prone and frequently during surgery the eyes, nose, and periorbital areas should be checked through the mirror to make sure that they are not compressed (Fig. 3).

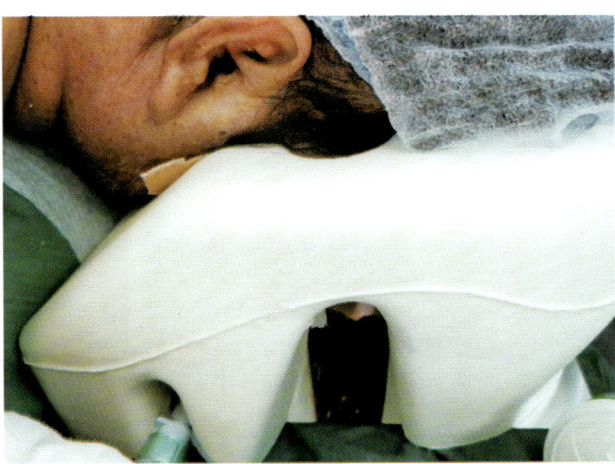

Fig. 3. Foam headrest with mirror in place

100% Oxygen should be administered before turning patient to prevent desaturation while ventilation is interrupted. Intravenous tubing and arterial line transducer tubing should be positioned along the patient's side to avoid dislodgement while turning. Monitoring cables may be disconnected for the turn but should be replaced as soon as possible.

The turning of the patient should be coordinated among the anaesthetist, the surgeon, and the other individuals helping with positioning. The breathing circuit should be disconnected at the last possible moment and for as briefly as possible. During the turn, the patient's neck should be kept in a neutral position.

Special attention should be paid to the endotracheal tube when positioning prone. After turning prone, the ability to ventilate, bilateral breath sounds and blood pressure should be confirmed immediately. Once the patient is prone, the breathing circuit should be supported to avoid traction on the endotracheal tube.

Maintenance of anaesthesia

The main aim of maintenance of anaesthesia is to provide a stable anaesthetic depth with stable hemodynamic parameters so that the intraoperative monitoring of somatosensory and motor evoked potentials can be performed reliably. The use of 60% nitrous oxide in oxygen with less than 0.5 MAC of sevoflurane/desflurane and titrated dose of opioids usually is compatible with the neurologic monitoring.

Fluid management

The aim is to keep patients euvolemic hence the balanced salt solutions are preferred. It is important to avoid excessive administration of crystalloids as it can lead to soft tissue oedema[5].

Blood pressure management

The overall aim is to avoid decreases in arterial blood pressures > 20% from baseline. In patients with myelopathy or trauma to the spine a mean arterial pressure should be maintained ≤ 80-90 mmHg.

Previously the induced hypotension technique was used to reduce intraoperative blood loss. The decreased blood loss is due to decrease blood flow at a site of surgery due to decrease in arterial blood flow. However, epidural venous plexus pressure and intraosseous pressure, both important determinants of blood loss in spine surgery, are independent of arterial blood pressure. Therefore, use of controlled hypotension is not recommended anymore.[1]

In fact, induced hypotension should be avoided as it can lead to end-organ ischaemia. The procedures like spinal instrumentation and distraction can reduce spinal cord perfusion and lead to ischaemia. It is important to maintain adequate arterial blood pressure during instrumented spinal surgery to avoid neurologic damage.

Major spine surgery can result in significant blood loss. The severity of blood loss depends on number of spinal levels fused. Other factors responsible for increased blood loss are obesity, increased intra-abdominal pressure in the prone position, surgery for tumours and the performance of transpedicular osteotomy[6].

The prophylactic use of tranexamic acid (10mg/kg bolus) should be considered for major surgery. But it should be avoided in patients with a history of thromboembolic events or patients suffering from malignancies.

Temperature management

Perioperative hypothermia is a phenomenon that happens often. Its manifestation during the anesthetic-surgical process is directly connected to the many disturbances the patients go through, including the occurrence of surgical wound infection. Thermoregulation may already be impaired in patients who have spinal cord lesions before surgery. Prolonged anaesthesia causes significant heat loss therefore it is mandatory to monitor temperature. To avoid hypothermia, use of warm air mattress device, i.v. fluids infusion warmers and covering exposed area with thin plastic sheet is recommended (Fig. 4).

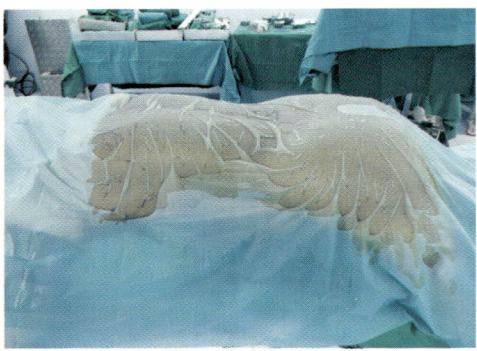

Fig. 4. Plastic sheet on exposed areas

The specific monitoring of spinal cord functions may be required intraoperatively in surgeries where the integrity of spinal cord may be affected like in spinal fusion surgery, deformity correction surgery where distractive forces are applied and in removal of spinal cord tumours and vascular lesions. The newer modalities like bispectral index system (BIS) have become available which can measure the electroencephalographic activity during the surgical procedure and can help in maintaining adequate depth of anaesthesia. The studies have shown that incidence of neurologic injury can be reduced significantly if intraoperative spinal cord monitoring is employed. The surgery can lead to dysfunction of sensory or motor functions of spinal cord which can be detected early by these monitoring techniques and corrective measures can be taken by the surgeons intraoperatively[4].

Commonly used spinal cord monitoring are Somatosensory evoked potentials (SSEP)

It involves electrical stimulation of a peripheral mixed nerve (posterior tibial, sural or peroneal nerve) and recording of the evoked potential at a distant site cephalad to the site of surgery. After obtaining the baseline values, a stable plane of anaesthesia is established and intraoperatively the integrity of somatosensory pathways is monitored by comparing the changes in amplitude and latency period of the evoked potentials with the baseline. A significant response is considered as a 50% reduction in amplitude and a 10% reduction in latency period. SSEP monitoring helps in detecting the change in integrity of the dorsomedial tract in the posterior part of spinal cord which is supplied by posterior spinal artery, so it does not detect any changes in the motor pathways which occupy mainly the anterior part of the spinal cord. Anaesthetic agents can have significant effect on the pattern of SSEP's. The inhalational agents along with nitrous oxide can decrease the amplitude and prolong the latent period of SSEP's in a dose dependent manner. However, an anaesthetic containing 60% nitrous oxide combined with 0.5 MAC sevoflurane is considered compatible with SSEP monitoring.

The amplitude of SSEP's is also reduced by intravenous opioids but to a lesser degree while neuromuscular blockers have no effect on monitoring of SSEP.

SSEP monitoring is a reliable technique with acceptable sensitivity and specificity in detecting intraoperative neurological damage during spinal surgery.

Motor evoked potentials (MEP)

It involves stimulation of the spinal cord or motor cortex cephalad to the site of surgery and recording the evoked potentials in motor tracts of spinal cord or the muscle distal to the site of surgery. Any damage to motor tracts by surgery results in reduction in amplitude and prolongation of latency of evoked potentials. The myogenic responses are obtained by summation of electromyographic responses of muscles stimulated and are influenced by the degree of neuromuscular blockade which should be continuously monitored. It is generally employed that an anaesthetic technique based on Propofol infusion and fentanyl or remifentanil can provide reliable monitoring of motor evoked potentials in majority of the patients.

Wake-up test

This test demonstrates the integrity of motor pathways of the spinal cord during intraoperative period. The procedure requires a preoperative counselling of the patient explaining that the patient would be asked to move fingers, hand, toes and legs intraoperatively. The surgeon normally informs the anaesthesiologist 30 minutes prior to test and during testing neuromuscular blockade is reversed and the plane of anaesthesia is lightened. It does not evaluate the integrity of sensory pathways. To achieve this the anaesthetic technique must be tailored in a fashion to allow for waking up of the patient. The drawback of this technique is patient can get agitated which can lead to leading to accidental extubation and injury too.

Postoperative care:

Main concern is neurological dysfunction, hence early regaining of consciousness in postoperative period is usually required for immediate neurological assessment by surgeons.

The adequate control of postoperative pain is a challenge in these patients as a large incision is usually present with lot of bone manipulation. A multi-modal approach involving parenteral analgesics combined with regional techniques is usually recommended. The drugs are used for pain relief are opioids and non-steroidal anti-inflammatory drugs (NSAID's).[7, 8]

The early postoperative complications following major spinal surgery include fluid deficit, neurological dysfunction, dural injury leading to leakage of cerebrospinal fluid, nausea and vomiting, atelectasis, pneumonia, urinary retention and venous thrombosis.

The incidence of thromboembolic complications following major spinal injury has been found to range between 0.39 to 15.5% suggesting importance of instituting prophylaxis against thromboembolism.

Another important complication related to spine surgery especially in prone position is perioperative vision loss which is of great medico legal importance. The most common cause remains to be perioperative ischemic optic neuropathy while central retinal artery and vein occlusion and occipital lobe infarction are other less common causes.

Postoperative visual loss (POVL) occurs in 1/60000–1/125000 operationsInitial careful positioning of the head and regular checks throughout the procedure in case of movement minimizes the risk. Documentation of these eye checks throughout the course of long procedures has been advised by the ASA. Horseshoe-shaped head rests should be avoided in prone patients as they have been implicated in cases of central retinal artery occlusion (CRAO).[1]

POVL caused by ischaemic optic neuropathy is associated with male gender, obesity, increasing blood loss and operative procedures > 6 hrs in length. In postoperative period if the patient complains of vision problems an early ophthalmic opinion is sought. Initial management should include optimization of arterial pressure, oxygenation and correction of anaemia. Treatment with agents such as acetazolamide has not been beneficial and there is rarely any useful improvement in vision with either injury, so attention should be focused on preventative measures. Careful positioning with the head at the same level as the heart, meticulous haemostasis and possibly staging prolonged procedures should be considered[3].

CONCLUSION

Spine surgery presents a wide range of challenges to the surgeon as well as the anaesthesiologist. The perioperative morbidity has been reduced by advancement in intraoperative monitoring of neurological functions which may be affected by the type of spinal surgery. The anaesthesiologist plays a dominant role in facilitating the Intraoperative neurologic monitoring and in managing the postoperative pain relief which may be challenging in these patients. A detailed preanaesthetic evaluation and intraoperative anaesthetictechnique facilitating neurologic monitoring and good postoperative pain relief are main anaesthetic concerns in spine surgery.

REFERENCES

1. Up-to-date [Internet]. [Place unknown]: Up-to-date, Inc; c2017. Anaesthesia for elective spine surgery in adults; [updated 2017 Feb 28 cited 2017 June]; [about 5 screens]. Available from: https://www.uptodate.com/contents/anesthesia-for-elective-spine-surgery-in-adults#H478155361.

2. Raw DA, Beattie JK, Hunter JM. Anaesthesia for spinal surgery in adults. Br J Anaesth. 2003;91(6):886-904.

3. Nowicki RW. Anaesthesia for major spinal surgery. BJA Education. 2014;14(4):147-152.

4. Bajwa SJ, Kulshrestha A. Spine Surgeries: Challenging Aspects and Implications for Anaesthesia. J Spine Neurosurg [Internet]. 2013 Jan [cited 2013 Jun 18]; 2:3. Available from: http://dx.doi.org/10.4172/2325-9701.1000114.

5. Ether Stanford Medicine [Internet]. [Place unknown]: Stanford Medicine; 2017. Guidelines for the intraoperative management of patients undergoing spine surgery; [updated 2017]; [about 5 screens]. Available from: http://ether.stanford.edu/policies/spine_surgery.html.

6. Miller RD. Anaesthesia for orthopaedic surgery. In: Miller RD, editor. Miller's Anaesthesia. 8th ed. [Place unknown]: Elsevier/Saunders; 2015. P. 2402-05.

7. Leemans M. Anaesthesia for spine surgery. In: Pollard BJ, editor. Handbook of Clinical Anaesthesia. 3rd ed. London: Edward Arnold (Publishers) Ltd; 2011. p. 322-325.

8. Crabb I. Anaesthesia for spinal surgery. Anaesthesia and intensive care medicine [Internet]. 2008 [cited]; Available from: http://www.anaesthesiajournal.co.uk/article/S1472-0299(08)00280-4/abstract#.

MULTIPLE CHOICE QUESTIONS

1. **Intraoperatively mean BP should be maintained**
   a. Above 60
   b. Above 70
   c. Above 100
   d. Above 80

2. **While shifting patient from supine head should be maintained in**
   a. Flexion
   b. Extension
   c. Neutral
   d. None of the above

3. **Intraoperatively eyes should be protected with**
   a. Clear plastic adhesive dressing
   b. Multiple gamzee pads
   c. Antibiotic cream
   d. None of the above

4. **In prone positioning arms should be abducted to**
   a. No more than 30 degree
   b. No more than 90 degree
   c. No more than 15 degree
   d. None of the above

5. **Awake intubation is usually indicated in patients with**
   a. Unstable cervical spine
   b. Lower thoracic fractures
   c. Patients with myelopathy
   d. None of the above

6. **Recommended spinal cord monitoring is**
   a. BSI
   b. Entropy
   c. SSEP/MEP
   d. Wakeup test

7. **SSEP monitoring done in spinal surgery**
   a. To measure the depth of anesthesia
   b. To monitor neuromuscular blockade
   c. Detecting neurological damage during spinal surgery
   d. None of these

8. **POVL can be prevented**
   a. By low blood pressure
   b. Fluid load
   c. Keeping head on horseshoe head rest
   d. Careful position of head with frequent inspection

9. **The effects of anesthesthetic agents on SSEP**
   a. No effect
   b. Minimal effect
   c. Significant effect
   d. None of the above

10. **The most common cause of POVL**
    a. Occipital lobe infarction
    b. Central retinal artery occlusion
    c. Central retinal vein occlusion
    d. Ischemic optic neuropathy

CHAPTER 15

ANAESTHESIA FOR NEURO - ENDOVASCULAR PROCEDURES

Sugandha A. Karapurkar

Introduction

In last three decades, neuro-radiological diagnosis and treatment of cerebro-vascular diseases, has undergone significant advances.

The risks encountered are the same as those faced by anesthesiologists during operative neurosurgery. The difference is that these procedures are done and in INR suite or catheter labs where there are no ideal conditions are available as in operation theatres. The working environment is totally different and on many occasions anesthetist must manipulate systemic and cerebral hemodynamics as per needs of patient as well as neuro interventionist[1,2]. The understanding of these challenges and their implications on INR procedures are vital for anesthesiologist.

Pre-Anesthetic assessment

A preop visit to patients undergoing INR procedures, is must for anesthesiologist. The assessment of relevant history of present and past complaints, physical examination of all systems. It includes neurological examination with

any involvement of cranial nerves to compare withany post procedure deficit. The co-morbidity like DM, Hypertension, IHD, Renal impairment should be optimized.

History of pregnancy; adverse reactions to contrast; patients on antiplatelet, anticoagulant and in elderly patients of history of backpain, arthritis should be noted. All patients should be kept fasting as per procedure.

Laboratory tests

It includes routine hematological; biochemical tests; electrolytes Na, K, Cl; and Mg levels are necessary. Many of these patients are on diuretics for BP, raised ICP and poor oral intake can lead to impairment in electrolytes balance.

Renal Functions: Serum creatinine is important as radio opaque dye is excreted by the kidneys. If the creatinine is high, patient should be hydrated with I.V. Saline, Acetyl cysteine (Mucomix) 600-1200 mg twice daily for 3 days before and after the procedure. On the day of procedure, soda bicarb is given intravenously to alkalinize the urine.

ECG and 2 D Echo

ECG and 2 D Echo should be done to know the cardiac status of the patient. As following SAH, ECG may show ST changes suggestive of "stunned myocardium" indicating sudden severe stress on the myocardium.The treatment of vasospasm requires "HHH" (Hypertension, Hypervolemia, Hemodilution) which may not be possible if cardiac function are impaired. The chemical or balloon angioplasty followed by "HHH" therapy may need to be continued for upto day 21 after SAH. In patients with poor cardiac function during angioplasty and stenting for carotid stenosis bradycardia and hypotension may not be tolerated.

Coagulation Profile

As many patients, are on antiplatelet, anticoagulant therapy, PT, PTT, INR – should be tested. The PT, PTT, INR may need to be corrected before to avoid hematoma formation at puncture site as during these procedures patient receives large doses of heparin.

Radiation Safety

Three sources of radiation in INR suite

Direct   - From X-ray tube

Leakage   - Through collimator's protective shielding.

Scattered - Reflected from patient and surrounding body part

The radiation exposure is inversely proportional to the distance from the source of radiation. All concerned peoples including anesthesiologists should station themselves away from the source and should wear lead aprons, thyroid shields, Radiation exposure badges, and use movable lead glass screen[3,4].

Intravenous access

It is advisable to put a large gauge cannula (No.18/20) on left hand and internal Jugular Vein (IJV) catheter is to be inserted before heparinization[5]. A 200 cm. extension tubing is required for infusion and monitoring lines to keep away from C arm[4.]

Arterial pressure monitoring

In patients with cardiac problem and during treatment of aneurysm continuous display of arterial pressure monitoring is advisable.The arterial cannulation should be done before heparinization and to be continued post procedure in ICU or if patient needs further monitoring.If arterial cannulation is difficult, then side port of the femoral artery introducer sheath, can be used to monitor arterial pressure.

Bladder Catheterization: is required in all major procedures to assists in fluid management as well as for patient comfort.

Temperature monitoring

Hypothermia does occur in the neuroradiology suite and measures should be taken to keep the body temperature near normal and core temperature measured, especially in children and old patients.

Anticoagulation

The management of coagulation is required to prevent thromboembolic complication during and after procedure.The activated clotting time (ACT) is recorded before patient is heparinized. Inj. Heparin 70 IU/kg is given to keep ACT two to three times the control and if needed additional doses of Heparin are given.

Intravenous fluids: Avoid fluids containing dextrose as high level of glucose can cause poor outcome. The Ringer lactate is usually preferred to fill capillary bed for better angiographic demonstration[6].

Premedication

In anxious patient mild sedative or anxiolytic medicine can be given. In case of altered consciousness and compromised airway patient avoid sedatives. The antihypertensive, anticonvulsants, corticosteroids, antiplatelet should be given in premedication after assessment of patient's status[1].

Preprocedural preparation: Ideally, INR suite should be like any standard operation room anesthesia machine with monitoring facility and check for all emergency& resuscitation drugs; anesthetic drugs; intravenous fluids; availability of emergency trolley for CP resuscitation;[1] equipment for access to airway, difficult airway equipment. The anesthesia machine must have double length circuit tubing's, to remain away from the C arm and imaging devices to rotate freely around the head. The iv fluid and drug infusion lines should be long enough so that injection of drugs becomes easy without interrupting the procedure.

Anesthesia technique

The choice of anesthetic technique varies from center to center as very little data is available to support as particular technique. One must consider the need for radiologist and procedure while choosing a technique. There is more and more trend to move towards general anesthesiabut it depends up to local practice and training[1, 4].

Advantage of General Anesthesia

Many neuro-radiologists prefer general anesthesia as opposed to sedation. As under general anesthesia, patient is comfortable, immobile; provides a good quality image[4] and better control on oxygenation, carbon di-oxide with hemodynamic stability.

Disadvantages of GA[4]

Inability to assess the patient neurologically during the procedure. The consequences of endotracheal intubation and extubation are hypertension and coughing, straining leads to increase ICP.

Intravenous sedation: The advantages of sedation just before procedure are easy to perform neurological assessment as there are no hemodynamic changes.

The disadvantages are the unprotected airway can cause risk of aspiration, respiratory depression and obstruction this can lead to hypoxia. The sudden movement of patient may mar the picture and repeated acquisitions may be required because of poor road map or images[4].

Procedures done in INR suite[7]

Diagnostic:

- DSA (Digital Substraction Angiography)
- Balloon test occlusion.

Therapeutics

- Acute Stroke
- Embolization of vascular malformation
- Intracranial AVM
- Dural AV Fistula
- Cerebral Aneurysm
- Carotid Cavernous Fistula (CCF)
- Spinal AVM, A V Fistula
- Angioplasty and Stenting-intra- and extracranial occlusive diseases
- Balloon Angioplasty for vasospasm following SAH, Sclerotherapy of venous angiomas.
- Embolization for epistaxis.
- Intra-arterial chemotherapy of head and neck tumors.

Goals of anesthesia during INR procedures[7]

- Immobile and physiologically stable patient.
- Easy manipulation of systemic blood pressure either hypo or hypertension as per neuro-radiologist's requirements. To have quiet breathing for good quality of pictures.
- Catastrophe can be handled better.

Problems during anesthesia

- Remote and unprotected area
- Inaccessible airway and venous lines
- Use of large doses of heparin.
- Quick and smooth recovery from anesthesia.
- Provide protection from hypothermia as temperature of INR suite is kept around 19-20⁰ C.
- Continuous infusion of irrigation fluid.

Anesthetic technique[8]

There is no clear conclusion regarding which mode of anesthesia is superior to another. The selection criteria, include complexity and length of procedure;

patient status;needsof interventionist while selecting anesthetic technique.

Awake patient

To allay anxiety and win patients confidence always explain about the type of procedure and having transient warm sensation in head and face while procedure.

These procedures are under LA, still all resuscitative measures and monitoring BP, SpO2, ECG are mandatory with secured intravenous access.

Advantage: Neurological assessment is easy.

Conscious sedation

Sedation and monitored anesthesia care (MAC)

In anxious, uncomfortable patients mild sedation is necessary.

In small children, compromised airway patients, restless patients procedure should be done under GA[9].

The selection of sedation to be decided anesthesiologist and availability of drugs[1]and should be ready for the potential risk of respiratory arrest and cardiorespiratory complications[1]. The shivering can interfere with image quality and in elderly, critical patient and small children care should be taken to prevent hypothermia.

Midazolam: 1mg IV bolus and repeat if needed.

Inj. Fentanyl 1-2 microg/kg followed by Propofol infusion 10-20 mg/kg/min is recommended.When properly titratedneurological assessment is possible. Strict vigilance is mandatory for airway obstruction and respiratory depression[1].

Dexmedetomidine: Alpha 2 agonist has good analgesic and hypnotic property with little effect on respiratory depression and patient is arousable, co-operative when stimulated[1,9]. Anesthesiologist should be prepared to convert MAC to GA[9].

General anesthesia with ETT: The advantages are to reduce motion artifacts; to improve the quality of image especially small children; for uncooperative patients and easy to create apnea, on radiologist request while taking road mapping.

Disadvantage: The neurological assessment is not possible until patient comes out of anesthesia and hemodynamic changes occur during intubation and emergence of anesthesia.

Monitoring: ECG, SpO2, NIBP., continuous arterial monitoring for aneurysm coiling and patient with poor cardiac status.

A good intravenous access isimportant before starting MAC or general anesthesia.The documentation of dose and timing of heparin must be done.

Intravenous Anesthetic Agents : Propofol, Pentothal are preferred for their properties of minimal hemodynamic changes and smooth rapid emergence if used with vigilance.

Inhalational anesthetic agents : Sevoflurane, Desflurane.In a study, Sevoflurane was associated with rapid recovery[4] and Desflurane can cause increased cerebral flow and loss of autoregulation[4].

Avoid sudden surge of BP during intubation and extubation of the patient. During Laryngoscopy MAP is reduced by 15- 20% of base line by taking patient in deep plane of anaesthesia[6,1].

Muscle relaxant: Atracurium is preferred to avoid delayed recovery and can be used as continuous infusion. In case of sudden termination of procedure for various reasons short durationof action of Atracurium helps to bring the patient outof anesthesia.

Nitrous oxide (N2O)

Use of N20 during general anesthesia depends upon the ICP. In SAH avoid N_2O if ICP is raised. The endotracheal intubation with intermittent positive pressure ventilation is usually preferred.

Laryngeal mask airway

LMA may be used as an alternative to endotracheal intubation for management of airway.

Advantage: It allows airway control with less hemodynamic changes and smooth emergence from anaesthesia.[4] There is insufficient evidence to consider its use in routine practice[8].

Complications during INR procedures[4]

CNS complications	Non-CNS complications
Hemorrhagic	
Aneurysm perforation	Contrast reaction
IC vessel dissection	Contrast nephropathy
Occlusive	Hemorrhage at puncture
Thromboembolic complications	site, groin hematoma
Migration of coil	Retroperitoneal hematoma
Coil fracture	
Vasospasm	

Complications during INR procedures can be rapid and serious. The management is separate for hemorrhagic or occlusivefor successful management.

Hemorrhagic complications

It is accompanied by abrupt rise in MAP and severe bradycardia.

Steps of Management are following:

- Neutralize Inj. Heparin by Protamine sulphate (1 mg Protamine for each 100 units of Heparin)
- Systemic BP is lowered by increasing depth of anesthesia, anti-hypertensive agents.
- Brain edema-give Osmotic diuretic I.V. Mannitol (0.5 to 1 gm/kg).
- Aneurysmal perforation is usually sealed by packing the coils.

Occlusive complications

Management:

Raise arterial pressure by increasing collateral circulation and maintenance normo-carbia[4].

Angiographically visible thrombus can be removed by mechanical thrombectomy.

Use of thrombolytic agents like Reoprob, RTPA.

Vasospasm – Vasospasm of IC vessels can be treated with intra-arterial injection of Nimodipine or Intra-arterial Papaverine infusion[4].

Triple H therapy – Hypertension, hypervolemia and hemodilution and is useful to treat vasospasm following SAH which normally occurs between 5 to 12 days. The risks are pulmonary edema, myocardial ischemia, electrolyte imbalance, cerebral edema to be recognized and managed.

Balloon angioplasty

Is also considered effective procedure must be done early, within 2 hours of symptoms[10].

Endovascular procedures

Endovascular treatment for cerebral aneurysms

Endovascular treatment of aneurysm ruptured or unruptured should be under full general anesthesia. There should be good control of airway and patient should be immobile.

Technique:1) GDC Coils; 2) Balloon assisted coiling; 3) Stent assisted coiling 4) Flow diverter.

Monitoring: Continuous display of arterial BP along with basic monitoring is very important.

Complications

Perforation of Aneurysm: 2.3 to 3% of ruptured aneurysm

: < 0.5% of un-ruptured aneurysm

Thrombus: at the tip of the catheter, guide wire or coil.

Coil unravelling and coil fracture

Parent Artery: Occlusion due to displacement of the coil – 2.5%

Protamine sulphate: Should be always kept ready to neutralize Heparin.

Endovascular treatment of AVM, AVF

AVM (Arteriovenous malformation): Consists of a vascular component with a nidus that is fed by one or more arteries and drained by one or more veins. Arteries and veins are connected with shunts. These are the patients present with hemorrhage, seizures or neurological problems.

Endovascular treatment of AVM[4,9]:

There are three options of treatment.

1. Surgical excision (2) Embolization (3) Stereotactic radiosurgery (4) Combination of all above.

Anesthesia for embolization

Embolization of AVM is always done under GA and patients are kept physiologically stable, totally immobile and temporary apnea is required for better visualization.

Post embolization: After embolization of AVM, patient is shifted to ICU. The systemic pressure is kept 15-20% below base line. The patient is kept paralysed and sedated for elective ventilation for 24 hours or sedated for elective ventilation for next 24 hours and observe for sudden IC hemorrhage.

In AVM feeding arteries supply some normal brain tissue so, abrupt restoration of normal systemic pressure in a chronicallyhypo perfused vascular bed may impair cerebral autoregulation and result in parenchymal hemorrhage.

Second possibility is there is occlusion of venous drainage in the brain surrounding the AVM followed by passive hyperemia and stagnation in feeding vein and artery. This leads to IC hemorrhage in post-embolization period.

AVF (Arterio Venous Fistula)

Pial Fistula– direct connection between artery and vein. Pial fistula is usually congenital.

Commonly found in: Vein of Galen Malformation (VOGM).

Carotid cavernous fistulas (CCF)

Spinal AVF

Dural AVF: Endovascular treatment is done under full GA as it is along procedure and for better visualization. Dural A.V. Fistula and venous hypertension can lead to IC haemorrhage[4, 3].

Spinal cord lesions : Intramedullary spinal AVM

Dural Fistulae

Tumors

Spinal angiography

Usually done under LA with MAC. The bowel preparation is important to reduce gases in intestine and better visualization of lesion.

Endovascular treatment: requires GA with muscle relaxant and sedation. The descent of diaphragm must be reduced for better visualization and temporary apnea is required during injection.

Caution: For lateral films, both arms are abducted and taken at head level and care of pressure points for over stretching of Brachial plexus. Inj. Buscopan IV to reduce the intestinal motility and to reduce spinal cord edema post procedure IV Methyl prednisolone is started prior to the embolization.

Vein of Galen Malformations: Are relatively uncommon. Usually present with high output cardiac failure, myocardial lesions, intractable seizures, hydrocephalus. To improve the outcome in neonate's, aggressive intensive care and medical management of cardiac failure before embolization,

secondary to VOGM. These babies after embolization, should be paralyzed, sedated and electively ventilated for 24 to 48 hrs.The systemic pressure is lowered to reduce break through bleeding.Milrinone has been used as peripheral vasodilator to improve CCF[3, 11, 12].

Pre-embolization, babies should be thoroughly investigated to know the cardiac status.

ECG - Right Ventricular hypertrophy

2D ECHO - Right Ventricular hypertrophy, Tricuspid insufficiency, PA pressure

To prevent severe brain injury caused by excess flow through AVM early intervention and aggressive management of CCF is required.

Tumor embolization

The tumors like meningioma, glomus, nasopharyngeal angiofibroma are embolized preoperatively to reduce the vascularity and to reduce blood loss during surgery. These procedures done under LA and MAC.

In compromised airway presence of tumor of tongue, skull base tumor should be observed for airway obstruction after embolization.

Carotid test occlusion

In patient having a large, unclippable aneurysm are treated by proximal vessel occlusion. A balloon test occlusion under LA with MAC before permanent occlusion and clinical evaluation is done every five minutes. If not tolerated the occlusion, then balloon is deflated and give 100% Oxygen, usually these patients recover quickly. The sensitivity test increases by reducing BP by 10% during BTO.

Carotid angioplasty and stenting

This procedure is done under LA with MAC and in aphasic and uncooperative patient general anesthesia is indicated. Since atherosclerosis is the main pathology of the carotid stenosis, patient can have multiple vessel disease like coronary, renal, peripheral. Often patients are diabetic and hypertensive. To know cardiac status ECG and 2D ECHO is done apart from routine laboratory tests.

Premedication : Antihypertensive continued

Antiplatelet – Aspirin, Clopidogrel

Anticonvulsants already on

Monitoring : Routine monitoring like ECG, HR, NIBP, SpO2.

In patients with poor cardiac function invasive arterial monitoring is done. During angioplasty with inflated balloon there is carotid body stimulation which leads to severe bradycardia or asystole. Hence before balloon inflation, IV

Atropine or I.V.Glycopyolate is given. After deployment of stent there may be hypotension which is treated with IV crystalloids or colloids.

There can be transient loss of consciousness or convulsions during balloon angioplasty in patient with bilateral lesions. Such case deflate balloon quickly and for brain protection, treat with large doses of steroid, Midazolam, Dilantin and intubate if needed.

Post procedure

After procedure, monitor for BP and HR in ICU and systolic BP should be below 120 mm Hg. Patient should be watched for rebound hypertension which can lead to break through bleeding and cause IC Hemorrhage or brain edema.The hypotension is treated with crystalloid or colloid fluids in severe hypotension treat with Noradrenalin infusion. Also withhold antihypertensives until blood pressure is stabilized.

Thrombolysis of Acute Ischemic Stroke (IS)[13, 14, 15]

Stroke is sudden loss of brain function due to loss of blood supply or cerebral hemorrhage. It is third leading cause of death in USA after CV disease and cancer. Co-morbities are systemic hypertension, diabetes, heart disease, hypercholesterolemia, alcohol abuse smoking, obesity and physical inactivity. 80 to 85% of strokes are ischemic and 15 to 20% hemorrhagic.

IS often starts at night during the period of inactivity progresses over hours. Stroke may be preceded by transient ischemic attacks (TIAs). Atrial fibrillation, following MI, Septal defect, Cardiomyopathy can lead to IS. 5% of hemorrhagic strokes are due to coagulopathy. Window for treatment of anterior circulation for IV Lysis (rTPA) is 3 to 4.5 hours and up to 6 hours for thrombectomy. Window for posterior circulation is up to 24 hours.

Investigations: Plain CT, Perfusion CT, CTA MRA.

Lab Investigations: RBS, Creatinine, PT, PTT

Management of BP, hydration, body temperature and blood sugar in acute IS essential. The tips are as follows:

- BP should not be lowered unless systolic BP is more than 200 mm Hg or diastolic BP is more than 120 mm Hg. As excessive lowering of BP can cause decrease perfusion inischemia.

- Maintain Glucose level is maintained below 150 mg%. Glucose level is maintained below 150 mg% as Hyperglycemia worsens stroke outcome, avoid solutions containing glucose.

- Use NS to prevent hyperglycemia.

- Patient should be kept slightly hypervolemia to maintain cerebral perfusion. Fever usually has worse outcome and should be treated aggressively.

Mechanical embolus removal in acute IS - MERCI device was approved by FDA for use in clinical practice in August 2004. Stentretriver is currently used for thrombectomy. Suction devices like Penumbra or ACE catheter are also used for thrombectomy.

Anesthesia for interventional procedure for acute IS monitoring : ECG, HR, Spo2 and NIBP.

If the patient is restless, unstable, non-cooperativeIA thrombus extraction should be done under full GA.

If patient is co-operative, quiet, thrombectomy is done under conscious sedation which is safe and fast[14]. Junssen et al studied 84 patients of acute IS underwent mechanical thrombectomy for anterior acute IS. 53 patients underwent general anesthesia and 31 patients had conscious sedation with standard cervical collar. They concluded that mechanical thrombectomy can be performed with conscious sedation with head immobilized with standard cervical collar. Recovery is fast and safe and early neurological assessment is possible. In MR, CLEAN multicentric randomized open label trial of IA thrombectomy vs no IA thrombectomy, GA was associated with better outcome resulting in reduction up to 51% treatment effect compared to non-GA[13].

CONCLUSION

Following therapeutic interventional procedures close monitoring of ICP, BP, level of consciousness is done for 24 to 48 hours in ICU. In paralyzed patientthe elective ventilation done with sedation. The systolic BP should be kept 15-20% below base line to keep ICP under control.

The choice of GA or sedation entirely depends up anesthesiologist and type of procedure.

REFERENCES

1. Aliya Ahmad; Anesthesia for Interventional neuroradiology, J. Ayrub Med Coll, Abbottabad 2007: 19 (3).

2. Kumar P, Anaesthesia for Interventional Neuro Radiology; Health &Medicine; 2nd June 2015

3. Hashimoto T, Gupta DK, Young W, Interventional neuroradiology – anaesthetic considerations ; Anaesthesiology Clinics of North America 2002; 20:347–359.

4. M.K. Varma, K. Price, V. Jayakrishnan, Manickam B & Kessell G; Anaesthetic considerations for interventional neuroradiology Br. J of Anaesthesia 2007; 99: 75–85.

5. Rosas AL; Anesthesia for Interventional Neuroradiology Part IV: Intraoperative management, Anticoagulation, Management of neurologic complications, conclusions. The Internet Journal of Anaesthesiology 1997; 1, 1–10.

6. Wolfson B, Hetrick WD, Dastur K: Anesthesia for Neuro Radiologic Procedures:in Anesthesia & Neurosurgery Ed. Cottrell JE, Turndorf H; Mosby CV, St Louis 1986: 104–113.

7. William L, Young MD, SpellmanJP Anaesthetic considerations for interventional neuro-radiology.Review article; Anaesthesiology, Vol 1994; 80, 427–456.

8. Young KW, Yang KH, Shun WJ, Song MH, Ham K Jung SCet al; Anaesthetic consideration for Neurointervention procedures. Neurointervention 2014:9:72–77.

9. Sinha PK, Neema PK, Rathod RC:Anaesthesia and Intra cranial AVM. Neurology India: Review article: 2004; 52:163–170.

10. Brothers MF, HolgateRC; Intra cranial angioplasty for treatment of vasospasm after SAH. Technique and modifications to improve branch access. Am J Neuroradiology 1990;11: 239–47.

11. Frawley GP, Dargaville PA,Mitchell PJ, Tress BM, Loughnan PClinical course and medical management of neonates with severe cardiac failure related to VOGM –Arch Dis Child Fetal Neonates - 2002:87:144 – 149.

12. Setton A, Berenstein A, Interventional neuroradiology current opinion Neurol Neurosurgery 1992:5: 870 – 80

13. Berkherm OA, Van den Berg LA, Fransen PS, Beumer D, Yoo AJ, Lingsma HF et al. Effect of Anaesthetic management during Intra ArterialThrombolysis for Acute stroke in MR CLEAN, Neurology 2016; 87: 656 – 64.

14. Janssen H, Buchholz G, Killer M, Ertl L, Bruckmann H, Lutz J   GA versus conscious sedation in Acute stroke treatment – The importance of head immobilization Cardio Vascular Interventional Radiology: 2016; 39 (9) 1239 – 44.

15. Sophia R. Stroke and cerebrovascular disorders, Sharfsten Manual of Critical Care – Ed. Suhail Raoof A, Liziamma George, Anthony Saleh, McGrawHill, NY, Chicago2009: 688–699.

MULTIPLE CHOICE QUESTIONS

1. **What are the principles of Anesthesia for Interventional Neuroradiology (INR)**
    a. Patient should be physiologically stable, immobilized with quiet breathing
    b. Keep cerebral perfusion pressure (CPP) high for better result
    c. No need for all above

2. **Why are renal functions important in patients undergoing INR**
    a. Muscle relaxants are excreted by the kidneys
    b. To know the urine output
    c. Radio-opaque dye is excreted by the kidneys and to prevent contrast nephropathy
    d. Not at all important

3. **What are the sources of radiation in INR suite**
    a. Only X-Ray tube
    b. Direct through collimator and reflected from patient
    c. Only from patient

4. **Which intravenous fluid is preferred and why?**
    a. 5% Dextrose is preferred for better brain function
    b. Crystalloids are preferred for better capillary filling and good radiological pictures
    c. Any fluid can be given

5. **What precautions will you take for INR procedures**
    a. Patient should receive anti-epileptics, anti-hypertensives, steroids, if he is on
    b. Patient should be given only anti-sialagog drugs
    c. No pre-op. medication

6. **What drugs are used for brain protection**
    a. Dopamine, Dobutamine, 5% Dextrose
    b. No need for brain protection
    c. Mannitol, Dexamethasone, Propofol

7. **What is triple "H" therapy in SAH induced vaso-spasm**
    a. Patient should be well hydrated
    b. Hypertension, hypervolemia, hemodilution
    c. Given to prevent brain edema
    d. None of the above

8. **Which monitoring is important in aneurysm coiling**
    a. Continuous display of arterial BP
    b. Capnography
    c. Oxygen saturation
    d. None of the above

9. **What is the antidote for heparin**
    a. Platelet transfusion
    b. Dopamine, dobutamine
    c. Protamine sulphate
    d. None of the above

10. **What is monitored during carotid artery stenting**
    a. Laryngeal spasm
    b. Heart rate, BP
    c. Temperature
    d. None of the above

11. **Which blood investigation is important and why**
    a. Complete blood count
    b. S. Electrolytes
    c. Blood sugar if > 150 should be teeated urgently for good outcome for stroke
    d. No blood tests are needed

12. **Patient on antiplatelet therapy needing urgent surgery is treated with**
    a. Just discontinue the medicines
    b. Discontinue the medicines and give platelet transfusion
    c. Patient can be taken up for surgery right away
    d. None of the above

CHAPTER 16

PAEDIATRIC NEUROANAESTHESIA

Swati Daftary, Madhavi Desai

Introduction

The primary goal of paediatric neuroanaesthesia is "*Primum non nocere*" meaning "first, do no harm'. In addition, the goals are providing of optimum operating conditions and rapid, safe emergence at the end of surgery to allow early neurological assessment. The children differ from adults in their neuro-anatomical and physiological features including altered drug distribution, metabolism and elimination due to immature hepatic and renal function. Hence thorough preoperative evaluation for extent of neurologic compromise and associated co-morbidities become very important for conduct of successful paediatric neuroanaesthesia. The perioperative maintenance of normal ventilation, fluid-electrolyte balance, body temperature and glucose level become essential to prevent secondary neurologic injury.

Applied paediatric neuroanatomy and neurophysiology[1,2]:

The fontanelle and open cranial sutures in neonates and infants provide space for the cranium to expand. The posterior fontanelle closes at 2-6 months of age; the anterior fontanelle closes by 1 year -18 months. Intracranial pressure (ICP) is low in premature infants, 2-6 mm Hg in full term infants and 0-15 mm Hg in children to adults. Intracranial Hypertension (ICH) is ICP > 15-20mmHg (Table1).

Table 1: Age appropriate intracranial pressures in children

Age (years)	Intracranial Pressure (mmHg)	Cerebral Perfusion Pressure (mmHg)
<3	5-15	40
4-8	15-20	40-50
8 -adolescent	<20	50- 60

In neonates and infants, slow rise in ICP keeps fontanelle open and cranial sutures separate to enlarge the intracranial space. Acute rise in ICP leads to life threatening ICH in infants. In children choroid plexus produces 0.35 ml/min (500 ml/day) of cerebrospinal fluid (CSF), which is resorbed through arachnoid villi and ependymal lines in the ventricles. Conditions which alter CSF flow and decrease CSF reabsorption will increase intracranial volume and pressure. According to the Monro-Kellie doctrine, this can lead to reduction in CBF.

The Cerebral blood flow (CBF) also depends on systemic blood pressure, pCO_2, pO_2, blood viscosity, and cerebral autoregulation. The auto-regulatory range of blood pressure in a normal newborn is between 20 and 60 mm Hg. This makes them very vulnerable to cerebral ischemia and intraventricular hemorrhage. Therefore, tight blood pressure control is essential in the management of neonates. The CBF constitutes 55% of total cardiac output in 2 to 4 year old patients, in them sudden blood loss or venous air embolus can rapidly deteriorate to cardiovascular collapse. Therefore, normovolemia should be maintained throughout the procedure.

The detailed pharmacological knowledge of drugs used for neuroanaesthesia in children is essential because of age related drug metabolism, effects on the CBF and ICP and drug interactions. Their effects on functional neurosurgery and minimally invasive procedures also must be known.

Perioperative issues[3, 4]:

Preoperative assessment:detailed history (including birth history, symptoms suggestive of raised ICP, latex allergy, previous sedation and anaesthesia) and examination (including airway examination) along with relevant investigations markedly reduce perioperative morbidity and mortality in children. The relevant investigation should be ordered based on the profile of the child and the surgery.The advice regarding the fasting guidelines and continuing antiepileptic (unless child is for epilepsy surgery) and corticosteroid medication should be given during preoperative assessment.

Monitoring: Should include precordial stethoscope, capnography, pulse oximetry, electrocardiography, temperature, NIBP, Neuro-muscular block, inspired O_2, ventilatory parameters and endotracheal tube (ETT) cuff pressure. In major surgeries invasive arterial pressure, urine output and central venous cannulation are helpful. Whenever available, neurophysiological monitors like EEG, somatosensory-evoked potentials (SSEP), motor-evoked potentials (MEP), and transcranial Doppler should be used to reduce morbidity by early detection of potential neurological injury. The precordial Doppler, TEE and ETN_2 monitoring play important role in early detection of venous air embolism.

Sedative premedication: In children with normal ICP, oral midazolam can be safely given to relieve preoperative anxiety. Midazolam is contraindicated in children with raised ICP and in child having epilepsy surgery with intraoperative seizure monitoring. Dexmedetomidine can be a safe alternative.

Positioning: Goals of optimum positioning for paediatric neurosurgeries are same as adults. Specific to children is increased incidence of airway obstruction secondary to macroglossia due totight throat pack or excessive flexion of neck causing obstruction of venous and lymphatic drainage. Also, use of Mayfield head frame with pins may increase risk of skull fracture, dural tear, and intracranial hematoma in small children.

Anaesthesia for operative cases is general endotracheal anaesthesia (GETA) with controlled ventilation.Inductioncan be either intravenous induction after securing IV line in an awake patient or inhalation induction. IV induction is preferred in cases of altered sensorium, full stomach. Inhalation induction is best for anxious / uncooperative child and patients with unsecured aneurysm. Unobstructed airway is provided byoptimum sized reinforced ETT. Anaesthesia is maintained with combination of inhaled and intravenous anaesthetics. Nitrous oxide is avoided because of PONV and unwanted effects on SSEPs and MEPs. Intraoperative goal should be to avoid hypoxia, hypotension, hyponatremic and glucose containing fluids, maintain cerebral perfusion pressure, normothermia, normocapnia, Hb → 8 gm% and urine output of 0.5-1 ml/kg/hour. Extubation must be smooth without coughing and straining. Prompt recovery helps in immediate postoperative neurological evaluation which decides further course of management.

Fluid management: Children can have rapid changes in intravascular volume from bleeding, osmotic diuretics, or diabetes insipidus. To maintain CPP in them, preserving intravascular volume, and preventing cerebral edema are very important. Hypotonic fluids containing glucose are avoided for maintenance. Blood glucose levels are monitored in newborns and neonates to prevent hypoglycemia. Blood loss estimation becomes difficult due to constant oozing and saline irrigation. In major surgeries, maximum allowable blood loss should be calculated in advance and adequate amount of fresh packed red blood cells (PRBCs) (< 2 weeks old) should be ordered and made

available in the OT. Hemodynamically stable infants of > 4 months of age, not actively bleeding should be transfused once Hb → 7g/dL. Infants < 4 months of age and those with cyanotic or other congenital heart disease, chronic lung disease, and haemoglobinopathies should have their Hb maintained at 10g/dL. Each 5cc/kg of PRBCs (Hct 70%)raises the hemoglobin concentration by 1g/dL.

Postoperative care: Extubation is avoided if surgery affects brain stem functions and lower cranial nerves or associated with massive blood loss and transfusion or child develops facial, tongue or airway oedema. Pain can be managed with Paracetamol and addition of NSAID after 24 hours. Postoperative observation in HDU /PICU/NICU is essential for small children and after major surgeries.

ANAESTHETIC CONSIDERATIONS FOR SPECIFIC NEUROSURGICAL CASES

Hydrocephalus and shunt procedures[5]

Hydrocephalus (water in the brain) is due to either over production or reduced drainage of CSF leading to increased CSF volume. This may be either congenital or acquired. CSF is drained externally in cases of infection / intraventricular hemorrhage / acute rise in ICP. In majority of the cases, CSF is diverted to one of the body cavity: peritoneum / pleura / right atrium using shunts. Ventriculoperitoneal (VP) shunts are the commonest. Alternatively, internal CSF drainage can be provided with an endoscopic third ventriculostomy in which a hole is made in the floor of the third ventricle to allow CSF to drain into the basal cisterns and subarachnoid space.

Anaesthetic implications in VP shunt:

- Premedication: anticholinergic (Cushing response), prokinetic (if full stomach), sedative drugs (oral midazolam in controlled environment, if normal ICP)
- Inhalational / IV induction: Primary goal is to minimize rise in ICP and prevent aspiration
- GETA with rapid sequence induction and intubation (RSI) and controlled ventilation
- Temperature maintenance: Continuous exposure of surgical field from head to toe causes hypothermia
- Hyperventilation and hypocarbia can make ventricular cannulation difficult
- Ventricular cannulation causes fall in BP
- Possibility of venous air embolism (VAE)
- Subcutaneous tunneling causes sympathetic stimulation
- Revision due to natural growth of the child / blockage/ infection / malfunction
- Removal of ventricular end can cause fatal hemorrhage (choroid plexus rupture)

Anaesthetic implications in Endoscopic third ventriculostomy (ETV):

- Basilar artery rupture and hypovolemic shock
- Irrigation with warm RL / NS, volume of fluid infused and drained should be measured to avoid rapid increases in ICP
- Manipulation / acute distension of third ventricle can lead to severe bradycardia

Neural tube defects: Meningocele, Meningomyelocele (MMC)[6], Encephalocele

The failure of the neural tube to close during the first trimester results in various anomalies from spina bifida to enencephaly. The lumbosacral meningoceles (herniation of dural elements) are the most common conditions that come for neurosurgery. When this defect in addition contains neural element it becomes meningomyelocele. Both these require surgical correction within 24–48 hours of birth to minimize the risk of dural sac rupture, infection and progressive neural damage and decreased motor function. Some centers do repair of meningomyeloceles in utero which reduces the incidence of hydrocephalus and the need for ventriculoperitoneal shunt[7].

Anaesthetic implications:

- Latex precautions to avoid early sensitization (30–70%)
- Large insensible loss from the exposed MMC, check and treat preop dehydration
- Problems of prematurity and Chiari type II malformation
- Encephaloceles can have difficult airway management, increased risk of VAE
- Careful positioning for induction & surgery, protection of the neuroplaque, pressure points
- Improper prone position can give rise to increased abdominal pressure, bleeding and venous congestion of face, tongue, and neck
- Large intraoperative losses: CSF loss, Blood loss due to dissection of skin flaps and heat loss
- For intraoperative sensory and motor nerve root mapping avoid muscle relaxants
- Good IV access and blood availability in extensive lesion
- Avoid sudden release of pressure from the sac and give head low position to prevent coning
- Water tight closure of dura can cause postoperative acute hydrocephalus
- Postoperative respiratory distress can happen after repair of thoracic MMC, child may require postop ventilatory support

Tethered spinal cord[8]

- Nerve Root monitoring to prevent inadvertent injury to functional nerve roots
- EMG electrodes in the anal and urethral (in females) sphincter for continuous monitoring of pudendal nerve (S2 to S4)
- Monitoring of Anterior tibialis and Sural muscles
- Muscle relaxation must be discontinued before stimulation
- Deep plane of anaesthesia required as direct nerve root stimulation elicits sympathetic response and pain

Surgical correction of craniosynostosis[9, 10, 11]

Infants < 1 year, weight < 5 kg and/or an associated syndrome increases perioperative morbidity and mortality. Optimal care is best achieved by team approach involving paediatric team consisting of neurosurgeon, maxillofacial surgeon, reconstructive surgeon, anaesthesiologist and intensivist.

- Difficult and shared airway
- Associated cardiac anomalies
- Prolonged procedure, intracranial approach
- Significant blood loss, antifibrinolytics have beneficial role[12]
- Possible VAE with manipulation of sagittal sutures
- Oculocardiac reflex—severe bradycardia from orbital manipulation
- Surgery below the orbital ridge is associated with excessive facial oedema and may involve the use of a rigid extraction device frame. This may make airwaymanagement difficult at the initial and subsequent surgeries. Occasionally, a preoperative tracheostomy may be required
- Neuroendoscopic strip craniectomy markedly reduces blood loss and surgical time and gives better postoperative recovery
- Postoperative management in ICU, may require ventilator support

Paediatric brain tumors[4,13]

Pilocytic astrocytoma (benign and most common) Medulloblastomas, Ependymomas, brainstem gliomas are the posterior fossa tumors in children. Embryonal tumors (earlier known as "Primitive neuroectodermal tumors") and choroid plexus tumors are the commonly found supratentorial tumors in children. Craniopharyngeoma is a benign tumor in supracellar region.

Preoperative evaluation, fasting guidelines, sedative premedication, general anaesthesia, application of Mayfield head clamp, positioning, monitoring, principles of management of intraoperative blood loss and concerns regarding extubation, postoperative analgesia in a patient having SOL are like adults and have been discussed earlier in this chapter.

Some specific considerations in children are:

- Avoid Inhalational induction in a child with raised ICP
- Local anesthetic at pin site during head clamp application
- 2 wide bore peripheral IV cannula. Consider central venous access if IV access is difficult
- Invasive arterial BP monitoring
- Blood loss during craniotomy itself may be more in small children as the scalp is vascular and children have relatively big head
- Meningiomas and choroid plexus tumors are known to bleed more
- Intraoperative Neuromonitoring: Is more challenging because of immature pathways(myelination and synapses). In children < 2 years recording SSEPs may not be possible because of incomplete myelination of tracts. Needle placement at or close to the anterior fontanelle should be avoided. For monitoring of MEPs, avoid inhalational and muscle relaxants. Can use Propofol 50-200 mic/kg/min with Fentanyl 0.5-2 mic/kg/hr or dexmedetomidine 0.2 mic/kg/hr without bolus infusion as in adults. Propofol infusion is now used widely and safely, for neuromonitoring with no adverse events reported.[13] Some guidelines do not recommend propofol infusion in children in view of propofol infusion syndrome.

The vein of Galen aneurysmal malformation (VGAM)[14,15]

VGAM is an arteriovenous malformation resulting from a persistent embryonic median vein of prosencephalon. VGAM shunt provides a low resistance conduit for intracerebral blood flow and is directly unloaded into the right atrium and pulmonary circulation, leading to pulmonary vasoconstriction and pulmonary hypertension. This results in right ventricle failure with or without central nervous system symptoms secondary to hydrocephalus, in the neonatal and pediatric population. It may have associated ASD,VSD, PDA. Neuroradiological intervention with Staged transcatheter embolization of the feeding arteries is preferred over surgical correction. One should be aware of some important periprocedural challenges:

- Anaesthesia to a neonate in Intervention radiology (IR) suite
- Neonatal difficult airway (in v/o associated hydrocephalus) in peripheral locations.
- Invasive arterial BP monitoring mandatory

- Maintaining temperature of a neonate in IR suit where temperature is lower than operating rooms
- Contrast boluses may add to fluid overload in a neonate with right heart failure
- Hypotension at induction (inhalation preferred over intravenous): treated with phenylephrine boluses
- Hypotension during trans arterial injection of Nimodipine
- Hyper perfusion injury of the brain, raised ICP, transient bradycardia after embolization
- Worsening of the congestive cardiac failure after embolization as the blood volume from the malformation suddenly adds to the venous drainage
- Intraprocedural Urine output my not be a reliable marker of perfusion because of contrast induced diuresis.

Traumatic Brain injury in children[16]

The water content of neonatal brain is 89%, which decreases to 77% in adults. The high-water content, less connecting tissues and lack of myelination makes the neonatal brain softer, and therefore more susceptible to acceleration-deceleration injury (Shaken baby syndrome). In the neonatal period, birth related injuries are noted with subdural hematoma (SDH) along the falx cerebri and tentorium cerebellum. The infant skull is less rigid, and the open sutures function as joints in infants. This translates into only a small degree of movement in response to a mechanical stress. Therefore, the pediatric skull can absorb the initial impact better. In infants, inflicted trauma is a major cause of TBI and is associated with skull fractures, SDH, Diffuse axonal Injury (DAI), and delayed hypoxic-ischemic injury. The larger head-to-body proportion, relatively more head weight, lack of air spaces in paranasal sinuses, and a thinner skull in infants and children compared to adults result in the high prevalence of impact injuries in them. The infants and toddlers have a protruding forehead and therefore are prone to more frontal injuries. Therefore Zygomatico maxillary, nasal, and Le Fort fractures are more common in older children.

Management of TBI in children[17,18]:

Main focus is preventing secondary brain injury to improve outcome.

- Glasgow coma scale assessment is done after adequate initial resuscitation and restoring hemodynamics if associated with shock.
- A child with a GCS score of < 9 or decreasing consciousness needs tracheal intubation for airway protection and ICP management
- Management of Airway-Breathing-Circulation. Measures for neck immobilization are mandatory (Hard collar, Manual in-line immobilization) until cervical spine injury ruled out

- 25% of children with TBI have TBI induced pituitary dysfunction in the acute phase. Consider adrenocorticotropic hormone (ACTH) deficiency in patients with refractory hypotension

- Fluids: RL or Normal Saline preferred. Colloids not routinely recommended. Albumin is shown to be deleterious.

- 30^0 head up and avoid head turn to prevent Internal jugular venous obstruction

- Sedation and Controlled ventilation to avoid coughing on tube and rise in ICP (Midazolam 0.05-0.3 mg/kg/hr, Fentanyl 0.5-2 mic/kg/hr, muscle relaxant). Propofol infusion is not recommended in children with the concern of Propofol infusion syndrome. Instead, ketamine can be considered[17].

- Anticonvulsants: Phenytoin 15 mg/kg for depressed skull fracture, seizures

- Ventilation: TV 6-8 mL/kg and rate to keep PCO2 30-40 mm Hg, Avoid hyperventilation

- Active measures to reduce fever: maintain temperature $< 37 \rightarrow$ (Paracetamol, tepid sponging, Cold saline wash through Naso-gastric tube and Foley's catheter) as fever increases CMRO2.

- Glucose > 70mg/dL < 180mg/dL, S Sodium > 140mEq

- Maintain Cerebral Perfusion Pressure 40-50 mmHg (Refer - Table 1)

- Maintain ICP < 20 mmHg (Refer-Table 1). The measures are

  Hyperosmolar therapy:

  - Hypertonic saline bolus 3% saline 5-10 mL/kg or Infusion 0.1-1mL/Kg/hr (to maintain plasma < 360 mOsm, S Sodium < 160 mEq/L) OR

    20% Mannitol 0.2ml/kg (maintain osmolarity < 320 mOsm). 2012 guideline support the use of Hypertonic saline. Mannitol is not studied in Paediatric TBI.

  - Consider surgical intervention: External Ventricular drain, Decompression Craniectomy

Paediatric spine injuries and spinal cord injury without radiological abnormality SCIWORA [17,18]

Children with TBI may have associated cervical spine (C-spine) injury. Young children have weaker neck muscles than adults and a relatively heavy the head. Their craniocervical stability is dependent more on the ligaments thanbones. These anatomical differences also increase the chances of cranio-cervical junction lesions in children. In small children, maximal movement of C-spine occurs at C1–C3, and after 12 years of age at C5–C6. Therefore, younger children have injuries to the upper cervical spine, while older children have lower ones.

SCIWORA refers to spinal injuries, typically located in the cervical region, in the absence of identifiable bony or ligamentous injury on radiographs or computed tomography. SCIWORA is responsible for 6 to 19% of spinal injuries in children. The majority of children with SCIWORA do have demonstrable injury of the spinal cord, spinal ligaments, or vertebral body end plate on magnetic resonance imaging. SCIWORA should be suspected in patients subjected to blunt trauma who present with early symptoms of neurologic deficit upon initial assessment.

Management: Main focus is to prevent the secondary injury.

- Airway-Breathing-Circulation (Endotracheal intubation if GCS < 9, Child needs intra/interhospital transfer, diaphragm paresis)

- In infants < 6 months, the head and cervical spine should be immobilized using aspine board with tape across the forehead and blankets of towels around the neck. In infants > 6 months, use small rigid cervical collar or the above mentioned methods.

- Cricoid pressure should not be applied vigorously as it can lead to subluxation at the injury site or laryngeal and tracheal compression and obstruction to ventilation.

- Neurogenic shock management and treatment goals: A systolic blood pressure BP of 70-90 mm Hg should be achieved. May require vasopressors.

- Role of anti-inflammatory medicines: Though Methylprednisolone bolus of 30 mg/Kg iv within 8 hrs of injury, followed by infusion at 5.4 mg/Kg/hr for the next 23 hrs was recommended; recent NICE 2016 guidelines clearly opine that the use of high-dose methylprednisolone should not be recommended for neuroprotection in acute Spinal cord Injury, in view of lack of clinically significant benefit together with the clinically significant increased risk of adverse events. High dose Dexamethasone and NSAIDs have no supporting evidence [19]

Anaesthesia for Magnetic Resonance Imaging (MRI): Special considerations in children [20,21]

- Examine the child and the accompanying relative for metal implants: Patient with cochlear implants, Automatic Implantable Cardioverter- Defibrillator (AICD), Pacemakers, Phrenic and Vagal nerve stimulators, deep brain stimulators are contraindicated in zone III and IV of MRI. Most of the chemo ports are MR safe

- Now a days Anaesthesia is preferred (Except in infants < 2 months) over oral sedation or intramuscular medications as the onset and recovery is immediate, the effects are predictable and the plane of anaesthesia can be titrated. Movements under anaesthesia are less or minimal. Therefore the quality of images is better.

- Anaesthesia:
  - Conscious sedation and TIVA: Lighter planes of Anaesthesia are acceptable and safer.

    With IV Propofol 25-100 mic/kg/min OR IV Dexmedetomidine: 0.2 μ/kg/hr.

    Propofol is near Ideal agent. Dexmedetomidine is safe but takes longer onset time. Avoid bolus infusion dose of Dexmedetomidine in remote locations and especially in children with brainstem lesions, raised ICP for its confounding effect of bradycardia.

  - Inhalational Anaesthesia using MR safe anaesthesia machine in zone IV or MR unsafe conventional machine in zone III.

- Chloral hydrate 30-50 mg/kg for infants < 2 months
- MR safe infusion pumps can be used in zone IV OR MR unsafe pump in zone III with long tubing
- LMA or Endotracheal tube(ETT) for airway management is standard practice: cuffed ETT and LMAs cause ferromagnetic interference to the images because of metal in their valves. MR safe LMA with plastic valve or I-gel being cuffless device are preferred for MRI.
- Monitoring: MR compatible monitors in zone IV and III. Pulse oximeter, Cardio scope, capnometer.
- Recovery room for postprocedure monitoring

Anaesthesia for Computed Tomography (CT)of Brain: Special considerations in children [21]

- Procedure time is typically 3-10 minutes
- Immobilization of child mandates anaesthesia
- Look for sign and symptoms of raised ICP-irritability, vomiting. Young children may not be able to complain of headache. In such cases it is better to electively intubate the patient before subjecting to MRI/ CT

- Short duration anaesthesia with Sevoflurane or Propofol with patient spontaneously breathing is preferred as it has instant onset and fast emergence with good recovery and ensures immobility of the child. Oral or Intravenous sedation (IV Midazolam 0.3-0.5mg/kg, IV Ketamine 0.5-1mg/kg, oral chlorhydrate 30-50 mg/kg for neonates and small infants in absence of raised ICP)
- Monitoring: Pusleoximeter, capnogram (capnograph with a nasal cannula for monitoring spontaneously breathing patient are available) cardioscope, BP
- Equipment's for definitive airway and resuscitation should be available.

Anaesthesia for radiotherapy of brain: Special considerations in children [21]

- Anaesthesiaat remote location. Parents or medical personnel cannot wait inside the radiotherapy suite. So, patient can be seen only through a camera in console.
- The radiotherapy regime is usually daily for 3-6 weeks
- Average procedure duration is 10 minutes
- Sedation, conscious sedation or lighter planes of Propofol anaesthesia, IV Ketamine 0.5-1 mg/kg with patient spontaneously breathing under oxygen mask is safe and preferred
- Caution in patients with raised ICP, lower cranial nerve palsies. The equipment's for definitive airway and resuscitation should be available.
- Securing intravenous access can be difficult for daily anaesthesia.
- Monitoring: Pusleoximeter, capnogram (capnograph with a nasal cannula for monitoring spontaneously breathing patient are available) cardioscope, BP.

CONCLUSION

Some of the important features of common neurosurgical diseases in children and their anaesthetic implications are summarized.

Table 2: Common neurosurgical diseases and their anaesthetic implications

Type of pathology	Extra information needed	Anaesthetic implications
Seizures	- Type, presentation, frequency - Medication for control, toxicity	- Increased requirement of anaesthetic agents if Phenytoin - Avoid epileptogenic agents like Ketamine, pethidine - Lab tests for haematologic and Liver functions
Hydrocephalus	- Symptoms and signs of raised ICP (nausea, vomiting, lethargy, irritability, poor feeding) - Vomiting: fluid electrolyte status - Congenital / long standing hydrocephalus can cause bilateral vocal cord palsy causing stridor	- Rapid sequence induction and intubation without rise in ICP - Prophylactic antibiotic to prevent shunt infection - May have fixed vocal cords with very small laryngeal inlet - Possible VAE
Traumatic Brain Injury	- Rule out cervical spine injury and other injuries - Extent of neurologic injury - Assess protective airway reflexes	- Spinal cord precautions - Avoid secondary neurological injury: rise in ICP, hypoxia, hypercarbia, hyperglycemia
Intracranial SOL	- Check for signs of raised ICP, electrolyte imbalance - Chemotherapeutic agents, toxicity	- Anticipate major blood loss - Intraoperative steroids - Look out for VAE
Hypothalamic / pituitary lesions	- Diabetes insipidus, Hypothyroidism, Adrenal insufficiency	
Meningomyelocele / encephalocele	- Look for associated hydrocephalus, Chiari type II malformation (80-90%) - Stridor, apnoea, swallowing difficulty, absent gag reflex - Look for VACTERL associations, prematurity - Assess sensory/motor level	- Latex allergy precautions - Avoid muscle relaxant if nerve root monitoring required - Careful positioning - Reduced need for opioid if defect below sensory level - Large intraoperative losses
Arnold-Chiari Malformation	- Swallowing difficulty, stridor, apnoea, absent airway reflexes	- May require postoperative ventilation
Craniosynostosis	- Presence of craniofacial syndrome: sleep apnoea, difficult airway - Check for raised ICP	- If syndromic, difficult mask ventilation, intubation - Anticipate rapid major blood loss, possible VAE - Avoid further rise in ICP
Aneurysm/AV Malformation	- Look for signs of high output cardiac failure in neonates	- Avoid straining, struggling at induction - Avoid hypertensive response before the lesion is secured

CHAPTER 17

TRAUMATIC BRAIN INJURY

Anita N. Shetty, Nirav Kotak, Divyadarshni Vadivel, Pallavi Gaur

Introduction

The Traumatic Brain Injury (TBI) is one of the most common neurosurgical emergencies. The main goal in the perioperative management of TBI patient is to prevent secondary brain injury. The anaesthesiologist plays a vital role in the perioperative care of patients with TBI. They are involved in multiple locations such as stabilization and resuscitation in the emergency room (ER), sedation and anaesthesia for neuroimaging in the radiological suite, craniotomy and decompressive craniectomy in the operating room (OR), extra cranial surgeries and intensive care management.

Epedemiology

TBI is the third leading cause of death and disability worldwide. In India the number of reported cases are approximately 1.6 million with around 2,00,000 deaths and around 1 million requiring rehabilitation every year[1].

Classifications

Head injury can be classified based on the level of consciousness which is assessed by Glasgow Coma Scale (GCS) (Table1). Reversible causes such as hypotension, hypoxia and alcohol intoxication should be corrected before assessing GCS.

Table 1: Glasgow coma scale (GCS)

Symptoms & signs	Score
Eye opening	
Spontaneous	4
Response to verbal command	3
Response to pain	2
No eye opening	1
Best verbal response	
Oriented	5
Confused	4
Inappropriate words	3
Incomprehensible sounds	2
No verbal response	1
Best motor response	
Obeys commands	6
Localizing response to pain	5
Withdrawal response to pain	4
Flexion to pain	3
Extension to pain	2
No motor response	1
Total	**15**

For the ease of therapeutic interventions and management goals TBI is also classified into primary and secondary injury[2].

Primary injury

This is because of direct mechanical impact and acceleration-deceleration between the skull and brain tissue leading to fractures of the skull and intracranial lesions. The lesions in the brain may be diffuse or focal.

- Diffuse brain injury is further classified as

  Brain concussion: Loss of consciousness lasting for < 6 hours

  Diffuse axonal injury: Loss of consciousness lasting for > 6 hours.

- Focal injury to the brain subdivided into:

  Brain contusion: Injury is below or opposite to the region of impact.

  Subdural haematoma (SDH): Caused by sheering of the bridging vessels. It is defined acute, subacute and chronic when the symptoms occur within 72 hours, 3-15 days and after 15 days respectively.

  Epidural haematoma (EDH): Caused by sheering of middle meningeal artery. It is characterised by a lucid interval. Lucid interval is temporary improvement in consciousness after TBI followed by rapid neurological deterioration due to the expanding haematoma.

Intracerebral haematoma (ICH): Consequence of coup - countercoup injuries and is located frequently in the frontal or temporal regions.

Secondary injury

The inflammatory and neurotoxic process due to primary injury leads to fluid accumulation. This vasogenic edema leads to increased intracranial pressure (ICP), hypo perfusion and cerebral ischaemia. The systemic factors such as hypoxemia, hypotension, anaemia, hypo/hypercarbia, pyrexia and hyponatremia can also contribute to secondary brain injury and must be aggressively treated.

Clinical evaluation and management

The management strategies in this chapter will be in accordance to the latest recommendations of the Brain Trauma Foundation (BTF). The recommendations are evidence based and form a basis to formulate protocols The 4th edition of the BTF[3] recommendations focus on three headings : treatment , monitoring and thresholds as described in Table 2.

Level of evidence:

Level I: based on a high-quality body of evidence.

Level II A: based on a moderate-quality body of evidence.

Level II B and III: based on a low-quality body of evidence.

Table 2: Recommendation of BTF for management of TBI

Sr No.	Topic	Recommendations	Level of evidence
1.	Decompressive craniectomy (DC)	According to the GOS-E score at 6 months post injury bifrontal DC does not improve outcomes in severe TBI with diffuse injury. However there was a reduction in ICP and ICU stay. A large fronto-temporo-parietal DC (not less than 12 x 15 cm or 15 cm diameter) is recommended to reduce mortality and improve neurological outcomes.	Level II A
2.	Prophylactic hypothermia	There was no improved outcome in patients with diffuse injury with early (within 2.5 h), short-term (48 h post injury) prophylactic hypothermia	Level II B
3.	Hyperosmolar therapy	Prior to ICP monitoring at a dose of 0.25 to 1 g/kg is effective to control raised ICP only in patients with tentorial herniation or progressive neurological deterioration	Recommendations from 3rd edition not supported by evidence meeting current standards
4.	Cerebrospinal fluid (CSF) drainage	Continuous drainage of CSF via an EVD system zeroed at the midbrain is recommended over intermittent drainage. In patients with an initial GCS <6, CSF drainage may be used to reduce ICP during the first 12 hours of injury	Level III

5.	Ventilation therapies	Prolonged prophylactic hyperventilation with $PaCO_2$ of <25 mm Hg is not recommended	Level II B
		If hyperventilation is used, SjO_2 or $BtpO_2$ measurements are recommended to monitor oxygen delivery.	
6.	Anaesthetics, analgesics and sedative	Administration of barbiturates for burst suppression of EEG, as prophylaxis against the development of intracranial hypertension is not recommended. High-dose barbiturate administration is recommended to control elevated ICP refractory to standard medical and surgical management. However haemodynamic stability is essential before and during barbiturate therapy. Propofol, to control raised ICP, is not recommended as higher doses are associated with significant morbidity	Level II B
7.	Steroids	There is no role of steroids in reducing ICP or improving outcomes. High dose methyl prednisolone is contraindicated	Level 1
8.	Nutrition	Feeding to attain basic caloric requirement by the 5th day and at least by the 7th day reduced mortality.	Level II A
		Trans jejunal feeding reduced Ventilator Associated Pneumonia (VAP)	Level II B
9.	Infection prophylaxis	Early tracheostomy is recommended to reduce overall days of mechanical ventilation; however it does not reduce the incidence of nosocomial infections. The use of povidine iodine for oral care does not reduce the incidence of VAP.	Level II A
		Use of microcidal impregnated can reduce catheter induced infection.	Level III
10.	Deep-vein thromboprophylaxis	LMWH or low-dose un-fractioned heparin may be used in combination with mechanical prophylaxis. Pharmacological therapy can be considered when benefits outweight risk and the TBI is stable. Evidence is insufficient to support recommendations regarding the preferred agent, dose, or timing of pharmacologic prophylaxis for deep vein thrombosis.	Level III
11.	Seizure prophylaxis	Prophylactic use of phenytoin or valproate is not recommended to prevent late Post Traumatic Seizures (PTS). Phenytoin is recommended to decrease the incidence of early PTS (within 7 days of injury). Insufficient evidence to recommend levetiracetam over phenytoin in prevention of early post-traumatic seizures and toxicity.	Level II A

12.	ICP monitoring	ICP monitoring decreases in hospital and 2 week mortality. ICP should be monitored in all salvageable patients with TBI (GCS 3-8 after resuscitation) and an abnormal CT scan. ICP monitoring is indicated in patients with severe TBI with a normal CT scan, if at admission: age >40 years, unilateral or bilateral motor posturing, or SBP <90 mmHg.	Level II B Recommendations from 3rd edition
13.	Advanced cerebral monitoring	Jugular bulb monitoring of arterio-venous oxygen content difference (AVDO$_2$) to aid in management decision, may be considered to reduce mortality and improve outcomes at 3 and 6 months post-injury.	Level III
14.	Cerebral perfusion pressure (CPP) Monitoring (MAP-ICP)	Management of severe TBI with CPP monitoring may decrease 2 week mortality	Level II B
15.	Systolic Blood Pressure (SBP) thresholds	Maintenance of SBP >100 mmHg for patients 50 to 69 years old or at > 110 mmHg or above for patients 15 to 49 or >70 years old may decrease mortality and improve outcomes.	Level III
16.	ICP thresholds	Treatment of ICP >22 mmHg is recommended	Level II B
17.	CPP thresholds	The recommended target CPP value for survival and favorable outcomes is between 60 and 70 mmHg Avoid aggressive attempts to maintain CPP >70mm Hg: Risk of poorer outcomes and respiratory complications	Level II B Level III
18.	Advanced cerebral monitoring thresholds	Jugular venous saturation of <50% may be threshold to avoid in order to reduce mortality & improve outcomes	Level III

* GOS – E : Extended Glassgow coma outcome scale

Table 3: Stepwise clinical evaluation of patient with TBI

APPROACH TO TBI

Initial evaluation and stabilisation as per ATLS protocols

Airway & breathing	Circulation	Disability	Exposure
Maintain PO$_2$ >100mmHg PaCO$_2$ 35-45mmHg Intubation if GCS <8, SpO$_2$ <97% Rapid sequence intubation with cervical spine immobilisation	Maintain SBP >90mmHg Fluid resuscitation with isotonic crystalloids Avoid glucose containing fluids Avoid albumin for resuscitation Low threshold for use of blood & blood product (Hb >7gm/dL)	A – Alert V – Verbal response P – Pain U – Unresponsive	Rule out intrathoracic and intraperitoneal injury in persistent hypotension Treatment of haemorrhagic shock priority over neurological intervention

Detailed neurological examination

Consciousness	Pupillary examination	Lateralizing signs	Neuroimaging
GCS to be assessed in adults & children >2 years Reassess to prognosticate	Check pupils for size, symmetry & reactivity to light Aids in locating the lesion *Unilateral fixed dilated pupil:* uncal herniation. *Bilateral fixed dilated pupil :* bilateral uncal herniation / midbrain compression. *Non reactive pupils:* Local trauma to the eye causing injury to the third nerve	Hemiparesis Motor weakness Anisocoria Facial deviation	*CT SCAN:* Imaging modality of choice Canadian Rules *High risk:* GCS <15 for >2hours Suspected open/depressed fracture Base of skull fracture Vomiting >2 episodes Age >65 years *Medium risk:* Amnesia before impact >30min High impact injury *MRI:* Logistically complex & time consuming, useful to quantify axonal damage, injury to tracts of white matter *X-ray:* Fracture skull in children

Indications for surgery

Surgical management is based on GCS and CT scan findings[4]

- EDH > 30 mL in volume regardless of patient's GCS score; or GCS score ≤ 8 and pupillary abnormalities (anisocoria).

- Acute SDH > 10 mm thickness or > 5 mm midline shift on CT regardless of patient's GCS score or if GCS score ≤ 8 or GCS score has decreased by ≥ 2 points from injury time to hospital admission, and/or patient having abnormal pupils, and/or intracranial pressure >20 mmHg.

- Traumatic ICH in the posterior fossa with significant mass effect.

- ICH involving the cerebral hemisphere with volume > 50 cm^3, or if GCS score is 6-8 with a frontal/temporal haemorrhage> 20 cm^3 with midline shift of minimum 5 mm and/or CT scan showing cisternal compression.

- For penetrating injury - Superficial debridement and dural closure to prevent CSF leak

- Open skull fractures, if depressed greater than the thickness of the cranium or if there is dural penetration, significant ICH, frontal sinus involvement, cosmetic deformity, wound infection or pneumocephalus

Anaesthesia management

In the OR, ongoing resuscitation process should be continued and rapid assessment of the patient to be followed. The assessment includes airway, breathing and circulation, followed by a rapid evaluation of neurological status and associated extra-cranial injuries. Neurological assessment is based upon GCS score and pupillary response.

Anaesthesia technique is modified based on patient factors and type of surgery.

Goals of anaesthesia management[3,4]

1) Optimization of CPP and prevention of intracranial hypertension;

2) Provide adequate anaesthesia and analgesia;

3) Prevention of secondary brain injury;

4) Provide optimal surgical condition.

Anaesthesia induction and Intubation

Most of the patients may already be intubated but some patients, especially those with extradural haematoma, may be conscious and breathing spontaneously. Airway management may be complicated due to blood, debris, vomitus in the oral cavity, laryngo-pharyngeal injury, base of skull fracture, full stomach, underlying cervical injury and depleted volume status. All TBI patients requiring surgery should be considered to have full stomach and possibility of underlying cervical spine injury.

Incidence of Cervical spinal injury is seen in 2% of victims of blunt trauma. The incidence is increased if the GCS score is < 8 or if there is a focal neurologic deficit[5].

Rapid sequence intubation with cricoid pressure and manual in-line stabilization is used for endotracheal intubation. The anterior portion of cervical collar may be removed when manual in-line stabilization is established to allow greater mouth opening and introduction of laryngoscope. The videolaryngoscope may be useful in patients with difficult airway. However, inspite of good glottic view, negotiation of tube through the glottis may be difficult and the intubation time prolonged[6].

The nasal intubation should be avoided in patients with base of skull fracture, severe facial fractures or bleeding diathesis.

The commonly used agents are Sodium Thiopental, Etomidate and Propofol and these agents decrease the cerebral metabolic rate for oxygen ($CMRO_2$) and prevent rise in ICP. However, Propofol and Thiopentone may cause hypotension, especially in the presence of uncorrected hypovolemia. Etomidate can be agent of choice in haemodynamically unstable patients but may cause adrenal suppression even after a single dose. Recent studies show that Ketamine does not increase ICP[7]. On the contrary, Ketamine might prove beneficial in haemodynamically unstable patients. For RSI, either Succinylcholine or Rocuronium are most commonly used. Succinylcholine can produce a transient increase in ICP, which can be attenuated by administration of a defasciculating dose of a nondepolarizing NMBA or with an adequate dose of induction agent.

In TBI patients during maintenance of anaesthesia, intravenous or inhalation anaesthetics can be used. There is not much evidence to support the use of one over the other. Intravenous agents reduce $CMRO_2$, CBF and ICP. The inhalational agents reduce $CMRO_2$ but increase CBF and ICP due to vasodilatation at more than 1 MAC. However, lower concentration has minimal effect on CBF. The Nitrous oxide (N_2O) can increase $CMRO_2$ as well as cause cerebral vasodilation and increase in ICP. In addition, patients with TBI may have associated pneumocephalus or pneumothorax and hence N_2O should be avoided or used cautiously.

Monitoring

Standard American society of anesthesiologists (ASA) monitors (electrocardiography, noninvasive blood pressure (BP), pulse-oximetry, capnography, and temperature) should be used for all patients. In addition, invasive arterial catheterization for beat-to-beat monitoring of Arterial Blood Pressure and regular analysis of arterial blood gases (ABG) and glucose is recommended. The central venous catheterization (CVC) for central venous pressure monitoring and administration of vasoactive drugs is useful. The Trendelenburg positioning should be avoided or minimized during placement of a CVC in the neck because the head-down position increases ICP. However, surgical evacuation of expanding intracranial haematoma should not be delayed for institution of invasive monitoring. The ICP monitoring is recommended by BTF guidelines for patients requiring non-neurosurgical intervention and in

intensive care unit. The indications for ICP monitoring are given in the table of BTF Guidelines.

The advanced or multimodal neuromonitoring are placed in the ICU. The jugular venous oximetry and brain tissue oxygenation ($PbtO_2$) can be used intraoperatively, whereas other techniques like transcranial doppler, cerebral micro dialysis and thermal diffusion flowmetry are used post-operatively.

Intraoperative management

Haemodynamic management

BTF recommends that the systolic blood pressure should be > 90 mmHg and the CPP between 50 and 70 mm Hg. CPP > 70 mmHg increases the risk of pulmonary edema and Adult Respiratory Distress Syndrome (ARDS) and < 50 mmHg increases risk of ischemia.

Patients with TBI associated with polytrauma are at risk for hypotension related to blood loss and other organ damage. Associated thoracic, abdominal, spinal and long bone injuries must be considered in differential diagnosis of new onset hypotension, anemia, haemodynamic instability or hypoxemia during anaesthesia and surgery. Sudden hypotension can occur in these patients following removal of the bone flap and dural incision, which is thought to result from sudden decrease in ICP. Paediatric patients may lose large amount of blood into intracranial or subgaleal haematoma or through skin laceration. Hypotension is associated with increased mortality and poor neurological outcome. Hence, systolic blood pressure < 90 mmHg should be avoided and corrected rapidly with volume expansion and vasopressors.

Intravenous fluids and vasopressors

The warm, non-glucose containing isotonic crystalloid solution is recommended for resuscitation and volume replacement. The role of colloid is controversial. In Saline versus Albumin Fluid Evaluation (SAFE) study[8], higher mortality rate and unfavorable neurological outcome at 24 months was observed when TBI patients were resuscitated with albumin. Hypertonic saline may be beneficial as resuscitation fluid for TBI patients because it increases intravascular fluid volume and decreases ICP.

If targeted mean arterial pressure is not achieved despite adequate fluid replacement, vasopressors can be used. Phenylephrine is vasopressor of choice as it has greatest increase in MAP and CPP.

Blood transfusion - The optimal transfusion trigger for patients with TBI is uncertain. Anaemia can cause secondary brain injury by reducing O_2 delivery to the brain. However, a liberal transfusion strategy[9] (>10 g/dL) did not result in improved outcome at six months compared with a Hb of 7 g/dL, and the 10 g/dL threshold was associated with a higher incidence of thromboembolic events. Transfusion should depend on ongoing bleeding, the clinical status of the patient and patient comorbidities, rather than a specific haemoglobin trigger.

Oxygenation - BTF recommends maintain a $PaO_2 > 60$ mmHg and O_2 saturation of > 90%. The hypoxemia is associated with increased mortality and poor neurologic outcome in TBI patients. Low levels of PEEP up to 10 cm of H_2O can be applied to maintain oxygenation in patients who have pulmonary contusions, central neurogenic pulmonary oedema or aspiration. High level of PEEP can increase ICP due to impedance to cerebral venous drainage and should be avoided.

Ventilation - Ventilation should be adjusted to maintain $PaCO_2$ of 35-45 mmHg. Prolonged hyperventilation to a $PaCO_2$ of 25-30 mmHg causes cerebral vasoconstriction and ischaemia. Hence, prophylactic hyperventilation is no longer recommended except as a temporary measure to reduce refractory intracranial hypertension or to relax brain during craniotomy. During prolonged hyperventilation, monitoring of cerebral oxygenation with jugular bulb oximetry or $PbtO_2$ is recommended.

Temperature management - Intraoperative normothermia is the goal for temperature management. Fever aggravates secondary brain injury and should be treated aggressively. Therapeutic hypothermia has not been shown to improve outcome in patients with TBI and is rather associated with complications. Thus, Induced hypothermia should be reserved for patients with refractory intracranial hypertension.

Glucose management - Hyperglycaemia and hypoglycaemia are both associated with poor neurological outcome. Hence blood glucose should be maintained between 140 and 180 mg/dL.

Antiepileptic drugs - Prophylactic administration of phenytoin or valproate is not recommended for late post traumatic seizures. It is recommended only in early post traumatic seizures (7 days) and is often administered intraoperatively. There is not much evidence to administer levetiracetam over phenytoin.

Intraoperative glucocorticoids - Routine administration of glucocorticoids is no longer recommended for reducing ICP or improving outcome. Corticosteroid randomization after significant head injury (CRASH) trial[10] showed increase in mortality in patients receiving steroids as compared to not receiving steroids.

Coagulopathy - Coagulation indices should be monitored, and abnormalities corrected since these patients can develop coagulopathy due to the release of tissue thromboplastin. It is associated with increased risk of haematoma enlargement and intraoperative bleeding.

Hyperosmolar therapy

Mannitol is most commonly used hyperosmolar agent in the dose of 0.25-1.0 g/kg[11]. During administration of mannitol, hypotension and increase in osmolarity more than 300 mosm/L should be avoided since it causes renal and neurological complications. Hypertonic saline is alternative to mannitol especially in hypotensive patients.

Emergence and transfer of care

Patients with good preoperative GCS and an uneventful intraoperative period can be extubated in the OR, if the extubation criteria are met. Emergence should be smooth, avoiding coughing and hypertensive response.

Intensive care management

The intensive care management involves the application of general critical care principles and recognizing, preventing and treating the multisystem sequel of severe TBI.

General critical care principles[12]

1. Maintenance of neutral position of head with elevation by 30° to 45° to improve venous drainage and reduce ICP.

2. Avoidance of tight tracheal tube fixation ties and cervical collars that can lead to compression of the jugular veins and impede cerebral venous drainage.

3. Use of short acting opioids for pain relief to aid in timely assessment of neurological status.

4. Maintenance of normothermia.

5. Care of eyes, mouth and maintenance of skin hygiene.

6. Implementation of evidence based antibiotic protocols for VAP prophylaxis and catheter induced infection prophylaxis.

7. Resumption of enteral feeding by 5th day or atleast by 7th day to attain basic caloric requirement.

8. Institution of ulcer prophylaxis and bowel care to prevent constipation.

9. Institution of thromboprophylaxis.

10. Institution of physiotherapy.

Management of multiorgan sequalae[12]

Cardiovascular complications:

TBI activates a cascade of inflammatory and sympathetic responses, which cause a hyper dynamic cardiovascular response resulting in tachycardia, hypertension and ECG changes that can progress to myocardial ischaemia. The ECG changes are usually transient and revert in 10 weeks. Takotsubo cardiomyopathy is characterized by acute, transient LV dysfunction and should not be confused with myocardial infarction. Elevated ICP causes hypo perfusion of the medullary centers resulting in vagal stimulation. This response is known as Cushing's reflex and is associated with hypertension and bradycardia.

Management: This involves serial monitoring of Troponin I levels and treatment of conduction abnormalities secondary to sympathetic dysregulation and electrolyte abnormalities hypertension must be treated using beta blockers (Metaprolol, Esmolol, Labetalol) as the first line of drugs. Vasodilators such as Nitroprusside and Nitroglycerine are avoided as they cause cerebral vasodilatation. Clevidipine is a safe and effective alternative to control blood pressure. Hypotension should be avoided.

Respiratory system complications:

Hypoxia in patients with TBI can occur as a separate entity due to increased pulmonary shunting of blood. Other reasons for hypoxia include neurogenic pulmonary edema, atelectasis, aspiration, and inability to protect the airway and associated lung injuries. The pathophysiology of pulmonary edema is an enigma but has been attributed to sympathetic over activity in response to raised ICP causing increased hydrostatic pressure and leaky pulmonary capillaries.

Management: Ventilatory strategies include endotracheal intubation in severe TBI and early tracheostomy with adequate sedation and paralysis. ARDS / ALI could benefit from lung recruitment maneuvers and PEEP. Institution of mechanical ventilation with moderate PEEP for management of neurogenic pulmonary oedema.

Hematological complications:

The patient with TBI can succumb to Disseminated Intravascular Coagulation (DIC) due to release of tissue thromboplastin from the brain.

Management: DIC is treated by replacement with FFP, cryoprecipitate and platelets to achieve fibrinogen level above 100 mg/dL, platelet > 50,000 /mm^3 and activated partial thromboplastin time almost normal. The antifibrinolytics like Tranexamic acid, Aminocaproic Acid and Aprotinin, recombinant factor VIIa and prothrombin complex concentrate (superior to rF VIIa) have been proved to be beneficial.

Metabolic system complications: There can be associated hyperglycemia and hypokalemia in response to stress and trauma. The beta-adrenergic response drives Potassium into the cells leading to hypokalemia. The hypokalemia due to stress and hyperventilation requires no treatment, as the total potassium levels remain the same. Diabetes Insipidus (DI) can be an effect of base of skull fractures or severe TBI involving the posterior pituitary gland. These patients can present with hyponatremia due to Cerebral Salt Wasting Syndrome (CSWS) or due to Syndrome of Inappropriate Antidiuretic Hormone (SIADH).

Management: Serum glucose is maintained between 140 and 180 mg/dL. Hyperglycemia is detrimental and strict glucose monitoring is required. The hyponatremia due to CSWS or SIADH require different modes of management. SIADH is managed mainly by fluid restriction and administration of loop diuretics. CSWS on the other hand requires repletion of intravascular volume losses and correction of hyponatremia with hypertonic saline. Management of DI involves replacement of free water losses and supplementation with Desmopressin or Vasopressin.

Endocrine system complications: Hypopituitarism occurs in 28 to 57% patients with TBI and can present as low T3 syndrome (euthyroid sick syndrome), DI or secondary hypoadrenalism.

Management: Hypoadrenalism requires additional supplementation of steroids.

Management of ICP: As per the BTF guidelines, treatment is required for ICP > 22 mm Hg.

Manoeuvres include:

a. Temporary Hyperventilation
b. $CMRO_2$ reduction by barbiturates (only recommended in cases refractory to medical and surgical treatment), Propofol, opioids, lidocaine.
c. Mannitol followed by furosemide
d. Hypertonic saline
e. CSF drainage (continuous preferred over intermittent)
f. Propped up position
g. Surgical intervention

Non-neurological extracranial surgery for the TBI patient: TBI patients may have associated extra cranial injuries, which may require emergent intervention[13]. The main goal of anaesthesia management is to prevent secondary brain injury during non-neurosurgical procedures[14].

TBI patients with extra cranial injuries fall into three categories[15]:

- Life-threatening injury, e.g. blunt trauma causing solid organ (liver, spleen, kidney) rupture requiring exploratory laparotomy
- Less serious, non-life-threatening condition, e.g. along bone fracture, maxillofacial fractures.
- Stable head injuries for elective surgery

The timing of surgery depends on the severity of these injuries and their effect on the ability to maintain cerebral perfusion and oxygenation. The goals of anaesthesia management for extra cranial surgeries are same as for neurosurgical interventions.

1) Head injury with a life-threatening extra cranial injury

Patients with hemodynamic instability not responding to fluid resuscitation may require exploratory laparotomy as it can be due to intra-abdominal pathology. In addition, patients presenting with depressed skull fractures and lateralization signs may undergo craniotomy along with laparotomy[15].

If the patient is haemodynamically stable in the presence of ongoing resuscitation, somatic and head CT scans for further evaluation should be done. These will aid in the surgical management of both cranial and extra cranial injuries. Once these patients have been haemodynamically stabilized, management of the head injury should take priority.

2) Head injury with a non-life- threatening extra cranial injury

Non-life threatening extracranial injury does not warrant immediate intervention, as stabilization of severe head injury is priority. Early (<24 hours) fixation of long bone fractures might worsen neurological outcome. A limb-saving vascular procedure may be considered as a matter of urgency in all trauma patients.

Long-bone fixation should probably be done when physiological parameters have stabilised, usually within 48-72 hours. Compound fractures can be cleaned and debrided as part of the resuscitative effort. Skeletal traction can be instituted until fracture fixation can be performed.

3) Management of patient for elective extra cranial surgery after stabilization of acute brain injury

Brain is vital organ vulnerable to damage even after several weeks after recovery from TBI. The ideal time frame has not been given for the elective surgeries after TBI but safest period that does not affect the brain process is after 6 months[16].

CONCLUSION

A goal directed and protocolised management of patients with TBI is required right from admission in the ER to intensive care management involving multidisciplinary approach. Evidence based management of TBI will help in improving the outcome. Avoidance of secondary brain injury is the main goal of management of both cranial and extracranial injuries.

REFERENCES

1. Shekhar C, Gupta L, Premsagar I, Kishore J, Sinha M. An epidemiological study of traumatic brain injury cases in a trauma centre of New Delhi (India). J Emerg Trauma Shock. 2015;8(3):131.

2. Qureshi H, Ezell J, Mithaiwala H, Maurtua M. Anesthetic Management of Traumatic Brain Injury. Clin Med Rev Case Rep. 2017;4(2):1-10.

3. Carney N, Totten AM, Reilly CO, Ullman JS, Bell MJ, Bratton SL. Guidelines for the Management of Severe Traumatic Brain Injury, Fourth Edition. Neurosurgery. 2016;0(0):1-10.

4. Hemphill JC, Phan N. Management of acute severe traumatic brain injury. pdf. UpToDate. 2014. http://www.uptodate.com/contents/management-of-acute-severe-traumatic-brain-injury? topic Key=NEURO/4826 & elapsed Time Ms=7 & view=print & displayed View=full.

5. Crosby E. Airway management in adults after cervical spine trauma. Anesthesiology. 2006;104(6):1293-1318.

6. Platts-Mills TF, Campagne D, Chinnock B, Snowden B, Glickman LT, Hendey GW. A Comparison of GlideScope Video Laryngoscopy Versus Direct Laryngoscopy Intubation in the Emergency Department. Acad Emerg Med. 2009;16(9):866-71.

7. Dinsmore J, Frca M. Traumatic brain injury?: an evidence-based review of management. Contin Educ Anaesthesia, Crit care Pain. 2013;13(6):189-95.

8. SAFE Study Investigators, Australian and New Zealand Intensive Care Society Clinical Trials Group, Australian Red Cross Blood Service, George Institute for International Health. Saline or albumin for fluid resuscitation in patients with traumatic brain injury. N Engl J Med. 2007;357(9):874.

9. McIntyre L, Fergusson D, Hutchison J, et al. Effect of a liberal versus restrictive transfusion strategy on mortality in patients with moderate to severe head injury. Neurocrit Care. 2006;5(1):4-9.

10. Group TC trial management, The CRASH trial collaborators. Final results of MRC CRASH, a randomised placebo-controlled trial of intravenous corticosteroid in adults with head injury-outcomes at 6 months. Lancet. 2005;365(9475):1957-59.

11. Sharma D, Vavilala MS. Perioperative Management of Adult Traumatic Brain Injury. Anesth Clin. 30(2):333-46.

12. Worah SH, Minokadeh A. Postoperative and Intensive Care Including Head Injury and Multisystem Sequelae. In: Cottrell JE, Patel P, eds. Cottrell and Patel's Neuroanesthesia. Vol sixth. USA: Elsevier Inc.; 2017:410-23.

13. Mantilla JHMM, Arboleda LFG. Anesthesia for patients with traumatic brain injury. Rev Colomb Anestesiol. 2015;3(S 1) : 3-8.

14. Chowdhury T, Cappellani RB, Daya J. Neuroanesthetic considerations for emergent extracranial surgeries: What to know? Saudi J Anaesth. 6(4).

15. Prabhu AJ, Matta BF. Anaesthesia for extra-cranial surgery in patients with trauma brain injury. Contin Educ Anaesthesia, Crit care Pain. 2004;4(5):156-8.

16. Jangra K, Grover VK, Bhagat H. Chapter 47 - Neurological Patients for Nonneurosurgeries A2 - Prabhakar, Hemanshu BT - Essentials of Neuroanesthesia. In: Essentials of Neuroanesthesia. Vol Academic Press; 2017:783-803.

MULTIPLE CHOICE QUESTIONS

1. **Following severe head injury all are true except**
   a. Cerebral blood flow can fall to 50% of normal
   b. Cerebral perfusion pressure should be maintained above 70 mmHg
   c. Hypo- and hyperglycemia worsen outcome
   d. Temperature above 37°C worsens outcome.

2. **What is the threshold to treat ICP?**
   a. 10-15 mm Hg
   b. 15-20 mm Hg
   c. 20-25 mm Hg
   d. 25-30 mm Hg

3. **A linear relationship of cerebral blood flow exists with?**
   a. ICP
   b. $PaCO_2$
   c. PaO_2
   d. CPP

4. **Symptoms and signs of elevated intracranial pressure may include all except**
   a. Nausea and vomiting
   b. Papilloedema
   c. Pupillary constriction
   d. Decerebrate posturing

5. **Level II or III recommendations for these patients include all of the following, except...?**
   a. Avoid Hypoxia with $SpO_2 < 90\%$
   b. Provide prophylactic Hyperventilation to PCO_2 of 25 mmHg
   c. Avoid Hypotension with SBP < 90 mmHg
   d. Avoid Hypoxia with $PaO_2 < 60$ mmHg

6. **Recommendations for Perioperative fluid management of head injury patients include all except**
   a. Non glucose containing isotonic saline
   b. Albumin can be useful over saline
   c. Hypertonic saline may be beneficial
   d. Role of colloid is controversial

7. **Surgical management of non neurological injury in a TBI patient is done immediately when**
   a. Life threatening injury including solid organ damage with hemodynamic instability
   b. Long bone fracture
   c. Maxillofacial fracture
   d. Hemodynamically stable head injury with abdominal injury

8. **All are beneficial during TBI management except**
   a. Prevention of hypoxia and hypotension
   b. Rapid evacuation of intracranial hematoma
   c. Use of steroid and hyperventilation
   d. Seizure prophylaxis

9. **Nitrous oxide is avoided as it causes all except**
   a. Raise ICP
   b. increases CBF
   c. Fall in $CMRO_2$
   d. Impairement of autoregulation of brain

10. **All of the following anaesthetic agents are advantageous in TBI except**
    a. Propofol
    b. Thiopentone
    c. Enflurane
    d. Sevoflurane

CHAPTER 18

BRAIN DEATH

Vaibhavi Baxi, Dwarkadas K. Baheti, Rajshree Deopujari

Introduction

It was in 1968 that the concept of brain death as death was proposed by an Ad Hoc Committee of Harvard Medical School.[1] In 1976, UK Royal Medical Colleges defined brain death as complete irreversible loss of brainstem function and specified clinical criteria to certify brain death. It led to a redefining of death – "An individual who has sustained either 1) irreversible cessation of circulatory & respiratory functions or 2) irreversible cessation of all functions of the entire brain, including the brain stem, is dead."[1]

Once the brain death is certified due to irreversible cessation of brainstem function, it enables intensivists and specialists working in Intensive Care to withdraw futile treatment (e.g. mechanical ventilation), on humanitarian, ethical and (coincidentally) utilitarian grounds.

Definition

The brain death which is equivalent to legal death is defined as an "Irreversible cessation of all functions of the entire brain, including the brainstem". The brain death is a relatively new concept originating in the 20th Century with the advent of Mechanical Ventilation & Organ Transplantation.

Mechanism of Brain Death:

Trauma to the brain or cerebrovascular injury produces brain oedema. Because the brain is covered with a rigid bony skull, oedema is accompanied with an increase in intracranial pressure, which if significantly high; exceeds arterial blood pressure. When cerebral circulation ceases, aseptic necrosis of the brain ensues. In 3-5 days the brain becomes a liquefied mass. The increased intracranial pressure compresses the brain stem, and this results in total brain infarction.

Clinical diagnosis of brain death:

Clinical determination of brain death involves four steps[2]:

1. **Clinical Evaluation (Prerequisites):**

   - Establish irreversible & proximate cause of coma
   - Exclude CNS Depressants & NMBs
   - Normal Temperature (>36°C)
   - Normal Systolic Blood Pressure (>100mmHg)
   - Neurologic Exam (2 exams 6 hours apart) after a 'sufficient' time period has passed since the injury
   - Although physicians can determine brain death; individual hospitals may require that it be a neurologist or neurosurgeon

2. **Neurologic Examination**

   - Unresponsive coma
   - Motor: No response to deep nail bed pressure in any extremity
   - Sensory: No motor or haemodynamic(tachycardia) response to pain.
   - No CN reflexes
   - Reflexes: Brisk reflexes do not exclude brain death. E.g. Babinski, Lazarus reflex.
   - Apnoea (PCO2 > 60mmHg, or >20 over baseline)

3. **Ancillary Testing:** such as EEG, cerebral blood flow study.

4. **Documentation**: Time of Death; Checklist; Contact organ procurement organization.

Diagnosis of brainstem death based on clinical tests should not be made unless the following pre-conditions have been met:

(A) Proof that the patient's condition is due to irreversible structural brain damage

In each patient the underlying neurological diagnosis which caused the severe neurological injury and the accompanying loss of brain stem reflexes must be apparent and must be well documented.

CT scan, angiography or MRI scan are usually done as supplementary proof of sufficient brain pathology. In patients with acute hypoxic-ischaemic brain injury clinical evaluation should be delayed for at least 24 hours after the cardio-respiratory arrest.

(B) Exclusion of reversible causes of coma

a) Toxins, poisons, sedative drugs and many other agents may cause coma when exposed to large quantities. The drug history and a toxicology screen should be obtained.

b) If sedative drugs have been used, adequate time must be allowed for residual effects to have worn off. A recent review suggests waiting four times the elimination half-life of the sedatives used.[3]

c) Antagonist agents may be used like flumazenil for benzodiazepines and naloxone for opioids. If muscle relaxants have been used, confirm that neuromuscular conduction is intact with a peripheral nerve stimulator.

d) Measurement of plasma concentration of drugs should reveal drug concentrations below the therapeutic range e.g. alcohol below the legal limit for driving. The median concentration of thiopentone permitting motor response is 12 mg[4] but there is considerable individual variation.

e) Hypothermia must be excluded. Core body temperature should be more than 35°C when clinical assessment of brain stem reflexes is carried out.

f) Metabolic or endocrine abnormalities may contribute to coma and must be excluded. Hypothyroidism, panhypopituitarism, adrenal dysfunction, uraemia and hepatic failure can profoundly decrease the level of consciousness. Disorders of sodium, phosphate, magnesium and glucose can affect the response to brain stem tests. The commonest metabolic abnormality in brain dead patients is hypernatremia, often related to diabetes insipidus. Serum sodium should not be grossly abnormal. (150 mmol/dl: upper acceptable limit for brain stem tests)

g) Severe hypotension. Blood pressure should be greater than 90mmHg systolic (MAP > 60mmHg) for brain stem tests. Infusion of fluid and vasopressor drugs are often needed to maintain blood pressure.

Formal clinical testing for brainstem reflexes:

The first formal examination is undertaken when the patient has been observed to have

a. Fixed pupils

b. Absent cranial nerve reflexes for at least four hours and fulfils the pre-conditions above.

1) **No motor response** - within the cranial nerve distribution in response to adequate stimulation of the trigeminal area and of the limbs. Trigeminal stimulation can be applied by pressure on the supraorbital notch or at the level of the temporomandibular joint. Reflex: afferent nerve V and efferent nerve VII.

2) **No pupillary response to light** - Each pupil on examination using a strong light in a dimmed light room, should be more than 4mm in diameter. The normal response is brisk constriction of the pupil. Rule out pre-existing pupil abnormalities and pupil surgeries like iridectomy. Round, oval or irregularly shaped pupils in mid position (4-to 6 mm) are compatible with brain death. Reflex: afferent nerve II and efferent nerve III.

3) **Corneal reflex** - Touching the cornea with a wisp of cotton wool or a sterile throat swab elicits blinking of the eyelids which is the normal response. Both eyelids must be observed. Reflex: afferent nerve V and efferent nerve VII

4) **Oculocephalic reflex** – (Doll's head eye phenomenon). Examiner holds the patient's eyes open and the head is turned suddenly from the middle position to 90 degrees on both sides. When the reflex is intact the eyes turn opposite to the side of head movement as if lagging. The reflex is absent when the eyes move with the head and do not move within the orbit. One must avoid this test in patient with unstable cervical spine injury. Reflex: afferent VIII and efferent III,IV,VI.

5) **Oculovestibular reflex (caloric testing)** – A soft catheter is introduced into the external auditory canal for gentle, slow irrigation with at least 50ml of iced water, with patient's head in midline and elevated at 30⁰(lateral semi-circular canal is vertical) while the eyes are held open by an assistant. The test is repeated in opposite eye in 5 minutes. A prerequisite for this test is an intact tympanic membrane confirmed by an auroscope. An intact oculovestibular reflex causes tonic (slow) deviation of the eyes towards the irrigated ear. During testing to confirm brain death, any movement of one or both eyes, whether conjugate or not, excludes a diagnosis of brain death. When the reflex is absent the eyes remain fixed. Reflex: afferent nerve VIII and efferent nerves III and VI.

6) **Pharyngeal (gag) reflex** - Each side of the oropharynx is stimulated using a tongue depressor and the patient is observed for any pharyngeal or palatal movement. Reflex: afferent nerve IX and efferent nerve X.

7) **Laryngeal (cough) reflex** - Carina is stimulated by passing a suction catheter into the endotracheal or tracheostomy tube and the patient is observed for any cough response or movement of the chest or diaphragm. Reflex: Afferent nerve IX and efferent nerve X.

8) **Apnoea test** - This test is an essential part of the confirmation of brain death and should be performed when all other brain-stem reflexes are absent.

The test has three parts

a) Disconnection from mechanical ventilation to allow arterial CO2 tension to build up to reach a critical point.

b) Prevention of hypoxia during this period.

c) Absence of spontaneous respiratory efforts during this period.

Ventilate the patient with 100% oxygenfor >10mins to ensure pre-oxygenation (PaO2>200mmHg). Ensure patient is hemodynamically stable. Check arterial blood gas to make sure the PaCO2 is within normal limits (34-45mmHg). Disconnect the patient from the ventilator. Deliver 100% oxygen through a narrow suction catheter inserted into the endotracheal tube to the level of carina at 6L/min. Inspect the reservoir bag to monitor respiration; also inspect the chest and abdomen for any movement.

At five-minute intervals, check arterial blood gases until the PaCO2 rises above 60 mmHg or higher (decreased sensitivity to high PaCO2 in COPD patients)[5] or increased by 20mmHg over baseline CO2. Oxygen saturation levels should be maintained within the normal range. Ensure that a Valsalva effect or barotrauma do not occur. Maintain normal blood pressure by increasing vasopressors. If there is no attempt of spontaneous breathing despite of hypercarbia and acidaemia the test is positive for brain death.

In patients with a high cervical cord injury (abolished phrenic nerve function), severe head and facial injuries etc can make it impossible to test all the brainstem reflexes. In such cases additional tests for e.g. demonstrating absent intracranial blood flow in four vessel cerebral angiography may be needed to confirm brain death; which is the 'gold-standard' test to confirm a diagnosis of brain death. Confirmatory test findings that maybe helpful but are not mandatory include isoelectric electroencephalogram, absence of brainstem auditory evoked potentials, and absence of cerebral perfusion as documented by angiographic, transcranial Doppler or radio isotopic studies.

Spinal reflexes

Body movements, secondary to spinal cord reflexes may persist until all circulation has ceased[6]. These movements represent only spinal cord activity. Movements noted include abduction or adduction of the arms, leg movements, head rotation (due to cervical muscle activity) and even a brief attempt of the body to sit up to 40-60 degrees (Lazarus sign).

Declaration of brain death:

Before declaring two sets of tests should be undertaken by different doctors. They could be a consultant neurologist, neurosurgeon, anaesthetist or intensivist. If organ donation is being considered, the doctors certifying brain death should not be involved in any proposed transplant procedure.

When organ donation is being considered, this is regarded as essential. A 'reasonable' period of time should intervene between the two sets of tests. The apnoea test is the final test to be done. If it is positive for the second time, the patient should then be declared dead and the time and date noted.

It is important to inform the family sensitively by the clinicians, usually the Intensive Care team that they may be asked to begin to consider what the patient would have wished in relation to organ donation if brain death is confirmed. After the first set of formal tests; if there is no sign of brain stem activity, it is advisable to inform the family of the findings and that confirmation of these findings on second testing (which is anticipated) will lead to a diagnosis of brain death.

Brain dead patients can survive for about a week or two after brain death. Most of them suffer cardiac death in about a week. If organ donation is not to be considered then after declaration of brain death, life support systems can be withdrawn. The family of the deceased should be given privacy and time for their religious beliefs and other ceremonies with due respect.

Donation after brain death

The discussion of organ donation begins with the diagnosis of brain death. Doctors who discuss organ donation with the patient's family should be different from those who perform the organ procurement. The anesthesiologist plays a significant role in organ procurement from the brain-dead patient, as hemodynamic, thermoregulation, intravascular volume status, and skeletal muscle paralysis require active management and are vital to the procurement of healthy organs. In the presence of brain death, spinal cord function is still intact and both somatic and visceral reexes remain.

Effective anaesthetic management of donation requires an understanding of the effects of brain death on each organ system. Every organ system is affected by brain death. Aim here is the normalization of donor physiology to maximize the long-term viability of organs for donation[7]. This should continue from the ICU into the operating room during donation surgery. Table 1 comprises a concise summary of the effects of brain death on each organ system along with recommendations for anaesthetic management.

Table 1. Effect of Brain death on each organ system and its anaesthetic management

System	Effect of brain death	Anaesthesia management
Cardiac	• Myocardial injury • Loss of vascular tone • Hemodynamic instability	• Restore intravascular volume • Vasopressors to maintain organ perfusion • Maintain SBP >100 mmHg MAP >70mmHg HR 60-120 beats/min
Pulmonary	• Increased pulmonary capillary permeability • Pulmonary edema	• "Lung-protective" ventilatory strategy: TV 6-8-mL/kg PEEP 8-10 cm H2O • Aim PaO2 >100mmHg Judicious IV fluids: CVP 4-8 (<10)
Hematologic	• Coagulopathy, which may progress to DIC	• Transfuse for Hb <7 or 8 g/dl for optimal oxygen delivery. Aim >10g/dl • Correct coagulopathy with clotting factors or platelets (if e/o ongoing bleeding)
Endocrine	• Pituitary infarction may lead to diabetes insipidus and obliteration of thyroid axis Hyperglycemia Hypernatremia	• Vasopressin to support hemodynamics and control polyuria • Insulin infusion to maintain serum glucose/ 180 mgdl-1 • Consider hormone replacement - thyroxine or T3 infusion, corticosteroid • Aim Na <155 Glucose <150 pH 7.3 - 7.5
Musculoskeletal	• Reflex somatic movements mediated by spinal reflexes	• Skeletal muscle paralysis

Role of anaesthetist in organ procurement

Anesthesiologists play a vital role in the management of organ donors. The intraoperative care may affect the outcome of the organ recipient. Donation after brain death procurement operations requires highly specic intraoperative management by an anesthesiologist. To manage the heart-beating brain-dead donor, the anesthesiologist must incorporate knowledge of the effects of brain death on each organ system as well as the effects of the preoperative measures that the donor required in the ICU. It is also important to know which organs are going to be procured so that specic goals can be established and strategies can be implemented (e.g., lung-protective ventilation or intraoperative glycaemic control) to optimize donor outcome. The success of the anaesthesiologist in physiological optimization of the brain-dead donor may eventually determine the outcome of the organ in the recipient.

CONCLUSION

Brain death is permanent cessation of all functions of brain, though individual organs may function without integrating function of the brain. The lack of consciousness, cognition and respiratory drive along with the neurologic examination confirm the diagnosis of brain death. Before the diagnosis of brain death, patients should be managed as appropriate for their underlying condition. After the diagnosis of brain death, treatment becomes orientated towards organs that may be transplanted rather than orientated towards protection of the brain. The timely diagnosis and declaration allows a brain-dead patient to be a potential organ donor and gift life to end stage organ failure patients.

REFERENCES

1. A Definition of Irreversible Coma: A Report of the Ad Hoc Committee of the Harvard Medical School to Examine the Definition of Brain Death. JAMA. 1968 Aug 5;205(6):337-40.

2. Wijdicks EF, Varelas PN, Gronseth GS, Greer DM; American Academy of Neurology. Evidence-based guideline update: determining brain death in adults: report of the Quality Standards Subcommittee of the American Academy of Neurology. Neurology. 2010 Jun 8;74(23):1911-8.

3. Wijdicks EF. The diagnosis of brain death. N Engl J Med. 2001 Apr 19;344(16):1215-21.

4. Cordato DJ, Herkes GK, Mather LE, et al. Prolonged thiopentone infusion for neurosurgical emergencies: Usefulness of therapeutic drug monitoring. Anaesth Int Care 2001; 29:339-348.

5. Australia and New Zealand Intensive Care Society. ANZICS Statement on Death and Organ Donation. 2008. www.anzics.com.au.

6. Saposnik G, Bueri JA, Maurino J, et al. Spontaneous and reflex movements in brain death. Neurology 2000; 54:221-3.

7. Dictus C, Vienenkoetter B, Esmaeilzadeh M, Unterberg A, Ahmadi R. Critical care management of potential organ donors: our current standard. Clin Transplant 2009; 23(Suppl 21): 2-9.

MULTIPLE CHOICE QUESTIONS

1. **Definition of Brain Death is**
   a. Irreversible cessation of all functions of the entire brain, including the brainstem.
   b. Reversible cessation of all functions of the entire brain, including the brainstem.
   c. Irreversible cessation of all functions of the entire brain, excluding the brainstem.
   d. Irreversible cessation of higher functions cortical functions of the brain.

2. **State if following statements are True or False**
   a. Establishing irreversible and proximate cause of coma is an important prerequisite to diagnosis of brain death.
   b. Presence of brisk reflexes for e.g. babinski, lazarus reflex; exclude brain death.
   c. Exclusion of CNS depressants and NMBs, normal temperature (>36°C) and normal systolic Blood Pressure (>100mmHg) should be followed by neurologic exam (2 exams 6 hours apart) for clinical diagnosis of brain death.
   d. Cranial nerve reflexes are preserved in braid dead patients.

3. **In patients with acute hypoxic–ischaemic brain injury clinical evaluation should be delayed for at least _____ hours after the cardio–respiratory arrest.**
   a. 6hrs
   b. 12hrs
   c. 18hrs
   d. 24hrs

4. **What should be the core body temperature when clinical assessment of brain stem reflexes is carried out.**
   a. more than 30°C
   b. more than 35°C
   c. more than 38°C
   d. more than 40°C

5. **The commonest metabolic abnormality in brain dead patients related to diabetes insipidus is**
   a. Hypernatraemia
   b. Hyperkalemia
   c. Hyponatraemia
   d. Hypokalemia

6. **In Oculocephalic reflex (examiner holds the patient's eyes open and the head is turned suddenly from the middle position to 90 degrees on both sides), when the reflex is intact**
   a. there is no eye movement at all
   b. the eyes turn opposite to the side of head movement as if lagging behind
   c. the eyes move with the head and do not move within the orbit
   d. the eyes move in opposite directions of each other

7. **All the below are parts of the Apnoea test except:**
   a. Prevention of hypoxia during this period
   b. Absence of spontaneous respiratory efforts during this period
   c. No disconnection from mechanical ventilation
   d. Allow arterial CO2 tension to build up to reach a critical point.

8. **State if following statements with respect to Apnoea test are True or False**
   a. At five minute intervals, check arterial blood gases until the PaCO2 rises above 60 mmHg or higher.
   b. Oxygen saturation levels should be maintained within the normal range
   c. Valsalva effect or barotrauma may occur and is acceptable
   d. If there is no attempt of spontaneous breathing despite of hypercarbia and acidaemia the test is considered to be positive for brain death

9. **Investigations that may help in confirming brain death include the following except**
   a. Cerebral Angiography
   b. Isoelectric EEG
   c. Absent brain stem auditory evoked potentials
   d. 2 D ECHO

10. **Clinical diagnosis and certification of Brain death may be done by the following doctors except**
    a. Neurologist
    b. Intensivist
    c. Transplant Surgeon
    d. Anaesthetist

CHAPTER 19

ACUTE ISCHAEMIC STROKE - ANAESTHESIA MANAGEMENT

Lalita D. Naik, Neeta V. Karmarkar

Introduction

Stroke is one of the three leading causes of death worldwide and is the most common life threatening neurological disease with long-term disability.

Stroke is a clinical form for the acute loss of perfusion to the vascular territory of the brain from ischaemic or haemorrhagic insults resulting in corresponding loss of neurological functions. Therefore, prompt recognition of these conditions and treatment is very crucial for rapid restoration of blood flow to the deprived areas.

Ischemic stroke   **Hemorrhagic stroke**

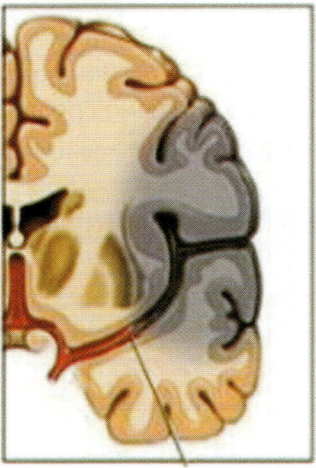 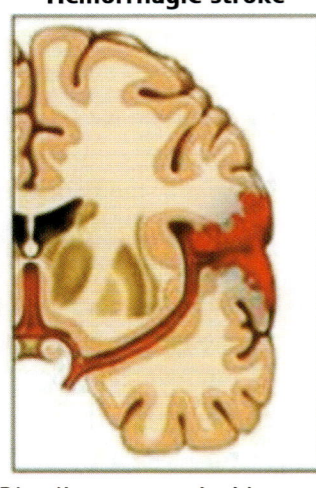

A clot blocking blood flow to an area of the brain   Bleeding occurs inside or around brain tissue (rupture of a vessel)

Fig. 1. Types of stroke

Acute ischaemic stroke accounts for 87% of all strokes. The World Health Organisation defines stroke as "rapidly developing clinical signs of focal or global disturbances of cerebral functions with symptoms lasting 24 hours or longer leading to death with no apparent cause other than vascular origin"[1].

Classification of acute ischaemic stroke:[2]

1) Thrombus: In situ obstruction of an artery.

2) Embolus: Particles of debris originating elsewhere that block arterial access to a particular region of the brain.

3) Systemic hypo perfusion: More of general circulatory problem manifesting itself in the brain and perhaps in other organs.

TOAST Classification:

1) Large artery atherosclerosis.

2) Cardiac embolism.

3) Small vessel occlusion (lacunar).

4) Stroke of other aetiology.

5) Undetermined e.g. cryptogenic.

Cerebral Arterial Territory

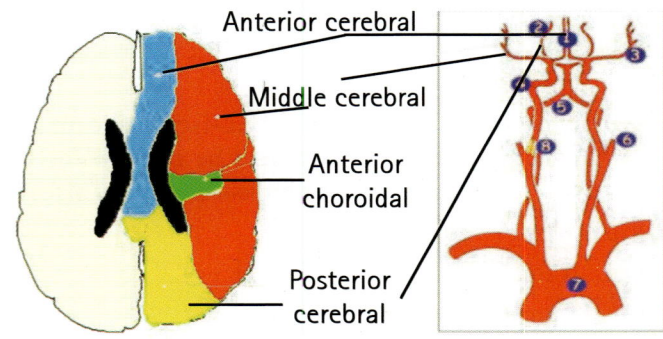

Anterior cerebral

Middle cerebral

Anterior choroidal

Posterior cerebral

Fig. 2. Cerebral blood supply

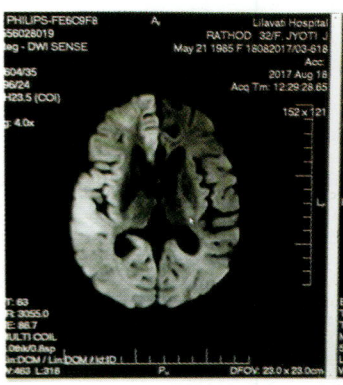 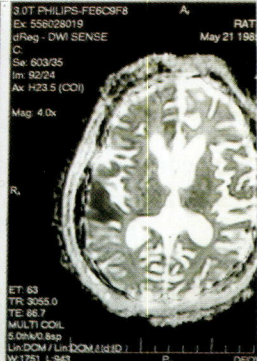

Fig. 3. Right MCA territory infarct

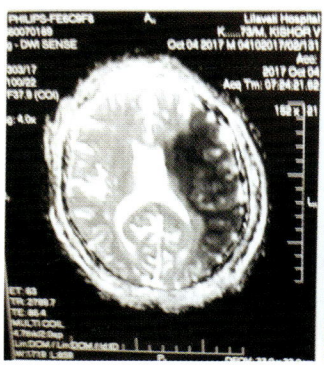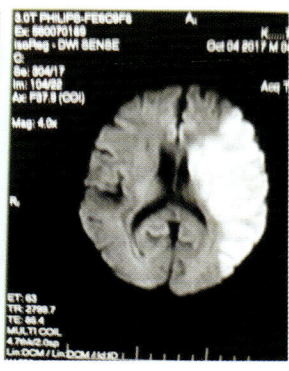

Fig. 4. Left MCA territory infarct

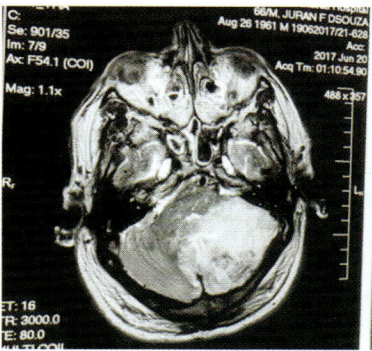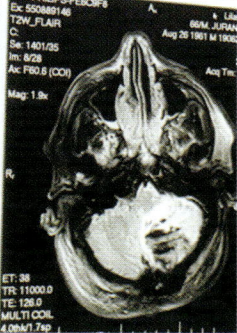

Fig. 5. Posterior circulation stroke

Based on symptoms:

1) Total Anterior Circulation Stroke (TAC)

2) Partial Anterior Circulation Stroke (PAC)

3) Lacunar Stroke (LAC)

4) Posterior Circulation Stroke (POC)

These four entities predict the extent of the stroke, area of the brain affected, the underlying cause and the prognosis.

Aetiology of AIS:

A) Thrombosis

Large vessels (extracranial /intracranial)

1) Atherosclerosis

2) Dissection

3) Takayasu arteritis

4) Giant cell arteritis

5) Fibromuscular dysplasia

6) Moya Moya syndrome (Intracranial vessels.) etc.

B) Cardiac embolic stroke

1) Atrial / LV thrombus

2) Atrial fibrillation

3) Recent myocardial infarction

4) RHD (Mitral / aortic valve)

5) Chronic myocardial infarction with EF < 25 %.

6) Dilated cardiomyopathy.

7) L V aneurysm.

8) Heart failure with EF < 30%.

C) Systemic hypoperfusion

E.g. Blood disorders like sickle cell anaemia, HIT syndrome and polycythaemia vera.

D) Small vessel disease

Lipohyalinosis, fibrinoid degeneration etc.

Pathophysiology of acute ischaemic stroke[2, 3, 4, 5, 6]

A sudden interruption of cerebral blood flow produces a gradient of hypoperfusion characterised by three zones-innermost zone of infarction surrounded by the zone of ischaemic penumbra and the outermost zone of oligaemia.

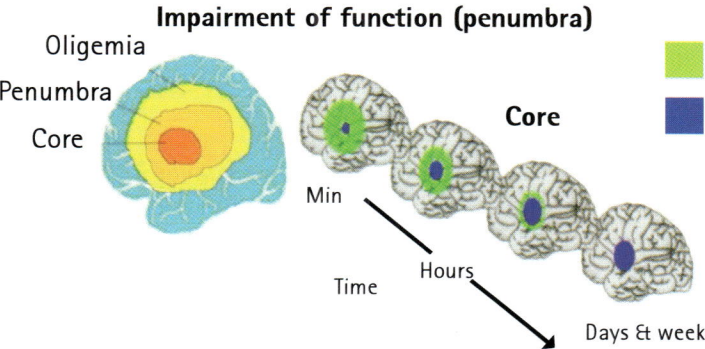

Fig. 6. Gradient of hypoperfusion stating the different zones of ischemia

In the zone of infarction severe hypoperfusion reduces metabolic activity resulting in irreversible cell damage and death, whereas the outermost oligaemic zone with milder hypoperfusion is not normally vulnerable to infarction & the central zone is the salvageable ischaemic penumbra.

The ischaemic penumbra – Around and as islands within the infarcted brain there is an ischaemic penumbra where the blood flow is less, functions are depressed, oxygen extraction fraction (OEF) is very high with impaired or loss of auto regulation.

It is threatened but salvageable tissue with "misery perfusion" where the metabolic needs of the tissues are not being met. The ischaemic penumbra is short lived lasting only for a few hours. The typical ischaemic stroke patients lose 1.9 million neurons for each minute they are untreated and the ischaemic brain ages by 3.6 years per hour without treatment. This tissue may die or recover depending on the speed and extent of restoration of blood flow by recanalization of the occluded artery.

This concept results in the "Therapeutic Time Window "[7] which is very short, during which rapid restoration of blood flow and or neuronal protection from ischaemic damage might prevent both cell death and recruitment of neurons into the zone of infarction and apoptosis and thus achieve better neurological outcome. Delayed recanalization may be detrimental as it might increase the perfusion pressure in the areas of impaired autoregulation resulting in hyperaemia, hyperperfusion, cerebral oedema, haemorrhagic transformation of the infarct, increased ICP resulting in transtentorial herniation and mass effect aggravating further cerebral ischaemia.

The normal cerebral blood flow (CBF) is 50 ml /100gm of brain / min, neuro electrical failure occurs at CBF of 16-18ml / 100 gm of brain / min and failure of membrane ion homeostasis occurs at CBF of 10 – 12 ml / 100 gm of brain / min which marks the threshold for infarct. Normally CBF depends on cerebral perfusion pressure (CPP) and cerebral vascular resistance (CVR). CBF remains constant when the mean arterial pressure is between 50 – 170 mm of Hg. The homeostatic mechanism to maintain a constant CBF in the face of changing CPP is autoregulation and beyond the autoregulatory level the CBF becomes pressure passive falling and rising with CPP.

In hypertensive patients, the autoregulatory range is shifted upwards, so that when CBF starts falling, ischaemic symptoms occur at a higher systolic blood pressure (SBP) than normal. Therefore, sudden lowering of blood pressure may exacerbate cerebral ischaemia and infarction in AIS patients. Most of the AIS patients present with hypertension due to excess release of catecholamines & cortisol to maintain collateral blood flow to the penumbra.

As seen in the diagram

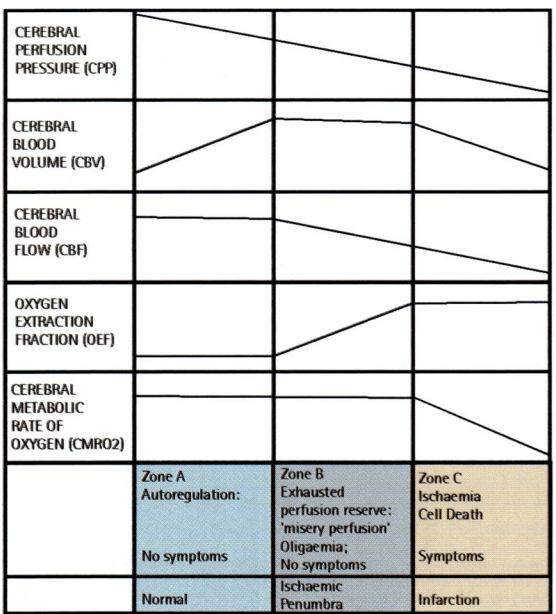

Fig. 7. Pathophysiology of acute ischemic stroke

Zone A: In the normal **"autoregulatory" range** when CPP falls, cerebral vascular resistance drops resulting in cerebral vasodilatation, increasing the cerebral blood volume (CBV) and thus CBF remains constant.

Zone B: In the **"ischaemic zone"** when vasodilatation is maximal and the CBV can rise no more, if CPP still continues to fall e.g. preoperative hypotension or hypotension during induction of anaesthesia or increased ICP etc., CBV starts falling along with fall in CBF resulting in exhaused of cerebral perfusion reserve, but the metabolic activity is maintained by increasing the oxygen extraction fraction (OEF). This is termed "misery perfusion".

Zone C: In the last **"stage of infarction"**, OEF can increase no more and if CPP still continues to fall, in the presence of exhausted perfusion reserves, metabolism becomes limited, CBF is inadequate to meet the metabolic needs of the tissue resulting in the onset of infarction. At around this time the patient becomes symptomatic.

The effect of hemodynamic fluctuations on penumbra

In the ischaemic penumbra autoregulation is impaired or lost & the CBF becomes pressure passive e.g. preoperative hypotension or during induction of anaesthesia results in severe cerebral ischaemia which should be corrected with vasopressors, volume replacement & the cause should be investigated. Whereas severe preoperative hypertension makes the patient ineligible for Recombinant tissue plasminogen activator (rtPA) therapy & hypertension following reperfusion of the occluded artery may result in hyperperfusion injury. Therefore both hypotension & hypertension are worse predictors of poor neurological outcome in AIS.

Effect of secondary insults: Ischaemic penumbra has impaired responsiveness to Pao2 and Paco2 which makes it very sensitive to secondary insults viz hypoxia, hypercarbia, hyperglycemia, hyperthermia, dehydration and seizures etc which exacerbate cerebral ischaemia.

Mechanism of ischaemic cell injury and death and role of hyperglycemia

The brain contains little or no energy stores and relies on uninterrupted blood supply for their delivery. Ischaemia results in deprivation of glucose and oxygen leading to anaerobic metabolism with depletion of ATP and accumulation of lactic acid.

Lactic acidosis results in loss of membrane ion homeostasis with intracellular influx of sodium and calcium ions. This initiates a cascade of deleterious events like cerebral oedema, release of free radicals, neuro excitatory chemicals, arachidonic acid metabolites, proteolytic enzymes, inflammatory responses and disruption of BBB with increased permeability. All these factors result in cell necrosis. Hyperglycemia (HG) augments the lactic acidosis induced events and consequences of ischaemia are exacerbated.

HG is most common in AIS patients (Glucose levels > 140 mg/dl) and it independently predicts:

1) Larger Infarct Size

2) Poor Clinical outcome.

3) Higher risk of mortality especially in patients with cortical infarction.

4) Poor clinical outcome in patients treated with IV rtPA.

5) Unsuccessful intra arterial (IA) thrombolysis unless HG is strictly controlled.

6) Poor outcome despite successful endo vascular (EV) recanalization.

7) Increased risk of parenchymal haemorrhage.

Studies have shown that favourable neurologic outcomes are seen with glucose values between 70-139 mg%

Therefore, glucose containing IV fluids should be avoided and blood glucose levels of < 140 mg% should be maintained in AIS patients.

Understanding pathophysiology of AIS raises 3 concepts:

1) "Therapeutic Time Window"

2) "Time is Brain"

3) Penumbra as the "target" for both endovascular therapy and for more scientific approach to the perioperative anaesthesia plan.

Time is brain concept and method to prolong the time window

The narrow time frame for the therapeutic action has impeded effective treatment for the majority of AIS cases. Further extending the time window for endovascular therapy is an important endeavour for increasing the number of stroke patients who might benefit from this treatment.

1. Recent studies have demonstrated that Penumbra imaging with advanced MRI (PWI /DWI) techniques can identify sub group of patients who are likely to improve following reperfusion and others at risk for haemorrhage and poor clinical outcomes.

   (This will maximise the benefit and reduce the risk of adverse events and poor outcome when used both early after stroke onset and at a later time). This has enhanced patient selection and extended the therapeutic time window.

2. DAWN TRIAL – "Thrombectomy effective up to 24 hrs. after AIS "(Medscape coverage from 3rd European Stroke Organization Conference ESCO – May 2017)[8].

   In this trial patients with large artery occlusion underwent CT perfusion or MRI diffusion weighted imaging and the results have shown that removal of clot by endovascular thrombectomy reduced the disability in the selected patients presenting upto 24 hours after the onset of symptoms.

3. By using neuro protective drugs.

   e.g. Free radical scavengers, anti-apoptotic enzyme inhibitors.

   e.g. Edaravone (free radical scavenger), Caspases inhibitors (Caspases is a key enzyme in apotosis).

   Using them preoperatively along with IV rtPA have shown to improve neurological outcome and extend the therapeutic time window.

Predictors of poor neurological outcomes

1) Time Delay in starting anaesthesia.

2) High NIHSS Scores. (National Institutes of Health Stroke Scale) for Neurological Impairment. NIHSS Score Range 0-42

   Mild 0-4, Moderate 5-15, Severe >15

3) Hemodynamic fluctuations under GA.

4) Hyperglycemia.

5) General anaesthesia.

6) Hyperthermia.

7) Baseline low SPO2 and hypercapnia.

8) Posterior Circulation stroke.

9) Total Anterior Circulation Stroke

10) More than 1/3rd MCA territory infarct.

11) Severe Hemiparesis

12) Old Age with Multiple Co-Morbidities

13) Carotid Terminus Occlusion.

14) Failed / Unsuccessful Recanalization.

15) Seizures.

16) Dehydration.

General Anaesthesia has been blamed for the poor neurological outcome in AIS patients mainly due to,

1) Delay in starting the case.

2) Hemodynamic fluctuations associated with GA.

3) Neuro toxicity of anaesthetic agents.

Factors causing delay in starting the case[9]

Logistic problems:

1) The endovascular suite is situated away from the main theatre complex making it difficult for the anaesthesia team to respond quickly especially during off hours.

2) Non-availability of experienced anaesthesiologist in managing stroke cases.

3) Anaesthesia team not familiar with endovascular suite, non – availability of equipments, monitors and medications.

4) Non-availability of specialized equipments required for difficult airway access.

5) Team not familiar with endovascular interventions and their specific anaesthesia requirements.

6) Uncontrolled co morbidities (e.g. Difficult airway access, COPD, bronchial asthma, cardiac problems, OSA, Severe Obesity etc.) taking much of the attention of the anaesthesiologist.

7) Less work force available during off hours.

8) Anaesthesia team not familiar with the guidelines, recommendations of management of AIS patients.

Patient problems:

1) Due to time constraints patient gets transferred to the endovascular suite from the emergency department without admission papers, informed consent and investigation reports.

2) Preoperative evaluation may be inadequate as patient may be aphasic, non-communicative or having severe neurological impairment and non-availability of relatives to get proper medical / surgical history and information regarding allergies & medications.

3) Uncontrolled co-morbid diseases which need to be addressed before administering anaesthesia (e.g. heart blocks, bronchial asthma, severe cardio-respiratory problems, difficult airways).

4) Time needed to collect all the specialised equipments, monitors and medications.

5) Patient not adequately starving.

The goal of early therapy in AIS is to rapidly restore perfusion to the Ischaemic Penumbra by recanalization of the occluded intracerebral vessel within 3 hrs of onset of the stroke symptoms. This prevents recruitment of this zone into the zone of infarction and apoptosis and hence achieves better neurological outcome.

If there is a delay in starting anaesthesia or the procedure the entire tissue at risk would have already progressed to an irreversible infarction zone and recanalization of the occluded artery at this stage will not be able to achieve good clinical outcome. In fact it may even cause harm by increasing the risk of haemorrhagic transformation of the infarct.

VARIOUS TREATMENT OPTIONS AVAILABLE FOR AIS[10,11]

1) All patients who present within 3 hrs of onset of symptoms and have no contraindications to IV rtPA therapy are treated with intravenous Recombinant tissue, Plasminogen activator (IV rtPA).

2) Patients who present between 3 and 4½ hrs after the onset of stroke and have no contraindications may be considered for IV rtPA therapy.

3) Patients who are not eligible for IV rtPA therapy e.g. delayed time for presentation, contraindications to IV rtPA therapy such as recent surgery or coagulopathies, patients with unsuccessful recanalization with IV rtPA therapy, large artery occlusion etc. can be considered for endovascular therapy.

   (e.g. Intra-arterial thrombolysis (IA), mechanical clot removal, mechanical thrombectomy, clot laceration, angiography, angioplasty and stenting). Intra-arterial thrombolysis must be performed within 6 hrs of onset of symptoms and mechanical thrombectomy upto 8 hrs of onset of stroke.

The endovascular treatment for acute ischaemic stroke provides a supplement or an alternative to systemic intravenous thrombolysis in carefully selected patients for recanalization of occluded artery to restore cerebral blood flow with better neurological outcome. The emergency delivery of endovascular therapy to an occluded intracranial vessel requires an excellent and effective teamwork, involving multi-disciplinary clinical specialities like neurologist, neurointerventionalist, neurosurgeon, anaesthesiologist experienced in stroke care, radiologist, dedicated neuro and stroke care intensivist and endovascular suite staff. This could be challenging and time consuming and may not be available in all the centres.

The institutions which have a dedicated stroke team have been associated with improved neurological outcomes in patients with AIS. The procedures are emergent in nature and the management of these patients requires multidisciplinary approach. Hence it is very essential to have a good communication amongst team members which should be timely and targeted at avoiding delays in the definitive treatment strategies e.g. blood pressure goals, glycemic control, preferred anaesthesia techniques, pharmacological aids, managing uncontrolled co-morbidities, monitoring, extubation criteria, vigilance to avoid predictable complications and continuous evaluation of the patients to detect deterioration.

The endovascular therapy offers a more direct approach to the occlusive lesion and depends upon micro navigation of catheters and devices into the cerebral vasculature which is easier and safer in a motionless patient for two reasons

1. Patient's movement creates imaging artefact resulting in angiographic images that are difficult to interpret. valuable time is lost repeating imaging to obtain a clear picture of the anatomy and occlusive site and this can add up to a significant delay.
2. Patient's movement during the critical parts of the procedure while the mechanical instrumentation is in the cerebral vasculature can lead to trauma, vessel injury and ICH.

Patients with AIS may have altered levels of consciousness, unable to communicate, unco-operative, restless and unable to remain motionless for a prolonged period of time. (This may affect the image quality and difficult to use the road map functions).

To address all these problems anaesthesia in the form of general anaesthesia (GA), conscious sedation (CS), or Local Anaesthesia (LA) is used depending on the condition of the patient.

There are several retrospective studies published evaluating anaesthesia techniques and outcomes for AIS patients undergoing endovascular therapy. They have suggested that all patients who received GA had a longer ICU stay, increased in hospital mortality, worse clinical outcomes and a larger infarct size. The patients with anterior circulation stroke who received local anaesthesia had relatively good outcome, lower death rate, higher perfusion rates and those who received GA for anterior circulation stroke had poorer outcome. But those who received GA had higher baseline NIHSS score, lower baseline arterial pressure and likely to have carotid terminal occlusion. They also found that those who had baseline blood pressure > 140 mmHg had a better outcome[12,13].

All these studies have shown that the major disadvantages of GA are time delay and hemodynamic fluctuations.

The disadvantages of general anaesthesia are:

1. Time delay in administering anaesthesia
2. Hemodynamic fluctuations associated with GA.
3. Unable to perform intra procedural neurologic assessment.
4. Prolonged intubation and its associated pulmonary complications.
5. Prolonged ICU stay
6. Increased in - hospital mortality
7. Increased size of the infarct.
8. Neurotoxicity of anaesthetic agents.
9. GA also requires an experienced anaesthesiologist & extra work force.

In contrast, patients receiving conscious sedation and local anaesthesia are more co-operative, have minimal neurologic impairment (low NIHSS score). Most of them have anterior circulation stroke, have no hemodynamic fluctuations, no time delay in reperfusion, well controlled co-morbidities, allow intra procedural assessment and hence are associated with better outcome.

The sedation required to produce a co-operative non-moving patient without respiratory or airway problems varies from patient to patient. These patients may not be adequately starving therefore this raises the concern of vomiting and pulmonary aspiration of gastric content in a sedated supine patient.

Over sedation could result in airway compromise or obstruction due to tongue fall or due to pre-existing airway problems e.g. OSA or due to decline in the neurologic status resulting in hypercarbia, hypoxia, increased ICP and hypotension. These secondary insults can further aggravate cerebral ischaemia.

The patient may become restless, agitated, uncomfortable lying motionless for a prolonged period of time. This could be unsafe with indwelling microcatheters in the cerebral vasculature. This not only results in poor image quality but also prolongs the procedural time.

All these factors may necessitate urgent conversion of CS & LA to general anaesthesia which can be difficult in the middle of the procedure especially if the patient has difficult airway access. This also necessitates the availability of an experienced anaesthesiologist.

Anaesthesia technique for Endo-vascular therapy in AIS.[15, 16, 17, 18]

The number of intracranial endovascular procedures for AIS are fast growing & therefore anaesthesiologists will be presented with these patients for various procedures & surgeries more frequently in the future[14].

It is therefore very essential for the anaesthesiologists to have a fair knowledge of

1) Patho physiologic mechanism of AIS;
2) "Time is Brain" & "save the penumbra" concept before planning anaesthesia management
3) Aetiology/ site of stroke/ vascular territory involved
4) Presenting signs & symptoms, NIHSS Scores
5) CT/ MRI findings
6) Predictors of poor neurological outcomes
7) IV rtPA details.
8) Various endovascular therapies available, their anaesthetic requirements.

9) Expected peri procedural complications & their management.

10) SNACC/ASA/AHA guide lines, recommendations etc.

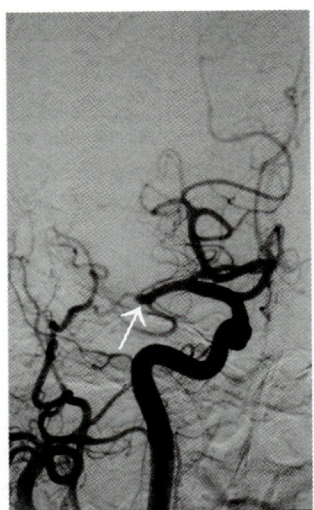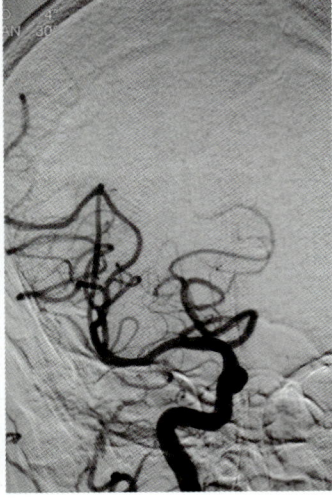

Fig. 8, 9 . DSA showing MCA occlusion (R) and good flow after thrombectomy

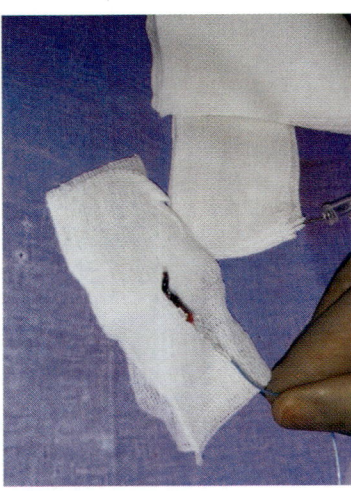

Fig. 10. Thrombus from MCA occlusion site with micro cathetar

All these informations will enable them to have a more scientific approach to the perioperative anaesthesia management plan to achieve better neurological outcome. Therefore, "Time is of essence" and "Ischaemic Penumbra is the, "Target" for peri-procedural anaesthesia plan.

Preanesthetic evaluation: should be done as quickly as possible to avoid delay in EV therapy. Anaesthesiologists should get involved in the patient management from the emergency dept. itself where, preoperative evaluation, interviewing the patient/ relatives for medical/ surgical history/ medications/ allergies/ contraindications to rtPA therapy/ management of Co-morbidities, cross referrals especially for cardiac problems, ordering investigations/ vascular access and obtaining

informed consent etc. can be taken care of even before the patient comes to the endovascular suite. Most of these requirements may be incomplete or not available. It should be documented on the patient's Chart & Communicated to the Neuro-interventionalist. Anaesthesia related procedures should be performed as quickly as possible to avoid delays. The anaesthesiologist must follow ASA standards for emergency procedure.

Preoperative investigations

As per AHA / ASA guidelines:

For all patients; 1) Non-contrast CT- Brain or MRI 2) Blood glucose level 3) O2 Saturation 4) Sr. Electrolytes, Sr. Creatinine/ Renal profile 5) CBC, platelets 6) Markers of Cardiac Ischaemia 7) PT/ INR/ PTT / ECG/ X-ray chest.

In special cases 1) TT / ACT if patient is taking direct thrombin or X a inhibitors 2) LFT 3) Toxicology screening 4) Blood alcohol test 5) Pregnancy test 6) ABG (if Hypoxia is detected 7) 2D Echo 8)TEE.

Anaesthesia technique

The choice of anaesthesia technique is tailored to each patient's clinical characteristics, neurological condition (NIHSS Score) and individualized.

General anaesthesia is preferred in

1) uncooperative agitated patients with severe neurological impairments (high NIHSS Score)

2) those who are already intubated for medical reasons

3) Posterior fossa circulation stroke and

4) Patients with signs of brainstem dysfunction

5) Patients with compromised protective airway reflexes or develop airway obstruction or respiratory depression under sedation & patients who have active nausea/ Vomiting.

Conscious sedation or local anaesthesia (LA) are feasible options for patients with anterior circulation stroke, conscious, co- operative patients (low NIHSS scores), who can protect their airway. The experienced anaesthesiologist must be physically present in the endovascular suite for all the procedures done under LA or sedation & should provide potential immobility in an agitated patient to enable smooth working conditions & is responsible for the airway management, proper oxygenation, ventilation & continuous monitoring, managing hemodynamics, glycemic control, and should avoid respiratory depression & its consequences. Anaesthesiologist should be prepared to rapidly convert LA/ CSinto GA if needed.

Before Starting GA, following parameters should be noted down.

1. Baseline SBP, DBP, MAP, Blood Sugar level, SPO2, Resp. rate, NIHSS score, body temperature, MRI/CT findings, Site & type of Stroke.

2. If Blood Sugar level is > 140 mg%, it should be corrected with Insulin infusion to maintain blood sugar level between 70-140 mg% & If it is < 50 mg%, hypoglycemia should be treated with dextrose containing fluids to achieve blood sugar level > 70 mg%. One hourly blood sugar estimation is recommended.

3. If Baseline SPO2 is < 92 %, ABG should be done & cause of hypoxia is ascertained.

4. Pre-operative hypotension or during the induction of anaesthesia is strictly not permissible and should be corrected with, volume replacement & vasopressors to achieve SBP > 140 mmHg.

5. Similarly, preoperative hypertension too should be treated to achieve blood pressure levels between 140 mmHg – 180 mmHg.

Periprocedural hemodynamic management

1. Hemodynamic monitoring & management should start as soon as the diagnosis of AIS has been made.

2. Both elevated & low blood pressures are associated with worse neurological outcome. There is a U-Shaped relationship between systolic pressure & both early and late death & dependency.

3. Continuous Intra arterial blood pressure measurement is mandatory. NIBP monitoring every 3 mins can be continued till such time the radial or femoral artery is secured.

4. SBP, DBP, MAP, HR, cardiac rhythm should be continuously monitored.

5. Blood pressure targets may be adjusted in Communication with the neuro-interventionalist following successful recanalization of the occluded artery to avoid hyperperfusion injury.

Control of peri-procedural hypertension

1. **For thrombolytic therapy (IVrtPA) in AIS** patients, SBP should be < 185 mmHg; DBP < 110 mmHg; MAP < 120mmHg. Antihypertensive treatment is withheld unless the SBP is > 220 mmHg; DBP > 120 mmHg. Blood pressure should be maintained below 180/105 mmHg atleast for 24 hrs after rtPA therapy.

Table 1 : Periprocedural haemodynamic management

Drug	Dose
Labetalol Bolus	i.v. 10-20 mg slowly over 2 mins. May repeat after 10-15 mins (max dose 300 mg) or start after the initial bolus
Labetalol infusion	2-8 mg/min (40 mg/ 40 ml NS) OR
Nicardipine - Infusion: (no bolus dose)	After the bolus dose of labetalol start infusion of Nicardipine 5 mg/hr, titrate up by 2.5 mg/hr every 5-15 mins interval to a maximum dose of 15 mg/hr
Hydralazine	Bolus 10-20 mg IV (over 2-3 mins) or IM. Repeat after 4-6 hours. Max 40mg. Infusion: 0.5-10 mg/hr
Enalapirate - (only bolus, no infusion)	i.v. 0.625-1.25 mg slowly repeat 6 hourly
Esmolol Bolus Esmolol Infusion	i.v. 150-500 mcg/kg over 2 min 50 mcg/kg/min (max 300 mcg/kg/min)
Sodium Nitroprusside (only in hypertensive crisis)	
Infusion	0.25 mcg-10 mcg/kg/min, max dose not more than 10 mins

Before the endovascular therapy, if SBP > 220 mmHg; DBP > 110–120 mm Hg, the management is same as above. In case of hypertensive crisis, (SBP > 230 mmHg; DBP > 120–130 mmHg; & MAP > 140 mmHg) & the blood pressure is not responding to the above management, consider Sodium Nitroprusside Infusion of 0.1–0.5 mcg/kg/min as an initial dose & then titrate it to achieve the desired level.

Aim for only 10% to 15% reduction in the blood pressure.

1. In chronic hypertensive patients drastic reduction of blood pressure to normal level is not recommended as their autoregulation is adapted at higher values & Cerebral Ischaemia can manifest at higher values of blood pressure.

The endovascular procedures may not require deep anaesthesia with the standard doses of intravenous and inhalational agents. Almost all the anaesthetic agent (except may be for etomidate) cause dose dependent

164

hypotension. Though propofol is supposed to preserve autoregulation, it sometime results in profound hypotension which is strictly to be avoided especially during induction of anaesthesia.

For the induction of anaesthesia, IV Midazolam for anxiolysis and IV Remifentanyl or fentanyl for analgesia, titrated doses of IV Etomidate and intermediate acting non-depolarizing muscle relaxant e.g. CisAtracurium, Vecuronium or Rocuronium are preferred choices of drugs along with local anaesthetic infiltration at the site of groin puncture.

Avoid Atracurium (tachycardia, histamine release resulting in hypotension and bronchospasm) & Nitrous oxide (as it may exacerbate venous air embolism entraining from the procedural site). Avoid secondary insults aggravating cerebral ischaemia. Maintain normocapnoea as hypocapnoea aggravates cerebral ischaemia & hypercapnoea increases ICP & cerebral oedema.

The standard protocol for early extubation for post procedural neurological assessment should be followed unless the patient is already intubated for medical reasons or has developed intra procedural complications eg; ICH, or does not meet standard extubation criteria. Emergence hypertension during extubation should be avoided using Esmolol or Labetalol bolus doses or infusions.

Monitoring : Continuous intra-arterial blood pressure monitoring is mandatory. NIBP monitoring is to be continued every 3 mins. till radial or femoral arterial line is secured

- **Continuous monitoring** of SBP, DBP, MAP, ECG, HR, Cardiac rhythm, SPO2, ETCO2, RR and body temperature is recommended so also, one hourly blood sugar estimation and ABG / electrolytes at regular intervals

TEE and TCD monitoring if indicated.

- **IV Fluids** – Maintain euvolemia, preferably with the balanced salt solutions. Avoid dextrose containing IV Fluids unless treating hypoglycemia

- Avoid dehydration

Glycemic control: Strict control of hyperglycemia (HG) is one of the most important goals of anaesthetic management of AIS patients.

- Measure Sr. glucose level on admission & estimate one hourly during endovascular therapy

- Insulin therapy should be initiated for glucose value > 140 mg %

- Protocol driven insulin infusion should be used to control HG rather than subcutaneous Insulin (SNACC)

- Maintain blood glucose levels between 70-140 mg %

- Avoid dextrose containing IV fluids unless the patient is hypoglycemic (aim for blood sugar level > 70 mg/%)

- Maintain **body temperature** between 35°C–37°C. Hyperthermia exacerbates cerebral Ischaemia. Hyperthermia should be treated with antipyretics & cooling devices

Anti-coagulation during EV therapy

The goals of peri-procedural anti coagulation and anti platelet therapy are to reduce catheter related, stent-related and thrombus & Embolic related events while minimizing the incidences of hemorrhagic events. Heparin is used to reduce Catheter induced embolic or thrombotic events.

- Anaesthesiologists must be prepared to administer heparin at regular intervals throughout the procedure as requested by the Neuro interventionalist. And they should be prepared to administer Protamine immediately to the patient in case of intra procedural ICH or Vascular trauma.

- Protamine should be kept loaded in a syringe.

Complications of endovascular therapy

- There is a risk of ICH associated with IV or IA thrombolysis and other Endovascular procedures.

- ICH can also occur due to hemorrhagic transformation of the infarct or iatrogenic through direct vessel trauma (Micro catheters, Mechanical thrombectomy)

- Symptomatic SAH may require urgent Ventriculostomy & increased ICP management.

- Heparin effect should be reversed immediately with protamine in case of intraprocedural ICH.

- Patients who have received IVrtPA, may require administration of FFP, Cryoprecipitate & Platelets.

Other acute complications include:

1. Catheter induced blood Vessel dissection.
2. Vasospasm
3. Puncture site hematoma
4. Limb Ischaemia
5. Thrombo - Embolism
6. Retro peritoneal hematoma
7. Haemorrhage at the puncture site
8. Pseudo aneurysm formation
9. Arterial dissection
10. Vaso- vagal reaction while removing the sheath
11. Arterial re-occlusion.
12. Anaesthesia related/ Sedation related complications.

Acute ischaemic stroke - anaesthesia management

Post-operative care

Patient should go to the dedicated ICU specializing in neurovascular/ stroke care. and personnel expertise in the management of critically ill neurological cases should take care of these patients.

1. Continuous invasive arterial pressure monitoring should be continued in the ICU.

2. Blood pressure goals & the decision to extubate the patient should be decided in communication with the neuro interventionalist.

CONCLUSION

In Acute Ischaemic Stroke (AIS), the goal of early therapy is to rapidly restore perfusion to the vulnerable ischaemic penumbra by recanalization of the occluded artery. Penumbra is the "target" for perioperative anaesthesia planning & endovascular therapy.

Time to perfusion & arterial pressure stability are the most important critical factors in maximizing the survival of ischaemic penumbra.

General anaesthesia is an independent predictor of poor outcome due to time delay in its administration, hemodynamic fluctuations associated with it & probably due to the neurotoxic effects of the anaesthetic agents. Time is of essence and the procedures are emergent in nature.

Therefore to achieve a better neurological outcome in acute ischaemic stroke patients, it is very essential to understand the pathophysiological mechanism of AIS, therapeutic time window & save the penumbra concept, predictors of poor neurological outcome, importance of strict hemodynamic & glycemic control, various endovascular therapies available, their complications & management, various guidelines & recommendations for the AIS management, and above all the importance of an excellent team work amongst the multidisciplinary specialities in the management of AIS.

REFERENCES

1) WHO – MONICA PROJECT (Monitoring and determinants in Cardio Vascular Diseases) a major international collaboration [WHO, MONICA PROJECT INVESTIGATORS] J. Clinic, Epidemiol. 1988: 41(2), 105-14.

2) CHARLES WARLAW Strokes, Transient Ichaemic attacks and Intracranial Venous Thrombosis Chapter27, Brain's "Disease of Nervous System "Edited by Micheal Donaghy 11th edition, Page 776 onwards.

3) Mustafa R.R., Baron J.C. Patho physiology of Ischaemic Stroke – Insights from Imaging and Implications for Therapy and Drug Discovery. Br. J. Pharmacol:2008:153: Suppl S44 to S54.

4) Saver J. L. – "Time is Brain"- Quantified. Stroke (2006) Vol: 37 (Page 263 to 6).

5) Astrup J. Siesjo B.K. Symon L. "Thresholds in Cerebral Ischaemia – The Ischaemic Penumbra. Stroke (1981); 12:723 to 725.

6) Heiss W.D. "Ischaemic Penumbra" – Evidence from Functional Imaging. J. Cereb blood flow: Metab (2000) 20:1276 to 1296.

7) Ginsberg MD; Pulsinelli W D – The Ischaemic Penumbra, Injury threshold and the therapeutic time window in Acute Stroke. Ann. Neurol (1994): 36:553–554.

8) Tudor Jovin. MD. Co-Principal Investigator; University of Pittsburgh Medical center; Pittsburgh; Pennsylvania. DAWN—Trial. Thrombectomy effective up to 24 hours after AIS. Medscape coverage from 3rd European Organization Conference in Prague, Czech Republic. ESCO May 2017. (Google search).

9) Michael T Froehler; Johana T Fifi, Arshad Majid et.al., Anaesthesia for endovascular treatment of Acute Ischaemic Stroke. Neurology; 2012;79; S167-S173.

10) Smith WS; Sung G; Saver J L et. al. Mechanical thrombectomy for Acute ischaemic stroke: Final results of the multi MERCI trial. Stroke: 2008: 39; 1205-1212.

11) Nogueira RG; Smith WS; Sung G et. al., Effect of time to reperfusion on clinical outcomes of Anterior circulation strokes treated with Thrombectomy. Pooled analysis of the MERCI & MULTI MERCI Trials. Stroke, 2011:42:3144-3149.

12) Abou-Chebl A, Lin R, Hussain MS et al. Conscious sedation versus general anaesthesia during endovascular therapy for acute anterior circulation stroke: Preliminary results from a retrospective multicentric study. Stroke 2010:41 (6): 1175-9.

13) Jumma MA, Zang: Ruiz-Ares G et.al., Comparison of safety and clinical outcomes in endovascular acute stroke therapy for proximal Middle cerebral artery occlusion with intubation & general anaesthesia versus nonintubated state. Stroke: 2010:41 (6): 1180-4.

14) Hughley AB, Lesniak MS, Ansari SA et al. What will be Anaesthesiologist be anaesthetising? Trends in Neurosurgical procedures usage. Anaesth. Analg.2010 :110 (6), 1686-97.

15) Pekka. O Talke: Deepak Sharma; Eric J Heyer: Sergio D Bergese; Kristine A Blackham; Robert D. Stevens. Republished: Society for Neurosciences in Anaesthesiology and Critical Care. Expert Consensus statement. Stroke: 2014; 45: e138-e150.

16) Alana M. Flexman; MD. FRCPC; Anne L. Donovan MD; Adrian W. Gelb, MBChB, FRCPC. Anaesthetic management of patients with acute stroke. Anaesthesiology Clin. 30 (2012);175-190.

17) Z.H. Anastasian Anaesthetic management of the patient with Acute Ischaemic stroke. Br. J. Anaesth. (2014) 113– (suppl 2) ii 9-ii 16.

18) Adams HP Jr; delZoppo G; Alberts MJ et.al., Guidelines for early management of adults with Ischaemic stroke. Stroke;2007: 38(5) 1165-711.

19) Edwards C. Jauch; J. L. Saver; Harold P. Adams et.al., Guidelines for early management of patient with Acute Ishaemic Stroke. Stroke L2013) 44; 870-947.

167

MULTIPLE CHOICE QUESTIONS

1. **Acute ischaemic stroke occurs due to**
   a. Rupture of MCA aneurysm
   b. Rupture of Anterior communicating artery aneurysm
   c. AV malformation bleed
   d. Sudden occlusion of an Intra cranial artery
   e. All of the above

2. **The ischaemic penumbra is**
   a. Within the zone of infarct
   b. Surrounding the zone of infarct
   c. Outer most zone
   d. Any of the above

3. **The target for Endovascular therapy is the,**
   a. Oligaemic zone
   b. Central infarct zone
   c. Penumbra

4. **In ischaemic penumbra the mechanism of cell death is**
   a. Apoptosis
   b. Necrotic
   c. Mechanical
   d. Toxicity due to free radicals

5. **Golden period for IV thrombolysis in AIS is**
   a. 12 hrs
   b. One hr
   c. Two hrs
   d. Three hrs
   e. Six hrs

6. **Drug of choice for IV thrombolysis is,**
   a. rtPA
   b. Urokinase
   c. Streptokinase
   d. Heparin
   e. Low molecular weight heparin

7. **Time lost is Brain lost is the slogan for initiating which modality of stroke therapy?**
   a. Anticoagulants
   b. Antiplatelets
   c. Thrombolysis
   d. Anti hypertensives

8. **Ischaemic penumbra has,**
   a. Impaired auto regulation
   b. Increased oxygen extraction
   c. Misery perfusion
   d. All of the above

9. **In AIS the systemic blood pressure should be lowered if it is**
   a. > 140/90 mm Hg
   b. > 185/110 mmHg
   c. > 165/110 mmHg
   d. >150/100 mmHg

10. **Cerebral perfusion pressure is**
    a. SBP - ICP
    b. DBP - ICP
    c. MAP - ICP
    d. MAP / ICP

11. **In AIS the TWO most critical factors in maximizing the survival of ischaemic Penumbra are,**
    a. Time to perfusion
    b. Endovascular therapy
    c. IV rtPA therapy
    d. Anticoagulant therapy
    e. Arterial pressure stability

12. **Following are the predictors of poor Neurological outcomes in AIS, except one**
    a. Delay in time to perfusion
    b. Hemodynamic fluctuations
    c. BP > 140/90 mmHg
    d. Hyperglycemia
    e. Posterior circulation stroke

13. **General anaesthesia is an independent predictor of poor neurological outcomes because of,**
    a. Delay in starting the case
    b. Hemodynamic fluctuations associated with GA
    c. Neuro toxicity of anaesthetic agents
    d. All of the above

14. **This blood sugar level is associated with good neurological outcome in AIS.**
    a. > 140 mg%
    b. 70 mg% – 140 mg%
    c. 160 mg% – 180 mg%
    d. < 200 mg%.

15. Hyperglycemia
a. Improves cerebral metabolism
b. Protects neurons from apoptosis
c. Aggravates lactic acidosis induced consequences
d. Decreases cerebral perfusion

16. Hyperglcemia predicts
a. Larger infarct size
b. Poor clinical outcome in patients treated with IV rtPA
c. Unsuccessful IA thrombolysis
d. Poor out come despite successful Endovascular therapy
e. Increased risk of paranchymal haemorrhge
f. All of the above

17. Following is responsible for the Auto regulation of the Cerebral blood flow
a. ACA, MCA, PCA
b. Circle of Willis
c. Microcirculation
d. All of the above

18. Post recanalization of the occluded artery, hyperperfusion injury is caused by,
a. Hypertension
b. Hypotension
c. Hyperglycemia
d. Heparin

19. Poor Neurological outcome in AIS is due to,
a. Hypotension, baseline or during induction of anaesthesia
b. Baseline low SPO2
c. Hyperthermia
d. Hypercapnea
e. seizures
f. All of the above

20. Best neurologic outcome in AIS is achieved by,
a. Rapid time to perfusion within the therapeutic time window
b. Hemodynamic stability
c. Strict Glycemic control
d. Avoiding Secondary insults
e. Excellent Team work with good communication
f. All of the above

CHAPTER 20

NEUROIMAGING IN ANAESTHESIA

Ritu Kashikar, Savi Kapila, Shrinivas B. Desai

Introduction

CT scan and MRI are radiological modalities used in neuroimaging. CT has several advantages in the form of easy availability and short scan duration and hence is modality of choice in patient with Craniocerebral trauma and early stroke to rule out haemorrhage. The disadvantages of CT scan however include radiation exposure and lack of ability to accurately diagnose and characterize various neurological disorders, particularly earlier during the disease.

MRI is the modality of choice for most neurological pathologies. It is a one stop shop providing diagnostic, metabolic and functional information regarding a myriad of pathologies. However, it is less readily available, requires longer scan duration and hence patient cooperation. It is more expensive than CT scan.

Relevant normal anatomy

The relevant normal anatomy of the brain on CT (Fig.1) and MRI along with important sequences have been discussed with the help of figures.

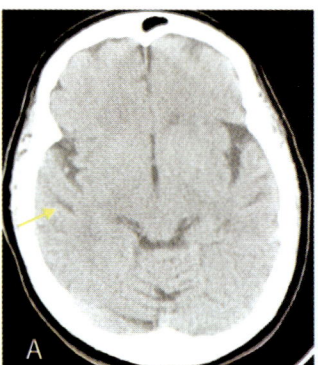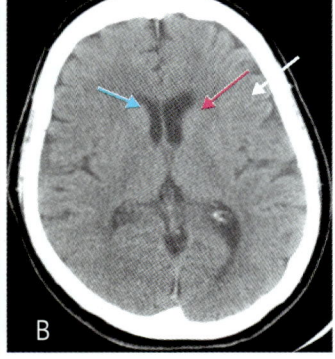

Fig. 1: Normal CT brain image (a) Showing sulcal spaces (yellow arrow)and (b) Normal ventricles (blue arrows) containing CSF, hence appearing hypodense (dark) compared to brain parenchyma. Also note that white matter (pink arrow) appears slightly dark compared to grey matter (white arrow).

The important MR sequences (Fig. 2 a–f) include T2 weighted (CSF bright) and FLAIR (fluid attenuated inversion recovery), which provide information regarding most pathologies, while T_1 weighted sequence (CSF dark), are good in depiction of normal anatomy. The diffusion weighted imaging (DWI) and ADC maps are excellent in detecting ischemic stroke and hypoxic changes. The susceptibility weighted images (SWI) help in picking up blood products and calcification, all of which appear hypo intense (dark)on this sequence.

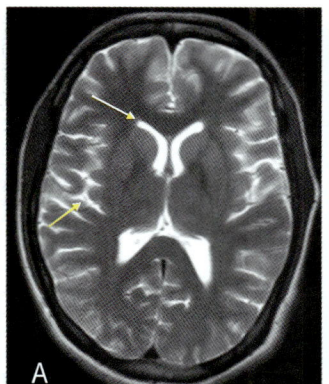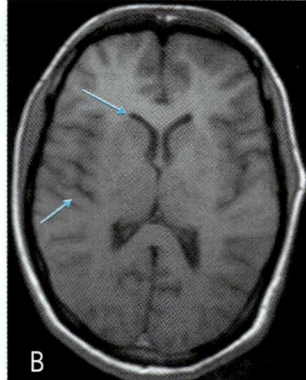

Fig. 2 : Normal MRI brain showing T2W1 images (a) In which fluid containing structures (CSF,sulcal spaces) appear hyperintense (bright) (yellow arrows). These images are useful in detection of pathologies, which usually appear bright on this sequence. T1W1 images (b) Showing hypointense (dark)fluid containing structures .(blue arrow). These images are good to study normal anatomy and aslo detection of blood products ,which sometimes appear bright.

This chapter has been structured into relevant clinical scenarios pertinent to the anaesthetist that merit neuroimaging.

Clinical Scenario – 1

Head injury

This subset of patients often requires neuroimaging in presence of neurological signs. The role of imaging in these patients is to detect trauma related intracerebral haemorrhage and features of raised intracranial tension including herniation. As previously mentioned CT is the modality of choice in this subset. The various hematomas encountered in trauma setting include subdural, extradural haemorrhages,contusions in the brain and subarachnoid haemorrhage. These are often associated with some form of mass effect in the form of oedema and /or herniations depending on the size and location.

Subdural hematoma

Subdural haemorrhage (SDH) is a collection of blood accumulated in the subdural space, the potential space between the dura and arachnoid layer of the meninges around the brain. SDH can happen in any age-group and is mainly due to head trauma. They are present in ~15% (range 10-20%) of all head trauma cases and occur in up to 30% of fatal injuries.[1]

Radiology

CT–The classic appearance of an acute subdural haematoma is a crescent-shaped homogeneously hyperdense extra-axial collection (Fig. 3).

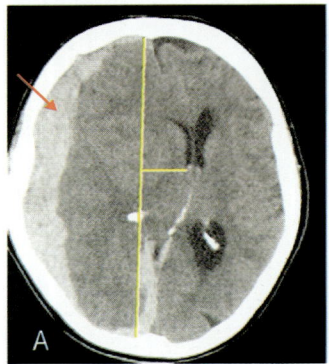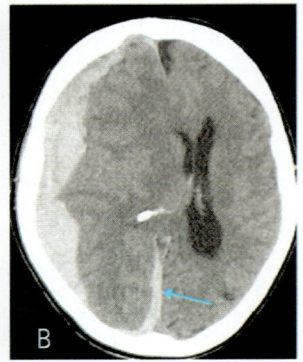

Fig. 3: Post contrast axial CT images reveal right fronto-parietal acute hyperdense concavo-convex subdural hematoma (Orange Arrows) with underlying sulcal effacement, effacement of right lateral ventricle and midline shift to left (yellow lines). Also seen subdural hematoma along the posterior aspect of falx (Blue Arrow)

MRI

The shape of the hematoma is like CT,while the appearance varies with the biochemical state of haemoglobin (explained later)which varies with the age of haematoma (Fig. 4).

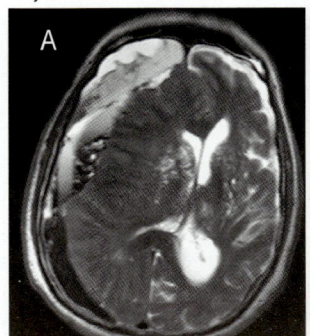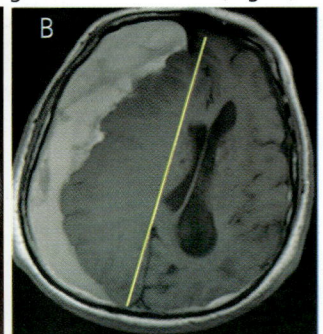

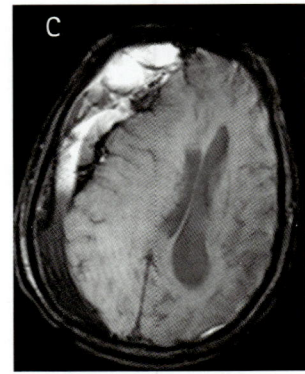

Fig. 4: Acute right fronto temporo-parietal concavo-convex subdural hematoma which shows blood fluid levels on T2W Fig. (A) as well as susceptibility weighted Fig. (C). It appears hyperintense on T1 W Fig. (B). Also seen effacement of right lateral ventricle and midline shift to left.

Treatment depends primarily on the amount of mass effect and neurological impairment caused by the collection, and thus correlates with the size of the subdural haemorrhage.

Extradural haemorrhage

Extradural haematoma (EDH), also known as an **epidural haematoma,** is a collection of blood that forms between the inner surface of the skull and outer layer of the dura, which is called the periosteal layer. They are commonly associated with a history of trauma and associated skull fracture. The source of bleeding is usually a torn meningeal artery. EDH is typically biconvex in shape and can cause a mass effect with herniation. They are unilateral in more than 95% of cases.[2]

CT–They are typically bi-convex (or lentiform) in shape, hyperdense, somewhat heterogeneous, and sharply demarcated (Fig. 5).

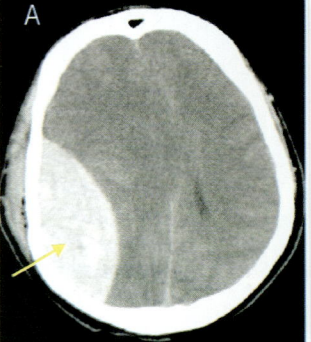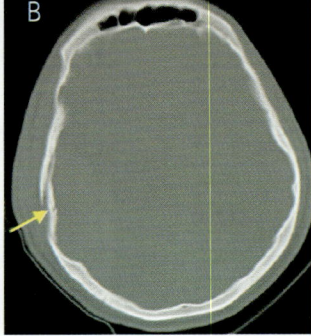

Fig. 5: Axial CT image (A) shows hyperdense biconvex epidural hematoma in right parietal region with underlying mass effect causing sulcal effacement. Bone window (B) showing depressed fracture in overlying bone (arrow).

MRI – Biconvex shaped with appearance depending on age of hematoma.

MRI can also demonstrate the displaced dura that appears as a hypointense line on T1 and T2 sequences which is helpful in distinguishing it from a subdural haematoma.

Haemorrhagic contusions

Cerebral haemorrhagic contusions are a type of intracerebral haemorrhage and are common in the setting of significant head injury.[3]

CT : Hyper dense foci in the frontal lobes adjacent to the floor of the anterior cranial fossa and in the temporal lobes. (Fig. 6).

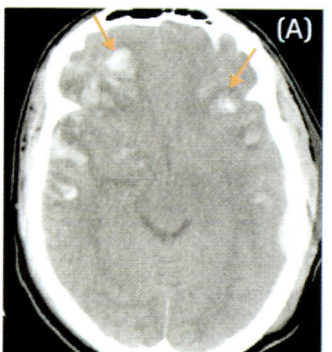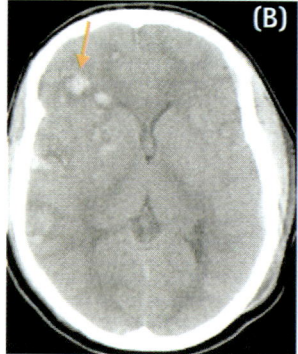

Fig. 6 : Axial CT figures show multiple hyperdense hemorrhagic contusions seen in bilateral frontal (right > left) and right temporal lob

MRI is far more sensitive to small contusions, especially when T2* sequences, i.e. SWI (susceptibility weighted Figs.) are used.

Signs of raised intracranial tension

Cerebral herniation, also referred to as **acquired intracranial herniation**, refers to shift of cerebral tissue from its normal location, into an adjacent space because of mass effect. Herniations can be seen in various CNS pathologies like trauma, tumours, infarctions and hemorrhages.[4]

There are number of different patterns of cerebral herniation which describe the type of herniation occurring:

- Subfalcine herniation
- Transtentorial herniation
- Downward: uncal herniation
- Upward: ascending trans tentorial
- Tonsillar herniation
- Transsellar herniation –ascending,descending

Subfalcine herniation, the most common cerebral herniation pattern, is characterised by displacement of the brain beneath the free edge of the falx cerebri due to raised intracranial pressure.

CT/MRI

The easiest method of evaluating for subfalcine shift is a straight line drawn in the expected location of the septum pellucidum from the posterior most aspects to the falx on axial images. The shift of the septum pellucidum from this midline can be measured in millimetres and compared over time to determine any change (Fig. 7).

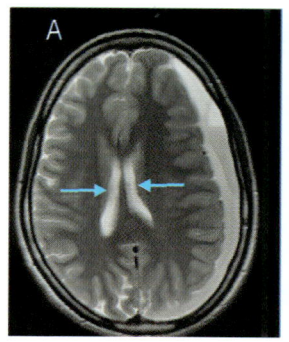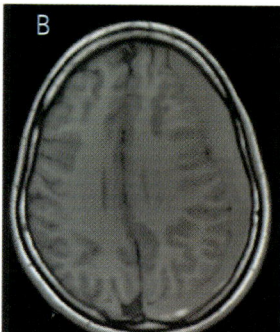

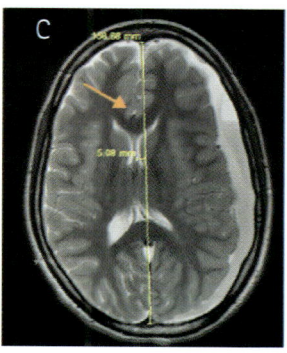

Fig. 7: Left Frontoparietal subdural hematoma which appears hyperintense on T2W (A), Isointense on T1W (B) There is resultant mass effect with cingulate gyrus displaced across midline under inferior free margin of falx with midline shift to right by 5mm (C) .

Complications

- Contralateral hydrocephalusue to obstruction of the foramen of Monro
- Anterior cerebral artery (ACA) territory infarct due to compression of ACA branches

Uncal herniation - is a subtype of trans tentorial downward brain herniation usually related to cerebral mass effect increasing the intracranial pressure.

Pathology - In uncal herniation, the uncus and the adjacent part of the temporal lobe glide downward across the tentorial incisura compressing the brainstem and the posterior cerebral arteries in the ambient cistern. Uncal herniation may be unilateral or bilateral

Uncal herniation can be suggested on CT, however, MRI is the gold standard.

Features of **unilateral** descending tentorial herniation include:

■ Medial displacement of ipsilateral uncus,para hippocampal gyrus and temporal horn of the lateral ventricle. The effacement of all basal cisterns seen. (Fig. 8)

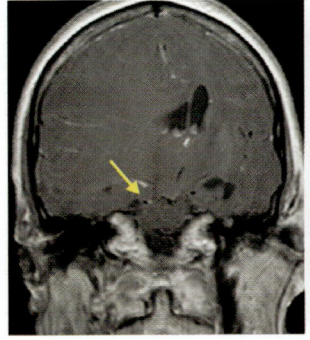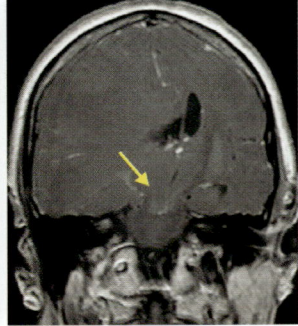

Fig. 8 : Coronal Post contrast T1W1 coronal images showing downward herniation of right uncus through tentorial incisura (arrows).

Bilateral trans tentorial herniation

■ Both temporal lobes herniate into tentorial incisura with complete obliteration of suprasellar cistern.The midbrain is effaced and displaced inferiorly.

Treatment and prognosis - Uncal herniation carries a bad prognosis due to the direct compression of the vital midbrain centres. They often require emergency neurosurgical decompression.

sending trans tentorial herniation – is a situation where space occupying lesions in the posterior cranial fossa cause superior displacement of superior parts of the cerebellum through the tentorial notch.

Tonsillar herniation - is a type of cerebellar herniation characterised by the inferior descent of the cerebellar tonsils below the foramen magnum.

It is a secondary sign of significant intra-cranial mass effect. Any intra-axial or extra-axial lesion (e.g. tumour, haemorrhage, stroke, abscess) exerting mass effect on the brain parenchyma can displace the posterior cranial fossa structures inferiorly. In doing so, the brainstem is compressed thereby altering the vital life-sustaining functions of the pons and medulla, such as the respiratory and cardiac centres.

Tonsillar herniation is seen on CT and MRI as effacement of the CSF cisterns surrounding the brainstem and as inferior descent of the cerebellar tonsils below the foramen magnum (Fig. 9).

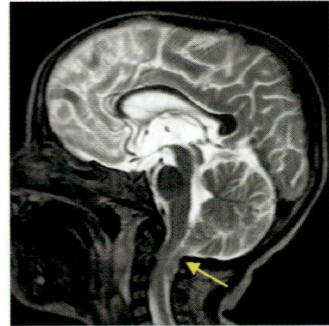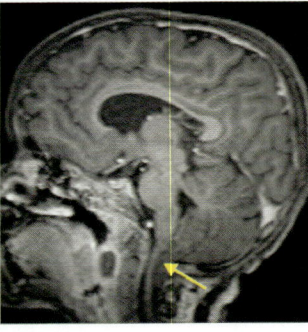

Fig. 9 : Sagittal MR images T2W1 (A) and post contrast T1W1 (B) showing cerebellar tonsils in the cervical canal (arrows).

Clinical Scenario – 2

Acute onset weakness

Stroke is a major cause of mortality and long-term disability. More than 80% of strokes stem from ischemic damage to the brain due to the acute reduction of the blood supply. Patients with large strokes may need urgent craniotomy/ craniectomy for decompression.

Ischemic stroke

Non-contrast CT remains the gold standard in ruling out intracranial haemorrhage in patients with acute onset weakness. It is an easily available, rapid technique to decide the further line of management.[5]

CT – Acute stroke may not be well seen on CT. There may be early signs such as subtle hypodensity, loss of gray white matter differentiation and hyper dense MCA. A well-established stroke appears hypodense on CT with developing mass effect causing ipsilateral oedema and may be associated with subfalcine or other herniation depending on size, degree of mass effect and location of infarct (Fig. 10). Such patients may warrant urgent decompression craniotomy /craniectomy.

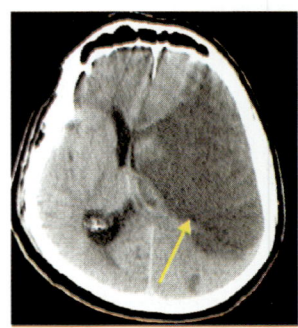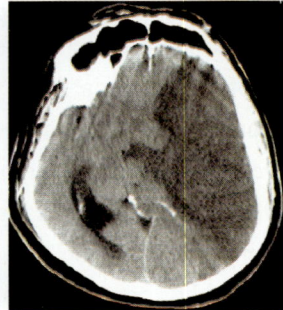

Fig. 10 : CT scan images reveal large hypodense large infarct in left fronto-parietal regions with effacement of left lateral ventricle and significant midline shift to right .

MRI – Although CT is the most commonly used modality for stroke imaging, partly because of its wide availability and faster acquisition time, some comprehensive stroke centres choose MR imaging. Diffusion-weighted imaging (DWI) provides the most specific way to image acute infarction. Acute infarct appears hyperintense (bright) on DWI with corresponding ADC drop[5] (Fig. 11).

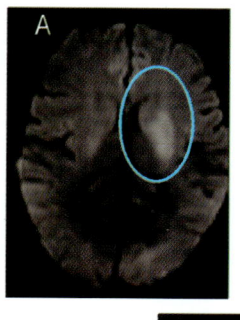
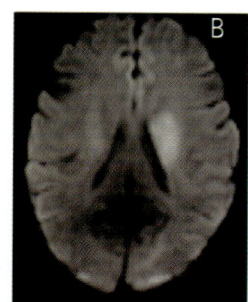
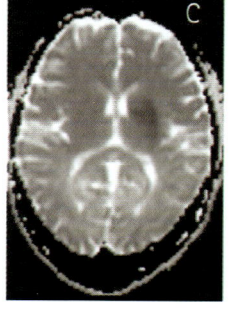

Fig. 11 : MRI Done immediately reveal left corona radiata restricted diffusion(bright)on DWI images (A, B) which appear hypointense on ADC (C).

Other MR sequences such as FLAIR, T2W1 are used to report the age of infarct. Infarcts typically appear hyperintense on these sequences. Susceptibility weighted images provide information regarding haemorrhagic transformation, which appears hypointense and can also show clot within an occluded vessel. The time of flight angiogram is a technique to study vasculature without administering contrast.

The signs of raised intracranial pressure and herniations are similar, to those described above; although MR has better ability to evaluate herniation related secondary complications.

Acute Intracerebral haemorrhage (Table-1) – Intracerebral haemorrhage accounts for 10-23% of strokes, with hypertension being the single most important risk factor in middle aged and elderly persons.

On CT scan, acute haemorrhage appears hyper dense (40-60HU) and density decreases over the period (Fig. 12).

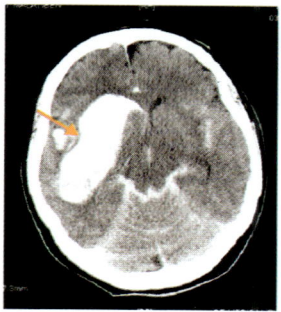
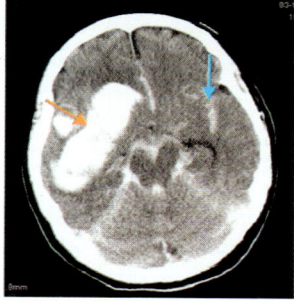

Fig. 12 : Plain CT images a and b in a known hypertensive showing large hyperdense hematoma (orange arrow) causing edema with subfalcine shift also note extensive subarachnoid hemorrhage (blue arrow) seen

On MRI, characteristics of blood are variable and depend on the age of blood (Fig. 13).

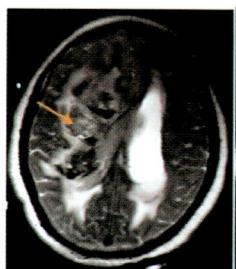
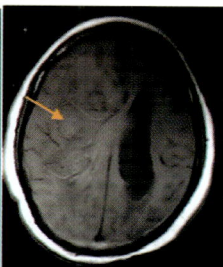
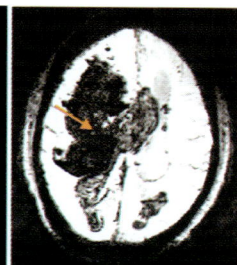

Fig. 13: Large intra-cerebral hemorrhage in the right gangliocapsular region and corona radiata with intraventricular extension and subfalcine shift. Hematoma appears hypointense on T2W image (A), isointense on T1 W image (B) with blooming on SWI image (C).

Table 1: Haemorrhage

Haemorrhage stage	Lesion Age	Brain Affected compartment	Involved magnetic susceptible substance	T1W MR	T2W MR
Hyper acute	< 24	Intracellular	Oxyhaemoglobin	Isointense	Slightly hyperintense
Acute	1-3 day	Intracellular	Deoxyhaemoglobin	Slightly Hypo intense	Hypo intense
Early Subacute	> 3 day	Intracellular	Methaemoglobin	Very hyperintense	Hypo intense
Late Subacute	> 7 days	Extracellular	Methaemoglobin	Very hyperintense	Very hyperintense
Chronic					
• Centre	> 30 days	Extracellular	Haemachromes	Isointense	Slightly hyperintense
• Rim		Extracellular	Hemosiderin	Slightly hypo intense	Very hypo intense

In case of cerebral haemorrhage secondary causes such as underlying vascular malformations, intertumoral haemorrhage, venous sinus thrombosis, blood dyscrasias need to be ruled out. The patients will have herniations like ischemic stroke depending on size and location. These patients usually warrant urgent neurosurgical decompression.

Large posterior fossa ischemic and haemorrhagic strokes may cause mass effect and sudden coning (tonsillar herniation) and often need posterior decompression.

Clinical Scenario – 3

ICU patient – acute hypoxic/hypotensive event

HIE is a brain dysfunction caused by a reduction in the supply of oxygen to the brain and other organs, compounded by low blood flow to vital organs leading to ischemia.[6]

Severe global hypoxic-ischemic injury in this population primarily affects the grey matter structures:

- Basal ganglia
- Thalami
- Cerebral cortex (the sensorimotor and visual cortices, although involvement is often diffuse)
- Cerebellum
- Hippocampus

Quick MRI usually requiring only Diffusion weighted sequences is the imaging modality of choice, (Fig. 14) as CT may miss the subtle changes earlier in course of ischemic event.

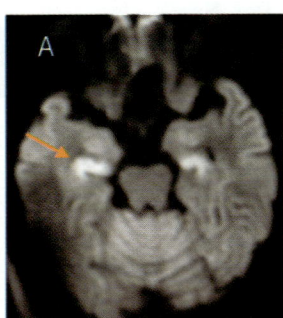
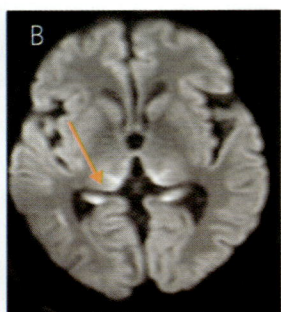
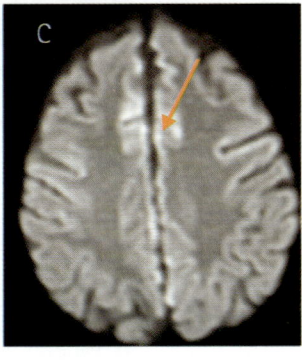

Fig. 14. Axial DWI images reveal restricted diffusion involving bilateral hippocampi, thalamus and cerebral sulci. These represent early changes of mild to moderate hypoxic brain damage.

Diffusion weighted MR imaging is positive, usually within the first few hours after a hypoxic-ischemic event due to early cytotoxic oedema. During the first 24 hours, there may be restricted diffusion in the cerebellar hemispheres, basal ganglia or cerebral cortex, (the peri-rolandic and occipital cortices) (Fig. 15). The thalami, brainstem or hippocampi may also be involved. Diffusion-weighted imaging abnormalities usually pseudo-normalize by the end of the 1st week.

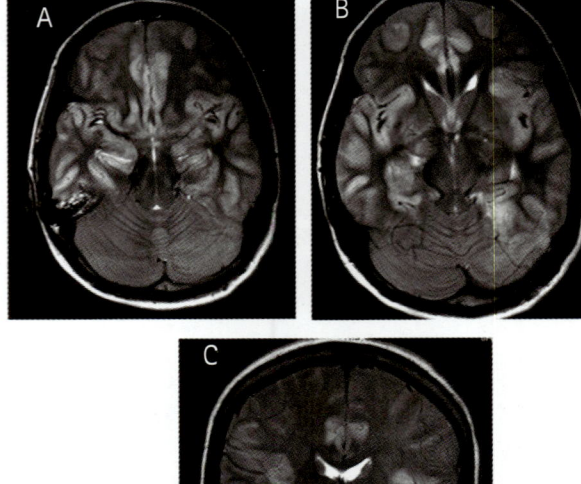

Fig. 15. Axial (a, b) and Coronal (c) T2W images reveal hyperintensity involving bilateral cerebral sulci basal ganglia, thalamus with descending transtentorial herniation. These represent changes of severe hypoxic brain damage with brain edema and herniation.

CT

May show diffuse cerebral oedema, hypo density in cerebral cortex, basal ganglia.

Clinical Scenario – 4

Suspected space occupying lesion

Patients with intracranial space occupying lesions often undergo neurosurgical removal. Urgent decompression surgeries may also be needed in case of mass effect on critical structures.

MRI is the modality of choice in this subset of patients as it best delineates the lesion, degree of surrounding oedema and mass effect on adjacent structures (Fig. 16).

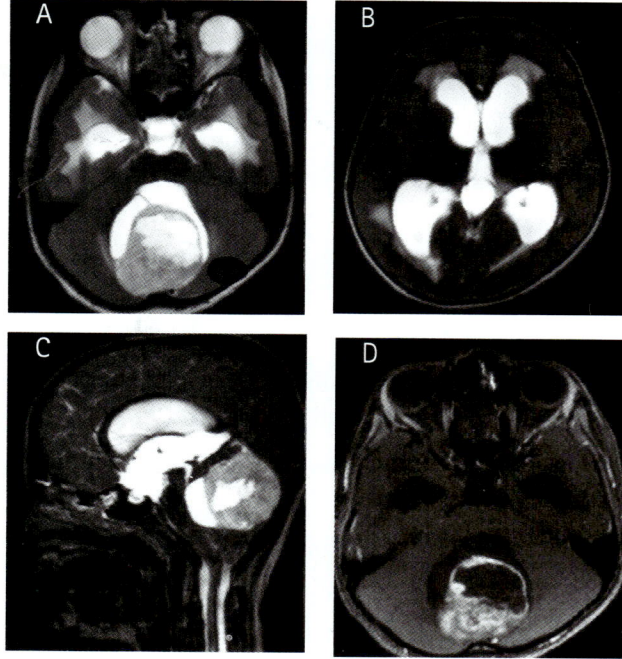

Fig. 16 : (A) Axial, (B) Sagittal T2W and (C) Coronal FLAIR images reveal heterogeneous mixed solid cystic lesion in the fourth ventricle which shows hetrogenous enhancment on (D) Sagittal Post contarst images.

Advanced MR imaging techniques

Functional magnetic resonance imaging (FMRI) – Enables the identification of the location, pattern, and time course of brain activity, in vivo, without the need for the administration of exogenous contrast agents or radioactive tracers.[7]

Principle

- FMRI is a technique that takes advantage of the differences in magnetic susceptibility between oxyhaemoglobin and deoxyhaemoglobin

- When a task is performed, oxygenated blood more than the amount needed (termed luxury perfusion) is delivered to the active area.

- The difference in magnetic susceptibility between deoxyhaemoglobin concentrations and oxyhaemoglobin concentrations creates the signal in functional imaging

Technique – The patient is required to perform a task depending on area of brain to be mapped. A paradigm generator is used for event related tasks (memory, language). The areas of brain getting activated during task can be seen after appropriate post processing (Fig. 17).

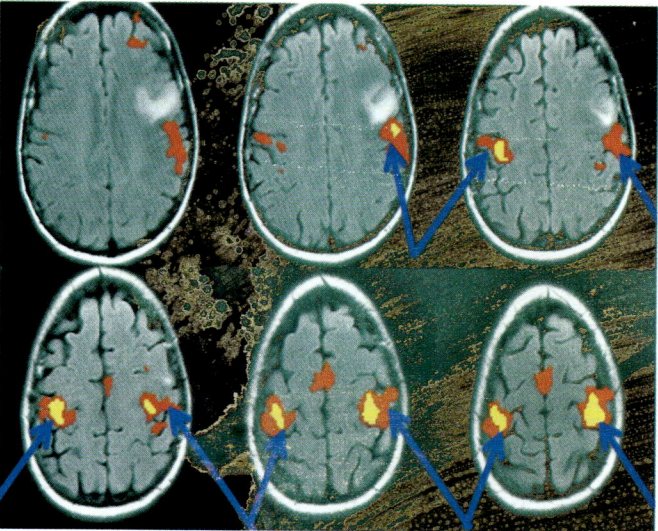

Fig. 17 : C/o infiltrative left frontal glioma. BOLD imaging localizing motor cortex for tongue and foot (red and yellow spots), seen posterior to tumour (yellow arrow).

Why may FMRI be useful for anaesthesia research? – FMRI is an established tool for pain research, shows promise in drug development, and more recently has been applied to the understanding of anaesthetic mechanisms, brain injury, and respiratory control.

Pain – FMRI is unparalleled for studying cognitive, complex emotional processes such as pain.

Drug development – FMRI can help understand mechanisms of drug action in the brain and thus can help the pharmaceutical industry decide whether it is worth investing in a compound for further development.

Anaesthetic mechanisms – It is used to identify where and how in the brain anaesthetics work. In human volunteers, FMRI has revealed how Propofol disrupts thalamic regulatory systems and their communication with higher cortical areas.

Respiratory control– Neural control of breathing is amenable to study with FMRI. The technique promises better understanding of opioid-induced respiratory depression, breathlessness, and potentially brain mechanisms pertinent to weaning from mechanical ventilation.

CONCLUSION

So, to summarize CT scan and MRI are essential tools in neuroimaging of critically ill patients in the appropriate setting. CT is the modality of choice in patients with suspected craniocerebral trauma because of its ability to detect haemorrhage readily. It is also the modality of choice in patients presenting with hemiparesis to rule out haemorrhage as a cause, which is absolute contraindication to initiation of thrombolytic therapy. MRI however is a more sensitive modality to detect early ischemic stroke and is superior to CT in diagnosis and characterization of all other pathologies. Newer MRI applications like BOLD (Blood Oxygen Level Dependence) imaging has been recently used in studying various centres in the brain and finding its application in evaluating central effects of neuroanesthetic agents.

REFERENCES

1. Osborn AG. Diagnostic neuroradiology. Mosby Inc. (1994) ISBN:0801674867.

2. Sullivan TP, Jarvik JG, Cohen WA. Follow-up of conservatively managed epidural hematomas: implications for timing of repeat CT. AJNR Am J Neuroradiol. 1999;20 (1): 107-13. AJNR Am J Neuroradiol (full text) - Pubmed citation.

3. D'avella D, Cacciola F, Angileri FF et-al. Traumatic intracerebellar haemorrhagic contusions and hematomas. J Neurosurg Sci. 2001;45 (1): 29-37. - Pubmed citation.

4. Laine FJ, Shedden AI, Dunn MM et-al. Acquired intracranial herniations: MR imaging findings. AJR Am J Roentgenol. 1995;165 (4): 967-73. AJR Am J Roentgenol (abstract) - PubMed citation.

5. Srinivasan A, Goyal M, Al azri F et-al. State-of-the-art imaging of acute stroke. Radiographics. 2006;26 Suppl 1: S75-95. doi:10.1148/rg.26si065501 - PubMed citation.

6. Huang BY, Castillo M. Hypoxic-ischemic brain injury: imaging findings from birth to adulthood. Radiographics. 28 (2): 417-39. doi:10.1148/rg.282075066 - PubMed citation.

7. Stippich C, Blatow M. Clinical Functional MRI, Pre-surgical Functional Neuroimaging. Springer Verlag. (2007) ISBN:3540244697. Read it at Google Books - Find it at Amazon.

MULTIPLE CHOICE QUESTIONS

1. **The classic appearance of an acute subdural haematoma on CT scan:**
   a. Crescent-shaped homogeneously hyper dense extra-axial collection.
   b. Crescent-shaped heterogeneously hypodense extra- axial collection
   c. Star shaped homogenous hypodense extra-axial collection
   d. Star shaped heterogenous hyper dense extra-axial collection

2. **The classic appearance of epidural haematoma on CT scan:**
   a. bi-concave in shape, hyper dense, heterogeneous and sharply demarcated
   b. bi-convex in shape, hyper dense, heterogeneous and sharply demarcated
   c. bi-concave in shape, hypodense, homogenous and poorly demarcated
   d. bi-convex in shape, hypodense, homogenous and poorly demarcated

3. **Which is the modality of choice to detect small contusions?**
   a. MRI - T1 images
   b. CT
   c. MRI - T2* images
   d. Both a and b

4. **Commonest Risk factor for acute intracerebral haemorrhage**
   a. Smoking
   b. Alcohol
   c. Hypertension
   d. Diabetes

5. **The gold standard means of detecting intracranial haemorrhage in acute stroke**
   a. Contrast CT
   b. MRI - T1
   c. Non- Contrast CT
   d. MRI - T2

6. **Magnetic susceptible substance in early subacute haemorrhage is:**
   a. Methaemoglobin
   b. Haemachrome
   c. Hemosiderin
   d. Deoxyhaemoglobin

7. **What is functional MRI?**
   a. fMRI is a technique that takes advantage of the differences in magnetic susceptibility between haemachrome and hemosiderin
   b. fMRI is a technique that takes advantage of the differences in magnetic susceptibility between oxyhaemoglobin and deoxyhaemoglobin
   c. fMRI is a technique that takes advantage of the differences in magnetic susceptibility between methaemoglobin and deoxyhaemoglobin
   d. None of the above

8. **Most common cause of Stroke**
   a. Ischemia
   b. Haemorrhage
   c. Hypoxia
   d. Hypovolemia

9. **Imaging modality of choice for Space occupying lesions:**
   a. PET scan
   b. CT scan
   c. MRI
   d. Ultrasound

10. **How does a hyper acute haemorrhage image view on T1W MR?**
    a. Isointense
    b. Hypo intense
    c. Hyper intense
    d. Very hyperintense

MCQs ANSWER KEYS

CHAPTER 1 :

1 – a , 2 – a, 3 – c, 4 – a, 5 – d, 6 – d, 7 – a, 8 – c, 9 – c, 10 – d.

CHAPTER 2 :

1 – c, 2 – b, 3 – d, 4 – d, 5 – a,   6 – c, 7 – a & d, 8 – c & d, 9 – b, 10 – c.

CHAPTER 3 :

1 – c, 2 – d,   3 – c,   4 – d, 5 – d,   6 – d, 7 – a, 8 – d, 9 – c, 10 – b.

CHAPTER 4 :

1 – c, 2 – b, 3 – c, 4 – b, 5 – b, 6 – d, 7 – d, 8 – a, 9 – b, 10 – a.

Chapter 5 :

1 – c, 2 – d, 3 – c, 4 – a, 5 – d, 6 – d, 7 – b, 8 – a, 9 – b, 10 – b.

CHAPTER 6 :

1 – b, 2 – c, 3 – a, 4 – d, 5 – c, 6 – d, 7 – d, 8 – a & b, 9 – b, 10 – b & c.

CHAPTER 7 :

1 – d, 2 – b, 3 – d, 4 – a, 5 – c, 6 – a, 7 – c, 8 – c, 9 – d, 10 – d.

CHAPTER 8 :

1 – b, 2 – a, b & c, 3 – a, b & c, 4 – b, 5 – a, b & e, 6 – a, b, c & d, 7 – a, b & c, 8 – a, b & d, 9 – c, 10 – a, b, c, d & e, 11 – d, 12 – a.

CHAPTER 9 :

1 – d, 2 – T.T.T.F., 3 – b, 4 – d, 5 – T.T.T.F., 6 – c, 7 – d, 8 – a, 9 – T.T.F.T., 10 – c.

CHAPTER 10 :

1 – b, 2 – a, 3 – a, 4 – a, 5 – d, 6 – c, 7 – d, 8 – d, 9 – a, 10 – b.

CHAPTER 11 :

1 – c, 2 – d, 3 – b, 4 – b, 5 – c, 6 – d, 7 – d, 8 – a, 9 – b, 10 – a.

CHAPTER 12 :

1 – c, 2 – a, b & c, 3 – e, 4 – c, 5 – d, 6 – a, b & c, 7 – a, c & d, 8 – a, b & c, 9 – b.

CHAPTER 13 :

1 – T, 2 – a, 3 – e, 4 – c, 5 – d, 6 – a, 7 – d, 8 – b, 9 – c, 10 – d.

CHAPTER 14 :

1 – d, 2 – c, 3 – a, 4 – b, 5 – a, 6 – c, 7 – c, 8 – d, 9 – c, 10 – d.

CHAPTER 15 :

1 – a, 2 – c, 3 – a, 4 – b , 5 – a, 6 – c, 7 – b, 8 – a, 9 – c, 10 – b, 11 – c, 12 – b.

CHAPTER 16 :

1 – c, 2 – e, 3 – c, 4 – d & e, 5 – b, 6 – b, 7 – a, 8 – a, b, 9 – c, 10 – a & b.

CHAPTER 17 :

1 – b, 2 – c, 3 – b, 4 – c, 5 – b, 6 – b, 7 – a, 8 – c, 9 – c, 10 – c.

CHAPTER 18 :

1 – a, 2 – T.F.T.F., 3 – d, 4 – b, 5 – a, 6 – b, 7 – c, 8 – T.T.F.T., 9 – d, 10 – c.

CHAPTER 19 :

1 – d, 2 – b, 3 – c, 4 – a, 5 – d, 6 – a, 7 – c, 8 – d, 9 – b, 10 – c, 11 – a & e, 12 – c, 13 – d, 14 – b, 15 – c, 16 – f, 17 – c, 18 – a, 19 – f, 20 – f.

CHAPTER 20 :

1 – a, 2 – b, 3 – c, 4 – c, 5 – c, 6 – a, 7 – b, 8 – a, 9 – c, 10 – a.

701